AF795036

Mādhava Nidāna

Ayurvedic System of Pathology

Indian Medical Science Series No. 7

Mādhava Nidāna

Ayurvedic System of Pathology

Translated into English
by
K.R.L. Gupta

Sri Satguru Publication
a division of
Indian Books Centre
Delhi-India

Published by:

Sri Satguru Publication
Indian Medical Science Series No. 7

a division of

Indian Books Centre
24/4/ Shakti Nagar,
Delhi-110007 (INDIA)

First Edition : Calcutta, 1892
Second Edition : Delhi, 1987, 1997, 2013

ISBN 81-7030-130-0

PRINTED IN INDIA

PREFACE.

"Old fashions please me best, I am not so nice
To change true rules for odd intentions."
Shakespere.

The tendencies and prejudices of the people are half revealed or not revealed to those who have not cared to watch with some interest the numerous editions and translations of ancient books that are printed off every month. What makes these possible ? Not certainly the increasing figures of population or the rising education of the people, but a reactionary feeling for encouraging the proper recognition of the genius of our sages. A revival has set in—a revival of the old faith for old institutions—especially for the old medical system. No one now puts it down as a huge sham—a pure product of fertile fancy. The people can now understand what a precious store house of medical knowledge is represented by the few old volumes that have descended to us. Even foreigners have not failed to admit, there are many things in them that were never dreamt of in the modern science of medicine. It is an established creed at present that the old system is the genuine creation of long experience and varied experiments and that it can be thus profitably made an excellent hand-maid to the modern one. When such a belief is once awakened, it is no wonder that editions and translations of a *Charaka* or a *Susruta* will spring up with a formidable rapidity. I myself have had the honour of appearing before the public as a translator of some of the oldest but noblest works of medicine and I have met with the greatest encouragement on every occasion. Relying on the same patronage of our people, I have undertaken to translate into English the Sanskrit treatise on pathology (compiled by Madhava Kar and generally known under the name of Nidana) giving a full account of the diseases known to the ancient Hindus. It contains many truths which have been recognised by several eminent scientists of Europe and it contains many other whose importance, a remote generation can alone realise. It is moreover a great aid to European scholars as supplying history of diseases which prevailed in past times but have now completely disappeared. The mere fact that it has been the text-book on medicine of native physicians from so long a time should not fail to recommend it to the public. "Our virtues lie in the interpretation of the time." Greatness is not greatness unless approved by time and age. Time has proved that there is infinite truth in the doctrines of Nidana. What higher testimony of its worth can there be than that a postirity separated by so many hundreds of years should still adore it and should not grudge to be guided by it. A translation of such a book can never be unwelcome. It has been already translated into Bengali. But an English translation is greatly calculated to make its use more general and I have therefore attempted to render it into English which is one day destined to be the language of the universe. The present work is not simply a literal translation of the Sanskrit text. It contains even much of the valuable information to be found in the commentary of Nidana by Bijoy Rakshit and Sreekanta Dutta. If the translation conveys an idea of the Hindu system of pathology to those who are unacquainted with Sanskrit and if it thus tends in any way to enhance the respect for those great men whose blood still runs in our veins, I shall think my labours amply rewarded.

KAVIRAJ RUSSICK LAL GUPTA.

CONTENTS.

NIDANA.

A SANSKRIT SYSTEM OF PATHOLOGY.

FEVERS, (*Jwara.*)

Fevers are first considered because it is said that man is born and dies with fever ; because it affects the whole body, the organs of senses, and the mind ; and is so severe that only man and gods can survive it, and by which various other diseases are produced.

Dakshya the father-in-law of *Shiva* did not invite him to a feast given to the gods, and spoke disrespectfully of him. His wife *Durgá* was present, and was so enraged, at the disrespect, that she considered it better to die than live under such a disgrace ; and while sitting, her spirit left her body. *Nundi* the ser-

---

ज्वरनिदानम् ।

दक्षापमानसंक्रुद्धरुद्रनिश्वाससम्भवः । ज्वरोऽष्टधा पृथग्द्वन्द्व संघाता गन्तुजः स्मृतः ॥ मिथ्याहारविहारस्य दोषा ह्यामाशयाश्रयाः । वहिर्निरस्य कोष्ठाग्निं ज्वरदाः स्युरसानुगाः ॥

स्वेदावरोधः सन्तापः सर्व्वाङ्गग्रहणन्तथा । युगपद् यत्र रोगे च स ज्वरो व्यपदिश्यते ॥ श्रमोऽरतिर्विवर्णत्वं वैरस्यं नयनप्लवः । इच्छाद्वेषौ मुहुश्चापि शीतवातातपादिषु ॥ जृम्भाङ्गमर्द्दो गुरुता रोमहर्षोऽरुचिस्तमः । अप्रहर्षश्च शीतञ्च भवत्युत्पत्स्यति ज्वरे ॥ सामान्यतो विशेषेण जृम्भात्यर्थं समीरणात् । पित्तान्नयनयोर्द्दाहः कफादन्नारुचिर्भवेत् ॥ रूपैरन्यतराभ्यान्तु संसृष्टैर्द्वन्द्वजं विदुः । सर्व्वत्र समलिङ्गञ्च सर्व्वदोषप्रकोपजे ॥

vant of *Durgá* seeing her die, went and informed *Shiva* of the event. He in grief for his loss, tore off one of his locks, and it fell into the fire, and a great devil named *Birabhadra* was produced from it. Others say that in his anger he heaved a deep sigh, and from his mouth the devil was produced. *Birabhadra* asked *Shiva* to be allowed to destroy his father-in-law. This was permitted, and after polluting the sacred fire of *Dakshya,* destroying many of his guests, and tearing his hair, he wrenched his head from his body. It was during the paroxysm of grief and rage of *Shiva* for the death of *Durgá* that the breath which proceeded from his nostrils, hot, and destructive, gave origin to fevers, which attack all persons, of all ages, and in all conditions.

The *cause* of all the principal varieties of fever, with the exception of five from accidents (*águntuka*), is using improper mixtures of food; as eating fish and milk; the want of seasoning in food; sleeping at improper hours; fighting with a strong man; exposure to the morning sun while fasting; eating voraciously of food of a very hot nature, when the body has been previously weakened by extreme hunger; and by fatigue, fear, grief, and watching. Fevers are also produced by poisons,

---

वेपथुर्विषमो वेगः कण्ठौष्ठपरिशोषणम् । निद्रानाशः क्षवस्तम्भो गात्राणां रौक्ष्यमेव च ॥ शिरोहृद्गात्ररुग्वक्त्रवैरस्यं गाढविट्-
कता । शूलाध्माने जृम्भणञ्च भवत्यनिलजे ज्वरे ।

वेगस्तीक्ष्णोतिसारश्च निद्राल्पत्वं तथा वमिः । कण्ठौष्ठमुख-
नासानां पाकः स्वेदश्च जायते ॥ प्रलापो वक्त्रकटुता मूर्च्छादाहौ मदस्तृषा । पीतविण्मूत्रनेत्रत्वं पैत्तिके भ्रम एव च ॥

स्तैमित्यं स्तिमितो वेग आलस्यं मधुरास्यता । शुक्लमूत्र-
पुरीषत्वं स्तम्भस्तृप्तिरथापि च । गौरवं शीतमुत्क्लेदो रोमहर्षो-
ऽतिनिद्रता । प्रतिश्यायोऽरुचिः कासः कफजेऽक्ष्णोश्च शुक्लता ॥

drinking stagnant water, in which withered leaves have fallen; taking a full meal without any appetite, or after delivery, especially if improperly treated. In other cases the first secretion of milk in the breast, produces fever, exposure to unseasonable weather, or to sudden vicissitudes of temperature; checked perspiration, long continued constipation; and living in wooded, ill ventilated valleys. Other causes of fever are the influence of bad stars, neglected adoration of saints or gods; visiting a new climate; the malign influence of evil spirits, and severe local diseases, or injuries. By such causes the air, bile, and phlegm are deranged, pass into the stomach (*ámishay*), and thus expel the internal heat. The humors stop also the chyle vessels, and derange the heat, which digests the food: in other words, whatever exposes our moral qualities, or bodily frame, to deviations from their natural and accustomed movements, produces fevers; and it requires remedies to drive back the heat, to its natural position, when the person is restored to health.

तृष्णा मूर्च्छा भ्रमो दाहः स्वप्ननाशः शिरोरुजा। कण्ठास्यशोषो वमथुरोमहर्षोऽरुचिस्तमः। पर्व्वभेदश्च जृम्भा च वातपित्तज्वराकृतिः॥

स्तैमित्यं पर्व्वणाम्भेदो निद्रागौरव मेव च। शिरोग्रहः प्रतिश्यायः कासः स्वेदाप्रवर्त्तनम्॥ सन्तापो मध्यवेगश्च वातश्लेष्मज्वराकृतिः। लिप्ततिक्तास्यता तन्द्रा मोहः कासोऽरुचिस्तृषाः। मुहुर्द्दाहो मुहुःशीतं पित्तश्लेष्मज्वराकृतिः॥

क्षणे दाहः क्षणे शीत मस्थिसन्धिशिरोरुजा। सास्रावे कलुषे रक्ते निर्भुग्ने चापि लोचने॥ सस्वनौ सरुजौ कर्णौ कण्ठः शूकैरिवावृतः। तन्द्रा मोहः प्रलापश्च कासः श्वासोऽरुचिर्भ्रमः॥ परिदग्धा खरस्पर्शा जिह्वास्रस्ताङ्गता परम्। ष्ठीवनं रक्तपित्तस्य

GENERAL SYMPTOMS OF FEVER.

The attack of fever commences with the person complaining of lassitude and fatigue ; he is continually yawning, and stretching; his skin loses its natural colour,and there is abad taste in his mouth; his eyes are watery, and he alternataly wants the application of heat, and cold to his body. Little, and much food distresses the person, as it is not digested; he has no appetite, the body is chilly and heavy, with dejection of mind ; and he is quarrelsome, and ready to fight with a much stronger person than himself.

These precursory symptoms are followed by heat of the surface,° cessation of perspiration, and pain affecting the whole body, but particularly the members. There is also pain in the chest, languor and drowsiness, loss of appetite, restlessness, heaviness of the abdomen with costiveness, and a copious flow of urine. These symptoms are always present in fevers ; but, when *air* is deranged, there is also much gaping ; when *bile* is affected the eyes feel hot, and when *phlegm* is deranged there is no appetite.

कफेनोन्मिश्रितस्र च। शिरसो लोठनं तृष्णा निद्रानाशो हृदि वय्रथा। स्वेदमूत्रपुरीषाणां चिराद्दर्शनमल्पशः॥ कृशत्वं नातिगात्राणां प्रततं कण्ठकुजनम्। कोठानां श्यावरक्तानां मण्डलानाञ्च दर्शनम। मूकत्वं स्रोतसां पाको गुरुत्वमुदरस्य च॥ चिरात् पाकश्च दोषाणां सन्निपातज्वराकृतिः॥

दोषे विवद्धे नष्टेऽग्नौ सर्व्वसम्पूर्णलक्षणः। सन्निपातज्वरोसाध्यः कृच्छ्रसाध्य स्ततोऽन्यथा॥ सप्तमे दिवसे प्राप्ते दशमे द्वादशेऽपि वा। पुनर्घोरतरो भूत्वा प्रशमं याति हन्ति वा॥ सप्तमी द्विगुणा चैव नवमेरकादशी तथा। एषा त्रिदोषमर्य्यादा मोक्षाय च बधाय च॥ सन्निपातज्वरस्यान्ते कर्णमूले सुदारुणः। शोथः सञ्जायते तेन कश्चिदेव प्रमुचय्रते॥

1st Variety of Fever. Bátik-jwara is that variety which is produced by a derangement of the air (*báyu*).

This fever commences with shivering, there is sometimes much at other times little heat ; the throat, mouth, and lips are dry. The patient has no sleep, does not sneeze, his skin is dry, with head-ache, and pain in the chest, as well as over the body. Whatever is taken into the stomach feels heavy, and creates uneasiness ; the stools are very hard ; pain in the abdomen ; flatulence as if much food had been eaten, and he is frequently yawning.

2nd form of Fever. When Bile is deranged, producing fever, it is called (*Paittika Jwara.*) This form of fever commences with a shivering fit, followed by a severe hot stage ; a frequent desire to go to stool, vomiting, a bitter taste in the mouth, and restlessness. Aphthæ form in the throat, lips, mouth, and nose ; the patient perspires freely, often speaks nonsense, and has sometimes fainting fits, and attacks of giddiness. Such a patient is very listless, his body is pale, with a burning sensation over the surface, he has great thirst, the stools and urine have a yellow colour, as well as the eye, which is often also red.

3rd form of Fever. Derangement of phlegm (*Kapha*), produces a fever named *shlaishmik-jwara*, or *kapha-jwara*. This

---

त्रयः प्रकुपिता दोषा उरःस्रोतोऽनुगामिनः। आमातिवृंद्धा ग्रथिता बुद्धीन्द्रियमनोगताः। जनयन्ति महाघोरमभिन्यासं ज्वरं दृढ़म्। श्रुतौ नेत्रे प्रसुप्तिः स्यान्न चेष्टां काञ्चिदीहते। नच दृष्टि-र्भवेत्त्वस्य समर्था रूपदर्शने। न घ्रानं न च संस्पर्शं शब्दं वा नैव बुध्यते। शिरो लोढयतेऽभीक्ष्ण-माहारं नाभिनन्दति। कुजति तुद्यते चैव परिवर्त्तनमीहते। अल्प प्रभाषते किञ्चिदभिन्यासः स उच्यते। प्रत्याख्यातः स भूयिष्ठः कश्चि-देवात्र सिध्यति॥

fever is ushered in by loss of appetite, and the symptoms of the hot stage is less marked than in the last form of fever. The person feels languid, and listless, with a sweet taste in his mouth. In this fever tho body feels cold, as if wrapped in a wet cloth, and the stools and urine are white. Such a person remains quiet and silent, does not eat; but feels as if he had eaten too much, his body is very heavy, eyes white, with nausea attended with cough. He is very sleepy, and there is a discharge of mucus from the eyes, mouth, and nose.

4th. Báta-paittika Jwara. This fever commences with giddiness, fainting and thirst: the body feels cold to another person, although he complains of his body being hot and burning: loss of memory, no sleep, pain in all the joints, head-ache, cough, throat and mouth dry, vomiting, goose-skin, no perspiration, low spirits, and yawning.

5th. Bata-shlaishmik Jwara. This form of fever is not very severe in its accession. The body feels cold, with slight shivering and pain in the bones; the person sleeps much, has pain in the head, with much saliva in the mouth, and running at the nose, with cough, a dry skin, and body hot.

अभिघाताभिचाराभ्यामभिषङ्गाभिशापतः। आगन्तुजायते दोषैर्यथास्वं तं विभावयेत्। श्यावास्यता विषकृते तथातीसार एव च। भक्तारुचिः पिपासा च तोदश्च सह मूर्च्छया। ओषधीगन्धजे मूर्च्छा शिरोरुग्वमथु स्तथा॥ कामजे चित्तविभ्रंश स्तन्द्रालस्यमभोजनम्। भयात् प्रलापः शोकाच्च भवेत् कोपाच्च वेपथुः॥ अभिचाराभिशापाभ्यां मोहस्तृष्णा च जायते। भूताभिषङ्गादुद्वेगो हास्यरोदनकम्पनम्॥

कामशोकभयाद्वायुः क्रोधात् पित्तं त्रयो मलाः। भूताभिषङ्गात् कुप्यन्ति भूतसामान्यलक्षणाः॥

6th. Bile and Phlegm, (Pitta-shlaishmik Jwara). The mouth is clammy and sour, with much saliva, in this form of fever. The person is always dozing, complains of faintness, and coughs; has no appetite, thirst, and is at one time hot, and at another time cold.

7th. Mixed Remittent or Synochus Fever, (Sannipât Jwara Bikâra). In this form of fever the air, bile, and phlegm, are deranged ; and it is always dangerous. At one time the patient is hot, at other times cold, with pains in the bones, and joints ; the eyes are watery, of a dirty yellow colour, and hollow ; the patient complains of ringing, and pain in the ears, with pain in the head, neck, and thorax ; is always dozing, but cannot sleep at night; has no memory, and is often delirious. Bodies seem to turn round, and sometimes he is laughing, crying, performs unnatural actions, is always coughing, has quick breathing, no appetite, the tongue is black like charcoal, and irregular like that of a cow, with pain. Blood, phlegm, air and bile flow from the mouth, the patient moves his head about continually, with thirst, watch-

---

दोषोल्पोऽहितसम्भूतो ज्वरोत्सृष्टस्य वा पुनः। धातुमनग्रतमं प्राप्य करोति बिषमज्वरम्॥ सन्ततं सततान्येद्युस्ततीयकचतुर्थकान्। सन्ततं रसरक्तास्थः सोऽन्येद्युः पिश्रिताश्रितः॥ मेदोगतस्तृतीयेऽह्नि अस्थिमज्जागतः पुनः। कुर्य्याच्चातुर्थकं घोरमन्तकं रोगसङ्करम्॥

सप्ताहं वा दशाहं वा द्वादशाहमथापि वा। सन्त्यत्या योऽबिसर्गी स्यात् सन्त्यतं स निगद्यते॥ अहोरात्रे सततको द्वौ कालावनुवर्त्तते। अन्येद्युष्कस्त्वहोरात्र एककालं प्रवर्त्तते॥ तृतीयकस्ततीयेऽह्नि चतुर्थेऽह्नि चतुर्थकः। केचिद्भूताभिषङ्गोत्थं ब्रुवते बिषमज्वरम् कफपित्तात्त्रिकग्राही पृष्ठाद्वातकफात्मकः। बातपित्ताच्छिरोग्राही त्रिविध स्यात्ततीयकः॥ चातुर्थको दर्शयति प्रभावं द्विविधं ज्वरः॥

ing, and pain in the breast. The urine is secreted in small quantities, with costiveness and no perspiration; great thirst, noises in the throat, so that there is a difficulty in comprehending what the sick person says; with round elevations, and central depressions of a blue and red colour, over the surface of the body. The person vomits blood, mixed with phlegm, and his abdomen diminishes in size. His body does not become thin, but his belly is heavy and enlarged. This kind of fever remains long, and much care and proper medicines are required for its cure. After the first stage, should the fever continue severe, it will be generally fatal; and at the last stage of the fever the lower part of the ear (the parotid gland) swells. This is supposed to be a fatal sign.

The 7th, 10th, 12th days, are always the days on which the fever is severe, or from these periods the symptoms diminish in severity.

In other books it is stated that the critical days are the 7th, 9th, 11th, 14th, 18th, 22nd; from which period the disease is diminished or increased. Those who live till the 22nd day generally recover.

जङ्घाभ्यां श्लैष्मिकं पूर्व्वं शिरस्तोऽनिलसम्भवः। विषमज्वर
एवान्यश्चातुर्थकविपर्य्ययः। मध्येऽह्नि ज्वरयतीत्यादावन्ते च
मुञ्चति॥

नित्यं मन्दज्वरो रुक्षः शूनकस्तेन सीदति। स्तब्धाङ्गः श्लेष्म-
भूयिष्ठो नरो वातबलासकी॥ प्रलिम्पन्निव गात्राणि घर्म्मेण
गौरवेण वा। मन्दज्वरविलेपी च सशीतः स्यात् प्रलेपकः॥

विदग्धेऽन्नरसे देहे श्लेष्मपित्ते व्यवस्थिते। तेनार्द्धं शीतलं
देहे चार्द्धचोष्णं प्रजायते॥ काये दुष्टं यदा पित्तं श्लेष्मा चान्ते
व्यवस्थितः। तेनोष्णत्वं शरीरस्य शीतत्वं हस्तपादयोः। काये
श्लेष्मा यदा दुष्टः पित्तञ्चान्ते व्यवस्थितम्॥ शीतत्वं तेन गात्राणां

There are thirteen kinds of mixed fever. In three kinds one of humours, that is the air, blie, or phlegm, are morbidly increased, or diminished beyond the others. In a second form two are increased or diminished. The thirteenth variety is that in which the three humours are morbidly increased.

1. *Bisfaraka Bátulbana.* When the air is increased, the usual symptoms of this form of fever will be accompanied with a bad taste in the mouth, difficulty of breathing, shivering, cough, yawning, giddiness, syncope, delirium, and pain in the sides of the belly.

2. *Pittulbana* or *Asukarí.* The peculiar symptoms of this form are looseness, giddiness, fainting, aphthæ in the mouth, red spots, and a burning sensation, over the body.

3. *Korupono* or *Kaphulbana,* is distinguished by a feeling of languor, a difficulty in speaking, sleeping much, eyes cloudy, and a sweet taste in the mouth.

4. *Pobru Bobru. Bátapittulbana.* When bile is increased the person feels as if he had taken narcotic medicines, complaining of thirst, dry mouth, drowsiness, flatulence, loss of appetite, cough, difficulty of breathing, giddiness, and languor.

5. *Bato Soleso, Ulbono,* or *Sigrokarí.* When the air and phlegm around the neck is stopped, fever comes on with shivering, fainting, sneezing, thirst, pains in the sides of the body and in the abdomen, and difficulty in breathing.

6. *Petu Soleso Bono Bolu.* Is distinguished by a burning sensation in the body with chilliness, much thirst, pain in the

---

उष्णत्वं हस्तपादयोः। त्वक्स्थौ श्लेष्मानिलौ शीतमादौ जनयतो ज्वरे। तयोः प्रशान्तयोः पित्तमन्ते दाहं करोति च॥ करोत्यादौ तथा पित्तं त्वक्स्थं दाहमतीव च। तस्मिन् प्रशान्ते त्वितरौ कुरुतः शीतमन्ततः॥ द्वावेतौ दाहशीतादिज्वरौ संसर्गजौ स्मृतौ। दाहपूर्व्वस्तयोः कष्टः कृच्छ्रसाध्यतमश्च सः॥

right side of the chest, head-ache, pain in the breast and throat, vomiting phlegm and bile, looseness, difficulty of breathing, hiccough, and drowsiness.

7. *Bato-Peto-Soliso-Ulbono* or *Kutopákolo.* In this form the three air, bile and phlegm are morbidly increased, and like thunder, fire and the sword, it kills quickly. The peculiar symptoms of this form of fever are, the patient breathes slowly and imperfectly, he is motionless, his eyes are fixed, and after three days he dies.

8. *Songonohohoko.* The peculiar symptoms of this variety are delirium, languor, faintness, shivering, giddiness, and paralysis of half the body. This is a very dangerous disease.

9. *Pákolo.* Faintness, delirium, stiffness of the neck, head-ache, cough, difficulty of breathing, giddiness, drowsiness, severe pain in the chest, hemorrhage from the mouth, and nose, and the eyes being fixed characterise this form of fever. The patient generally dies within three days.

10. *Jammo.* In this variety severe pain in the chest, and abscesses form in the liver, spleen and lungs; and both the patient's stools, and the matter vomited contain blood and pus.

11. *Korkotoko.* Is accompanied with a burning sensation internally, the person cannot speak, his face and eyes become red, he cannot expectorate the phlegm from his throat, has severe lancinating pains in the breast, with drowsiness, difficulty of breathing, and hiccough. These symptoms increase daily; the patient's tongue becomes black and rough, his throat becomes covered with prickles, involuntary evacuations follow; he

---

गुरुता हृदयोत्क्लेशः सदनं छर्द्यरोचकौ। रसस्थे तु ज्वरे लिङ्गं दैनन्द्यास्योपजायते॥ रक्तनिष्ठीवनं दाहो मोहश्छर्दनविभ्रमौ। प्रलापः पीड़का तृष्णा रक्तप्राप्ते ज्वरे नृनाम्॥ पिण्डिकोद्वेष्टनं तृष्णा सृष्टमूत्रपुरीषता। उष्मान्तर्दाहविक्षेपौ ग्लानिः स्यान्मांसगे ज्वरे। भृशं स्वेदस्तृषा मूर्च्छा प्रलापश्छर्दिरेव च।

moans much, like the cooing of a pigeon; his mouth, lips, and palate are dry, he sleeps much, and he cannot speak, with convulsions, or nausea and vomiting.

12. *Boidáriko.* In this fever there is pain in the loins, the body is cool, and during the accession the body feels cold, with diarrhœa, giddiness, languor, head-ache, drowsiness, pain in the neck and chest, cough, difficulty of breathing, and insensibility.

13. *Abhinyása Jwara.* Is characterized by dryness of the mouth, by the patient being always sleepy, and his body feels as if it belonged to another person; he speaks very little, and with great pain, is stupid, and breathes with difficulty. His internal heat is diminished, he feels an internal burning sensation accompanied with weakness, and a dead-like feeling of the skin.

8th. *Accidental fever, (A'gantuka.)* The causes of this order of fevers are injuries; such as wounds, &c. They may also be produced by the evil designs of an enemy, or a devil, by the passions; by the curses of a guru, a bráhman, or a prophet; by poison, or by the effects of air mixed with deleterious matter, as that proceeding from a kind of poisonous trees which are supposed to come from the east. These causes derange the air, bile, and phlegm, and thus produce fever.

Adultery, grief for parents, friends, &c. derange also the air, anger deranges bile, and devils derange both air, bile, and phlegm.

When a man wants to kill another, or to remove an obnoxious individual to another country; or to have command of

---

दौर्गन्ध्यारोचकौ ग्लानिः मैदस्थे चासहिष्णुता ॥ भेदोस्थ्नां कूजनं श्वासो विरेकश्छर्दिरेव च। विक्षेपणञ्च गात्राणामेतदस्थिगते ज्वरे ॥ तमः प्रवेशनं हिक्का कासः शैत्यं वमिस्तथा। अन्तर्दाहो महाश्वासो मर्म्मभेदश्च मज्जगे। मरणं प्राप्नुयात्तत्र शुक्रस्थानगते ज्वरे ॥ शेफसः स्तब्धता मोक्षः शुक्रस्य तु विशेषतः ॥

him, certain *mantras,* and directions are given in the *Tantra Shástra* for accomplishing these. But should he err in any of the injunctions enjoined, the person himself will be attacked with the fever, and he will not have power to injure the other. In some such cases the two front teeth are extracted to prevent the person blundering in pronouncing *mantras*

When the fever is produced by poisons the tongue is white, or black in the middle, the person has frequent stools, and fainting fits, and has no appetite, or memory, and complains of thirst, and pain over the body. By improper medicines this fever is sometimes produced with swooning, head-ache, and vomiting.

When it is produced by the passion of love there is no memory, the person dozes, is lazy, and delirious.

When produced by the curses of a good man, or by the sorcery of another, want of memory and thirst are the peculiar symptoms present; and when an evil spirit produces it, the person alternately is sorrowful and laughing; and at other times he cries and laughs.

9th. Intermittent fevers (Bishama Jwara). This is another form of fever, which occurs before and after attacks of other kinds of fever; by the derangements of the humours of the

---

वर्षाशरद्वसन्तेषु वाताद्यैः प्राकृतः क्रमात्। वैकृतोऽन्यः स दुःसाध्यः प्राकृतश्चानिलोद्भवः। वर्षासु मारुतो दुष्टः पित्तश्लेष्मान्वितो ज्वरं॥ कुर्य्यात् पित्तञ्च शरदि तस्य चानुबलः कफः। तत्प्रकृत्या विसर्गाच्च तत्रनानशनाद्भयम्॥ कफो वसन्ते तमपि वातपित्तं भवेदनु। काले यथास्वं सर्व्वेषां प्रवृत्तिर्वृद्धिरेव वा। निदानोक्तानुपशयो विपरीतोपशायिता॥

अन्तर्दाहोऽधिकस्तृष्णा प्रलापः श्वसनं भ्रमः। सन्ध्यस्थिशूलमस्वेदो दोषो वर्च्चो विनिग्रहः। अन्तर्व्वेगस्य लिङ्गानि ज्वर

body. The essential parts of the body such as chyle, blood, muscles, fat, bone, semen, and marrow, in the order now mentioned may be affected. One or more are sometimes deranged, and form so many types of fever.

These are *Santata, Satata, Anyejyuka, Tritíyaka, Cháturthaka.* The general symptoms of intermittent fever are as follows: when the paroxysm occurs at uncertain periods the patient feels first cold, then hot, and afterwards perspires.

The following five varieties are described :

1. *Santata* continues for several days without an intermission.
2. *Satata* has two paroxysms daily.
3. *Anyejyuka* occurs daily, at the same hour.
4. *Tritíyaka* occurs on alternate days.
5. *Cháturthaka* occurs every fourth day.

The following varieties of this class of fevers are described by Ancient Medical writers.

1. *Santata-jwara* affects the chyle and blood ; and it continues for 7, 10, or 12 days ; followed by an interval and again occurs, and remains for several days.

2. *Satata* has two paroxysms daily, one at night and another during the day,

Others say there are two kinds of this fever, one of which commences with a cold fit, and another with a hot fit. The first gives much uneasiness, and is cured with difficulty.

3. If the paroxysm of fever recurs at the same hour daily, it is called *Anyejyuka*.

सैतानि लक्षयेत्। सन्तापो ह्यधिको वाह्य स्तृष्णादीनाञ्च मार्द्दवम्। बहिर्व्वेगस्य लिङ्गानि सुखसाध्यत्वमेव च॥

लालाप्रसेको हृल्लासो हृदयाशुद्ध्यरोचकाः। तन्द्रालस्याविपाकास्य वैरस्यं गुरुगात्रता॥ क्षुन्नाशो बहुमूत्रत्वं स्तब्धता बलवान् ज्वरः। आमज्वरस्य लिङ्गानि न दद्यात्तत्र भेषजम्॥

4. When the fever returns at an interval of one day it is called *Tritíyaka*. These are the following three varieties of this fever:

a. When *phlegm* and *bile* are deranged in this fever, before the accession, pain is felt at the nape of the neck.

b. When *spirit* and *phlegm* are deranged, the patient first feels pain in the loins.

c. When *air* and *bile* are deranged, the fever is introduced with head-ache.

5. In *Cháturthaka*, the paroxysms of this fever occur every fourth day. When the paroxysm continues for two days, there is no paroxysm on the first and fourth day, the fever is that called *Cháturthaka Biparjyaya.*

This fever presents the following symptoms. It commences with shivering, dryness, and swelling. The patient has no strength, so as not to be able to walk. He evacuates much bile, air, and phlegm which are particularly affected.

When the body is heavy, with perspiration, and little fever and stools, it is called *Proapiko.*

When half the body is hot, and the other cold; when what is eaten is not digested, and does harm; the deranged bile and

---

भेषजं ह्यामदोषस्य भूयो ज्वलयति ज्वरम् ॥ ज्वरवेगोऽधिकस्तृष्णा प्रलापः श्वसनं भ्रमः । मलप्रवृत्तिरुत्क्लेशः पच्यमानस्य लक्षणम् ॥ क्षुत्क्षामता लघुत्वञ्च गात्राणां ज्वरमार्द्दवम् । दोषप्रवृत्तिरष्टाहो निरामज्वरलक्षणम् ॥

बलवत् स्वल्पदोषेषु ज्वरः साध्योऽनुपद्रवः । हेतुभिर्बहुभि र्जातो बलिभिर्बहुलक्षणः॥ ज्वरः प्राणान्तकृद् यश्च शीघ्रमिन्द्रियनाशनः । ज्वरः क्षीणस्य शूनस्य गम्भीरो दैर्घरात्रिकः ॥ असाध्यो बलवान् यश्च केशसीमन्तकृत् ज्वरः । गम्भीरस्तु ज्वरो ज्ञेयो ह्यन्तर्द्दाहेन तृष्णया । आनद्धत्वेन दोषाणां श्वासकासोद्गमेन च । आरम्भा-

phlegm have produced these morbid symptoms. When the bile of the body is deranged, and the phlegm of the arms and legs, the body is hot and the hands and feet cold. When the phlegm of the body is deranged, and the bile of the hands and feet, the body is cold, and the hands and feet are hot.

The fever is also modified, as the essential parts are deranged. Thus the air may be deranged in the blood, flesh, bone, marrow and semen; and the supposed danger increasing in the order above stated, until the last, the semen, when the fever is considered always fatal.

The type of the fever varies also according to the season of the year. Each of them forms two lunar months; during June and July, the rainy season (*Barshá*), air predominates, and the fevers takes on the characters of deranged air. The season called *Sharata*, autumn, or sultry months (Sept. and Oct.), the bile and the phlegm predominate; *Basanta* or spring (Feb. March and April), the phlegm is in excess, and is succeeded by derangement of the air and bile, followed by fever.

A'haka-jwara, (Nakra or *Násá-jwara.)* We are subject to this peculiar form of intermittent fever. The description of it is not contained in the more ancient medical works. It is produced by a swelling of the Schniderian membrane, and is

---

विषमो यस्तु यश्च वा दैर्घरात्रिकः । क्षीणस्य चातिरूक्षस्य गम्भीरो यस्य हन्ति तम् । विसंज्ञस्ताम्यते यस्तु शेते निपतितोऽपि वा ॥ शीतार्द्दितोऽन्तरुष्णश्च ज्वरेण म्रियते नरः । यो हृष्टरोमा रक्ताक्षो हृदि संघातशूलवान् ॥ वक्त्रेण चैवोच्छ्वसिति तं ज्वरो हन्ति मानवम् । हिक्काश्वासतृषायुक्तं मूढ़ं विभ्रान्तलोचनम् ॥ सन्ततोच्छ्वासिनं क्षीणं नरं क्षपयति ज्वरः ॥ हतप्रभेन्द्रियं क्षीणमरोचकनिपीड़ितम् ॥ गम्भीरतीक्ष्णवेगार्त्तं ज्वरितं परिवर्ज्जयेत् ॥

said to be caused by the air and phlegm deranging the blood of the part. It is accompanied with pain over the body, but particularly in the neck and back, and other symptoms of fever.

It is of frequent occurrence in Bengal; attacks adults alone, between the age of 20 and 40 years of age.

DYSENTERY, (*Atisár.*)

Dysentery is produced by a variety of causes; such as exposure to cold, eating very cold articles of food in considerable quantities, eating much ghee and oily articles, very heavy or hot substances, or very thin or dry articles of food; eating several articles of food with contrary qualities, such as milk and fish, &c., or any kind of indigestable food, causes this disease. In other cases it is produced by the food not being properly boiled or mixed, or being eaten at improper times; or when not properly seasoned, or in unusually small or large quantities. In some cases the disease is produced by poisons, great fear, or grief; by unwholesome drinking water; by much wine, and peculiar food which thus affects certain persons; and

---

दाहः स्वेदो भ्रमस्तृष्णा कम्पविड्भेदसंज्ञिता। कूजनञ्चास्य वैगन्ध्यमाकृतिर्ज्वरमोचणे॥ स्वेदो लघुत्वं शिरसः कण्डुः पाको मुखस्य च। चवथुश्चान्नलिप्सा च ज्वरमुक्तस्य लक्षणम्॥

अतीसारनिदानम्।

गुर्व्वतिस्निग्धरूक्षोष्ण द्रवस्थूलातिशीतलैः। विरुद्धाध्यसनाजीर्णै र्विषमैश्चापि भोजनैः॥ स्नेहाद्यै रतियुक्तैश्च मिथ्यायुक्तैर्विषैर्भयैः। शोकाद्दुष्टाम्बुमद्यातिपानैः सात्म्यर्त्तुपर्य्ययैः॥ जलाभिरमणैर्व्वेगविघातैः क्रिमिदोषतः। नृणां भवत्यतीसारो लक्षणं तस्य वक्ष्यते॥ संशम्यापां धातुरग्निं प्रवृद्धः शकृन्मिश्रो वायुनाधः

by irregular or sudden changes in the seasons. Remaining long in the water while bathing, worms, deranged or constipated alvine, or other excretions, sometimes produce the disease. The symptoms are explained by the internal fire being diminished by morbid watery secretions, or phlegm generated in the intestines; this is mixed with the fæces, and is carried off downwards by the air of the part. Hence the production of watery stools, &c. In some cases the fever occurs first from the derangement of air, bile, and phlegm; in other cases the dysentery precedes the fever, and sometimes both occur together. In these cases abstinence from eating and drinking is to be observed, and such medicines are to be given as prepare the food that is in the abdomen. If dysentery is present such medicines are to be used as will dry up and stop this discharge, and the physician is to decide in each case which sort of remedies are to be given, whether they should be to cure first the fever or the diarrhœa.

There are six varieties of this disease, as when the air, bile, and phlegm are deranged, it forms so many kinds; when the

---

प्रवृत्तः। सरत्यतीवातिसारं तमाहुर्व्याधिं घोरं षड्विधं वदन्ति॥ एकैकशः सर्व्वशश्चापि दोषैः शोकेनान्यः षष्ठ आमेन चोक्तः। हृन्नाभिपायूदरकुक्षितोदगात्रावसादानिलसन्निरोधाः॥ विट्संग आध्मानमथाविपाको भविष्यतस्तस्य पुरःसराणि॥

अरुणं फेनिलं रूक्षं अल्पमल्पं मुहुर्मुहुः। शकृदामं सरुक्शब्दं मारुतेनातिसार्य्यते॥ पित्तात् पीतं हरितं लोहितं वा तृष्णा मूर्च्छा दाहपाकोपपन्नम्। शुक्लं सान्द्रं सकफं श्लेष्मणा तु विस्रं शीतं हृष्टरोमा मनुष्यः॥ वराहस्नेहमांसाम्बुसदृशं सर्व्वरूपिणम्। कृच्छ्रसाध्यमतीसारं विद्याद्दोषत्रयोद्भवम्॥ तैस्तैर्भावैः शोचतोऽल्पाशनस्य वाष्पोष्मा वै वह्निमाविश्य जन्तोः। कोष्ठं गत्वा क्षोभ-

three are deranged together, when produced by grief, and when caused by mucus in the abdomen. *Dhanantwari* says, there are many other varieties as the symptoms vary from time to time.

Before this disease developes itself a sharp pain is felt in the chest, umbiliacus, and anus, and in the abdomen under the false ribs, which is succeeded by want of appetite, languor, and lassitude of the body; no air passed by the anus, the patient is costive, the abdomen swelled, and every thing taken remains undigested. When air produces the disease it commences with great pain; the dejections are of a dark yellow colour, frothy, dry and frequent, and in small quantities mixed with the indigested substances, which have been eaten, pain is felt in the anus on the expulsion of air, and the urine is scanty.

2. When bile is deranged, the dejections are expelled with an effort. They have a bad smell, are hot, and of a red yellowish colour, like the water in which flesh had been steeped. In other cases they are of a blue or red colour, and are accompanied with thirst, dozing, heat of body, free perspirations, and tenesmus at the time of the evacuation. There is often in such cases inflammation of the rectum with violent fever.

येत्तस्य रक्तं तच्चाधस्तात् आकषन्ती प्रकाशम् ॥ निर्गच्छद्वै विड्-विमिश्रं ह्यविड् वा निर्गन्धं बा गन्धवद्धातिसारः। शोकोत्पन्न-दुश्चिकित्स्योऽतिमात्रं रोगो वैद्यैः कष्ट एष प्रदृष्टः। अन्नाजीर्णात् प्रद्रुताः क्षोभयन्तः कोष्ठं दोषा धातुसङ्घान्मलांश्च। नानावर्णं नैकशः सारयन्ति शूलोपेतं षष्ठमेनं वदन्ति॥ संसृष्टमेभिर्दोषैस्तु न्यस्तमप्स्ववसीदति। पुरीषं भृशदुर्गन्धि पिच्छिलञ्चामसंज्ञितम् ॥ एतान्येव तु लिङ्गानि विपरीतानि यस्य वै। लाघवञ्च विशेषेण तस्य पक्वं विनिर्द्दिशेत् ॥

पक्वजाम्ववसङ्काशं यकृत्पिण्डनिभं तनु। घृततैलवसामज्जवेश-

3. When phlegm is deranged, the person dozes, the dejections are white, thick, and constipated, mixed with phlegm. He has no appetite, complains of languor and lassitude with dozing, and has frequent calls to stool, which are passed without any noise.

4. When the above three humours are deranged the dejections are of different colours. The patient is very thirsty with languor, dejection of mind, and drowsiness.* This kind of dysentery is fatal when children and old people are attacked; and in all cases it is difficult to cure, and will cause much vexation to the physician. The symptoms will vary according as one or other of the above forms predominate. The cause of the disease will likewise vary the symptoms.

5. When grief produces dysentery, the person has the internal fire of *pakasia* deranged by the watery vapours, which are formed by grief, and passing into *pakasia* mixes with the fire, and deranges the bright blood of the part. This blood is mixed with the dejections, often becomes putrid, and is expelled with them. In other cases it is discharged by itself. Some-

---

वारपयोदधि ॥ मांसधावनतोयाभं कृष्णं नीलारुणप्रभम्। मेचकं स्निग्धकर्वुरं चन्द्रकोपगतं घनम्। कुणपं मस्तुलुङ्गाभं सुगन्धि कथितं वहु। तृष्णा दाहतमःश्वासहिक्कापार्श्वास्थिशूलिनम्। संमूर्च्छारतिसंमोहयुक्तं पक्ववलीगुदम्। प्रलापयुक्तञ्च भिषग्वर्जयेदतिसारिणम्। असंवृतगुदं क्षीणं दुराध्मातमुपद्रुतम् ॥ गुदे पक्के गतोष्माणमतिसारकिणं त्यजेत ॥ श्वासशूलपिपासार्त्तं क्षीणं ज्वरनिपीड़ितम। विशेषेण नरं वृद्धमतीसारो विनाशयेत।

पित्तकृन्ति यदात्यर्थं द्रव्याण्यश्नाति पैत्तिके। तदोपजायतेऽभिक्ष्णं रक्तातीसार उल्वणः। वायुः प्रवृद्धो निचितं बलासं गुदत्यधस्तादहिताशनस्य। प्रताहतोऽल्पं बहुशो मलाक्तं प्रवा-

times it has a bad smell, in other cases it has not. The cure is tedious, and physicians are vexed by its obstinacy. If the dejections are frequent, the cure will be very difficult.

6. The sixth form is when it is produced by mucus, which deranges the stomach and is discharged frequently of various colours.

There are also two forms of dysentery, one being acute (*A'maapáka*) or crude, and the other chronic (*Pákátisár*) or mature.

Acute Dysentery (*A'maraktátisár*).

This form is known by the dejections sinking in. water, and being very fœtid. In the *páka* variety the opposite symptoms to the above are most prominent, and the abdomen does not feel heavy.

The unfavourable symptoms are a stiffness of the body, dejections of a dark bluish colour, like the ripe rose-apple ; in other cases the colour of the dejections is like that of the lime,

---

ह्विकां तां प्रवदन्ति तज्ज्ञाः। प्रवाह्विका वातकृता सशूला पित्तात् सदाहा सकफा कफाच्च। सशोणिता शोणितसम्भवाच्च ताः स्नेहरूक्षप्रभवा मतास्तु। तासामतीसारवदादिशेच्च लिङ्गं क्रमञ्चामविपक्वताञ्च। यस्योपचारं विना मूत्रं समम्वायुश्च गच्छति॥ दीप्ताग्ने र्लघुकोष्ठस्य स्थिततस्योदरामयः॥

ग्रहणीरोगनिदानम्।

अतीसारे निवृत्तेऽपि मन्दाग्नेरहिताशिनः। भूयः संदूषितो वह्निर्ग्रहणीमभिदूषयेत॥ एकैकशः सर्व्वशश्च दोषैरत्यर्थमूर्च्छितैः। सा दुष्टा बहुशो भुक्तमाममेव विमुञ्चति॥ पक्वं वा सरुजं पूति·

of ghee, or of oil, of tallow or marrow; in other cases they are like milk or curds; or like water in which flesh had been washed; or black, blue, or yellow; or like the colour of these three mixed together in different proportions; or like the water of Madar. In other cases they are very thin, of a fœtid smell, and cold; or of the colour of peacock's feathers, or that of the rainbow, or dry and hot. Sometimes the dejections are consistent, or like the brain, or like the refuse of well washed and beaten bark (fibrous), or its decoction, and are evacuated in large quantities. When the sick person is thirsty and hot, breathes through the nose, has hiccough, and pain in the side, and skin, with loss of memory, dosing and stupor, the disease will be fatal. Such a person has no inclination to do any thing, and remains stupid and complains of pain in the anus, like that of a ripe boil. He speaks incoherently and becomes insensible, with an involuntary discharge from the anus: such persons will not live. When the person is very much reduced in flesh, is cold and the abdomen distended, with pain in the anus: such a person should not be attended by the practitioner, as the disease is incurable.

मुहुर्ब्बद्धं मुहुर्द्रवम। ग्रहणीरोगमाहुस्तमायुर्व्वेदविदो जनाः॥ पूर्व्वरूपन्तु तस्येदं तृष्णालस्यं बलक्षयः। विदाहोऽन्नस्य पाकश्च चिरात कायस्य गौरवम॥

कटुतिक्तकषायातिरूक्षसंदुष्टभोजनैः। प्रमितानशनात्यध्ववेगविनिग्रहमैथुनैः॥ मारुतः कुपितो वह्निं संछाद्य कुरुते गदान्। तस्यान्नं पच्यते दुःखं शुक्तपाकं खराङ्गता॥ कण्ठास्यशोषः क्षुतृष्णा तिमिरं कर्णयोः स्वनः। पार्श्वोरुवङ्क्षणग्रीवारुगभीक्ष्णं विसूचिका॥ हृतपीड़कार्श्यदौर्व्वल्यं वैरस्यं परिकर्त्तिका। गृद्धिः सर्व्वरसानाञ्च मनसः सदनन्तथा। जिर्णे जीर्य्यति

The physician should be able to distinguish the symptoms of *A ma*, or acute, from those of chronic dysentery. Without this he will not be able to treat the disease properly.

Diarrhœa, (*Grihinî.*)

By the use of improper food the internal fire is weakened, which deranges the place where it is situated, between the stomach and place of the chyle. When any thing is eaten, which is not properly digested, and is frequently discharged, with or without pain, sometimes liquid, at other times consistent, sometimes it is evacuated without air, and at other times it is fœtid, it forms this disease. Before it commences the patient complains of lassitude and weakness of the body, accompanied with noise in the intestines, sour and bitter eructations, and a bad taste in the mouth. When a singing of the ears, œdema in the hands and feet, with pain in the joints, vomiting, fever, thirst, loss of appetite, and a heaviness and

---

चाध्मानं भुक्ते स्वास्थ्यमुपैति च। न वातगुल्महृद्रोगप्लीहाशङ्की
च मानवः॥ चिराद्दुःखं द्रवं शुष्कं तन्वामं शब्दफेनवत्। पुनः
पुनः सृजेद्वर्चः कासश्वासार्दितोऽनिलात्॥

कट्वजीर्णविदाह्यम्लक्षाराद्यैः पित्तमुल्बणम्। आप्लावयद्धन्त्य
नलं जलन्तप्तमिवानलम्॥ सोऽजीर्णं नीलपीताभं पीताभः सार्यते
द्रवम्। पूत्यम्लोद्गारहृत्कण्ठदाहारुचितृडर्दितः॥

गुर्व्वतिस्निग्धशीतादिभोजनादतिभोजनात्। भुक्तमात्रस्य
च स्वप्नाद्धन्त्यग्निं कुपितः कफः॥ तस्यान्नं पच्यते दुःखं
हृल्लासच्छर्द्यरोचकाः। आस्योपदेहमाधुर्यं कासष्ठीवनपीनसाः॥
हृदयं मन्यते स्त्यानमुदरः स्तिमितं गुरु। दुष्टो मधुर उद्गार

burning sensation of the body occurs, in old cases, the prognosis should be guarded. These symptoms are varied when either the air, bile, or phlegm, or their peculiar symptoms are present.

Another form of Diarrhœa is called *Sangraha Grihiní;* from *Sangraha*, (a collection,) and *Grihiní*, (place of internal fire;) in which there is much noise in the stomach, with laziness, weakness and lassitude. The stools are unnatural, irregular, and evacuated with noise; sometimes they are thin, and in other cases they are consistent or hard, and of a pale colour like indigested food. Some people remain ten or fifteen days, or even one month, without any fecal discharge; other patients feel well during the day, but have frequent dejections during the night. The prognosis of this form of disease is unfavourable, as it is obstinate and is cured with much difficulty.

सदनं स्त्रीषहर्षणम ॥ भिन्नामश्लेष्मसंश्लिष्टं गुरुवर्च्चप्रवर्त्तनं । अकृशस्यापि दौर्व्बल्यं मालस्यञ्च कफात्मके । पृथग्वातादिनिर्द्दिष्ट हेतुलिङ्गसमागमे । त्रिदोषं निर्द्दिशेदेवं तेषां वक्ष्यामि भेषजं ॥

अन्त्रकूजनमालस्यं दौवल्यं सदनन्तथा । द्रवं शीतं घनं स्निग्धं सकटिवेदनं शकृत् । आमं बहु सपैच्छिल्यं सशब्दं मन्दवेदनम् ॥ पक्षान्मासाद्दशाहाद्वा नित्यं वाप्यथ मुञ्चति ॥ दिवा प्रकोपो भवति रात्रौ शान्तिं व्रजेच्च सा । दुर्व्विज्ञेया दुश्चिकित्सा चिरकालानुबन्धिनी ॥ सा भवेदामवातेन संग्रहग्रहणी मता ।

अर्शोनिदानम् ।

पृथग्दोषैः समस्तैश्च शोणितैः सहजानि च । अर्शांसि षट् प्रकाराणि विद्याद्गुदवलित्रये ॥ दोषास्त्वङ्मांसमेदांसि संदुष्य विविधाकृतीन् । मांसाङ्कुरानपानादौ कुर्व्वन्त्यर्शांसितान् जगुः ॥

Arsa (*Piles.*)

There are six varieties of this disease according as it is produced from deranged air, bile, phlegm, the three humours deranged at the same time, diseased blood, and the last form is congenital or hereditary.

That part of the rectum called *guda* is five and a half fingers breadth in length, has three spiral turns called *Prabáhiní*, which accelerates or assists in expelling its contents. The second is called *Bisarjiní*, or that which expells; and *Sambariní*, or sphincter. Piles are usually situated in these parts, the causes producing them are as follows: The improper mixtures of food, excessive venery, the unnatural position of the body when long indulged in; horse riding, and the want of attention to the calls of nature. By these causes the humours are deranged in the anus and produce tubercles, or piles.

कषायकटुतिक्तानि रूक्षशीतलघूनि च। प्रमिताल्पाशनं तीक्ष्णं मद्यं मैथुनसेवनम्॥ लङ्घनं देशकालौ च शीतौ व्यायामकर्म्म च। शोको वातातपस्पर्शो हेतुर्व्वातार्शसां मतः। कट्वम्ललवणोष्णानि व्यायामाग्न्यातपप्रभाः॥ देशकालावशिशिरौ क्रोधो मद्यमसूयनम्। विदाही तिक्ष्णमुष्णञ्च सर्व्वं पानान्नभेषजम्। पित्तोल्वणानां विज्ञेयः प्रकोपे हेतुरर्शसाम्॥ मधुरस्निग्धशीतानि लवणाम्लगुरूणि च। अव्यायाम दिवास्वप्न शय्यासनसुखे रतिः॥ प्राग्वातसेवा शीतौ च देशकालावचिन्तनम्। श्लैष्मिकानां समुद्दिष्टमेतत् कारणमर्शसाम॥ हेतु लक्षणसंसर्गाद्विद्याद्द्वन्द्वोल्वणानि च। सर्व्व हेतु स्त्रिदोषाणां सहजे लक्षणैः समम्॥

विष्टम्भोऽन्नस्य दौर्ब्बल्यं कुक्षेराटोप एव च। कार्श्यमुद्गारबाहुल्यं स क्थिसादोऽल्पविट्कता॥ ग्रहणीदोष पाण्डुर्त्तेराशङ्का चोदरस्य च। पूर्व्वरूपाणि निर्द्दिष्टान्यर्शसामभिवृद्धये॥

When *air* is deranged it affords the following signs ; round the anus small tumors form, which are dry, slightly painful, red, and irregular like the *kadamba* fruit. The disease is accompanied with constipation, pain in the back, loins, penis, anus, and umbiliacus ; and is occasionally accompanied with pain in the breast, want of appetite, cough, and noise in breathing ; sometimes the appetite is good, at other times it is much impaired. The blood is often evacuated by a small orifice from time to time. The skin, eyes, face, mouth, teeth, and nails appear dirty and yellow with unhealthy yellowish dejections, and urine. Symptoms likewise appear like *Gulma* or spleen, or it even produces these diseases. In other cases the piles produce *Astila*, a kind of hysterical ball.

When bile is deranged the swelling has an erysipelatous appearance ; at other times it has a blue, yellow, red, or black colour, with orifices in its surface, like the mouths of leeches. The blood evacuated is very thin, and there is a considerable discharge, with pain in the part, accompanied with fever, thirst, and fainting.

When phlegm is deranged the tumors are pendulous, near each other, hard, round, shining, and of a white colour, like

---

गुदाङ्कुरा बह्वनिलाः शुष्का श्चिमचिमान्विताः । म्लानाः श्यावारुणास्तब्धा विषादा परुषाः खराः ॥ मिथो विसदृशा वक्रा स्तीक्ष्णा विस्फुटिताननाः । बिम्बीखर्ज्जूरकर्कन्धुकार्पासीफलसन्निभाः । केचित् कदम्बपुष्पाभाः केचित् सिद्धार्थकोपमाः । शिरः पार्श्वांस कट्यूरुवङ्क्षणाद्यधिकव्यथाः । क्षवथूद्गारविष्टम्भः हृद्ग्रहारोचकप्रदाः । कासश्वासाग्निवैषम्य कर्णनाद भ्रमावहाः ॥ तैरार्त्तो ग्रथितं स्तोकं सशब्दं सप्रवाहिकम् । रुक्फेनपिच्छानुगतं विबद्धमुपवेश्यते । कृष्णत्वङ्नखविण्मूत्रनेत्रवक्त्रश्च जायते । गुल्मप्लीहोदराष्ठीला सम्भवस्तत एव च ॥

the paps of the cow. There is no discharge, they are cold, itchy, heavy, remain stationary, and the stools are mixed with mucus, and appear like water in which flesh had been washed. In some cases the disease is accompanied with swelling of the extremities, with feverishness, loss of appetite, heaviness and pain of the head; and the skin, nails, eyes, face, urine, and fæces becomes white. In these diseases there is a great discharge of urine, the person often becomes impotent, and digestion is impaired, with vomiting. Those diseases which impair digestion, produce this disease. When the three humours are diseased, the symptoms of the three separate diseases are present.

When blood produces the disease, the pain is like that of a needle thrust into the skin, and symptoms appear like those of deranged bile. The tumors resemble the hanging roots of the banian tree, or the *kunch* seeds, small red seeds with black spots, or they are like coral. When costiveness occurs it is accompanied with a free and rapid discharge of blood, which is hot, and produces the usual effects of a great and sudden loss of blood; the person with this disease remains yellow, like the

---

पित्तोत्तरा नीलमुखा रक्तपीतासितप्रभा। तन्वस्रस्राविणो
विस्रा स्तनवो मृदवः श्लथाः। शुकजिह्वायकृत्खण्डजलौक
वक्त्रसन्निभाः। दाहपाकज्वरस्वेद-तृण्मूर्च्छारुचिमोहदाः। सोष्माणो
द्रवनीलोष्णपीतरक्तामवर्च्चसः। यवमध्या हरित्पीतहारिद्रत्वङ्
नखादयः।

श्लेष्मोल्बणा महामूला घना मन्दरुजः सिताः। उत्सन्नोपचित
स्निग्धाः स्तब्धवृत्तगुरुस्थिराः। पिच्छिलाः स्तिमिताः श्लक्ष्ण
कण्ड्वाढ्याः स्पर्शनप्रियाः। करीरपनसास्थ्याभा स्तथा गोस्तन
सन्निभाः। वङ्क्षणानाहिनः पायुवस्तिनाभिविकर्षिणः। सश्वास
कासहृल्लासप्रसेकारुचिपीनसाः। मेहकृच्छ्रशिरोजाड्य शिशिर

yellow frog; weak, silent, and sad; his skin is dirty, and all his senses perform their office imperfectly or they are depraved. The dejections are gray, like smoke, dry and hard, and in others they are thin, yellow, and frothy.

The last form of this disease is produced by hereditary disposition, from the taint being mixed in the semen and female blood. The tumors in this form become rough, of a white unnatural colour, with internal openings. The patient cannot eat much, his body has large veins over the surface, and his voice is low. He is impatient, is easily roused, has little appetite, is afflicted with diseases of the eyes, ears, nose, and head, and is always complaining of diseases of the stomach and intestines.

When piles are external they are easily cured, but when situated internally they are cured with difficulty, or are incurable. Tumors like those of piles sometimes form in the cavities of the ear, nose, mouth, vagina, and upon the penis.

When affecting the internal ear, they produce deafness, pain, and a fetid discharge from the organ. In the eyes they

---

ज्वरकारिणः। क्लैव्याग्निमार्द्दवः छर्द्दिरामप्राय विकारदाः। वसाभ सकफप्राज्य पुरीषाः सप्रवाहिकाः। न स्रवन्ति न भिद्यन्ते पाण्डु-स्निग्धत्वगादयः। सर्व्वैः सर्व्वात्मकान्याहु लक्षणैः सहजानि च।

रक्तोल्बणा गुदे कीलाः पित्ताकृतिसमन्विताः। वटप्ररोह-सदृशा गुञ्जाविद्रुमसन्निभाः॥ तेऽत्यर्थं दुष्टमुष्णाञ्च गाढ़विट्क प्रपीड़िताः। स्रवन्ति सहसा रक्तं तस्य चातिप्रवर्त्तितः॥ भेकाभः पीड्यते दुःखैः शोणितक्षयसम्भवैः। हीनवर्णबलोत्साहो हतौजाः कलुषेन्द्रियः। विट्श्यावं कठिनं रुक्षमधोवायुर्न वर्त्तते। तनु चारुणवर्णञ्च फेनिलञ्चासृगर्भसाम्। कट्यूरुगुदशूलञ्च दौर्व्बल्यं यदि चाधिकम्। तत्रानुवन्धो वातस्य हेतु यदि च रुक्षणम्।

cover the eyelids; and sometimes destroy the sight of the organ. When in the mouth, they are attached to the throat, lips, and palate, they impair the voice and taste, and produce other diseases of the mouth. When in the nostrils they produce difficult breathing, a fetid smell, a change of voice, pain in the head, and a considerable discharge from the nose.

The deranged humours produce the disease on the surface of the body when they form tumors of different sizes, which are called *Charmkíla.* When the air is deranged the disease is accompanied with throbbing; when phlegm, the colour of the tumor is the colour of the skin and hard. When bile and blood are deranged, producing the disease, the tumors become black and rough. Those piles which form externally are curable, as also those in the first and second convolutions of the rectum, but

---

शिथिलं श्वेतपीतञ्च विट्स्निग्धं गुरु शीतलम्। यदर्शसां घनञ्चासृक् तन्तुमत् पाण्डुपिच्छिलम्। गुदं सपिच्छं स्तिमितं गुरु स्निग्धञ्च कारणम्। श्लेष्मानुबन्धो विज्ञेय स्तत्र रक्तार्शसां बुधैः॥

पञ्चात्मा मारुतः पित्तं कफो गुदवलीत्रयम्। सर्व्व एवं प्रकुप्यन्ति गुदजानां समुद्भवे॥ तस्मादर्शांसि दुःखानि बहुव्याधिकराणि च। सर्व्वदेहोपतापीनि प्रायः कृच्छ्रतमानि च॥

बाह्यायान्तु बलौ जातान्येकदोषोल्बणानि च। अर्शांसि सुखसाध्यानि न चिरोत्पतितानि च॥ द्वन्द्वजानि द्वितीयायां बलौ यान्याश्रितानि च। कृच्छ्रसाध्यानि तान्याहुः परिसंवत्सराणि च॥ सहजानि त्रिदोषाणि यानि चाभ्यन्तरां बलिम्। जायन्तेऽर्शांसि संश्रित्य तान्यसाध्यानि निर्द्दिशेत्। शेषत्वादायुषस्तानि चतुष्पादसमन्विते॥ याप्यन्ते दीप्तकायाग्नेः प्रत्याख्येयान्यतोऽन्यथा हस्ते पादे मुखे नाभ्यां गुदे वृषणयोस्तथा॥ शोथो हृत्पार्श्व

in the third the disease is incurable, and also after they have existed for upwards of a year.

Ajirna (*Indigestion.*)

This disease is divided into three varieties, *A'ma Ajírna Bistabdha Ajírna,* and *Bidagdha Ajírna.* When digestion is good, the food is properly prepared for the use of the body, the eructations are free and without taste, and the dejections are natural, the body is light and elastic, and the person is inclined to exertion, he has a good appetite and the food is tasty, and is accompanied with thirst.

When digestion is imperfect the person's temper becomes bad, he is subject to anger, is fearful, and becomes covetous. The food of persons with a bad and hasty temper is not properly digested. When indigestion occurs, there is a disinclination to exertion, with giddiness; the body is heavy, the

---

शूलञ्च यस्यासाध्योऽर्शसो हि सः। हृत्पार्श्वशूलं संमोहश्छर्दिरङ्गस्य रुग्ज्वरः॥ तृष्णा गुदस्य पाकश्च निहन्युरर्गुदजातुरम्। तृष्णारोचकशूलार्त्तमतिप्रस्रुतशोणितम्॥ शोथातिसारसंयुक्तमर्शांसि क्षपयन्ति हि।

मेढ्रादिष्वपि वक्ष्यन्ते यथास्वं नाभिजानि च। गण्डूपदास्यरूपाणि पिच्छिलानि मृदूनि च।

अथाग्निमान्द्याजीर्णविसूचिकालसकविलम्बिका-
निदानम्।

मन्दस्तीक्ष्णोऽथ विषमः समश्चेति चतुर्व्विधः। कफपित्तानिलाधिक्यात्तत्साम्याज्जाठरोऽनलः॥ विषमो वातजान् रोगान् तीक्ष्णः पित्तनिमित्तजान्। करोत्यग्नि स्तथा मन्दो विकारान्

colour of the skin bad, and there is no passage of air; such a person does not like his food, his understanding is impaired, and his bowels are either constipated or there are copious dejections.

The unfavourable symptoms of this disease are fainting, delirium, vomiting, a copious discharge of saliva from the mouth, with languor, and giddiness.

A'ma Ajírna. In this disease the body feels heavy, with a flow of saliva and phlegm from the nose. The eyelids swell, and there are eructations of the substances eaten, some time before.

In *Bistabdha Ajírna,* the air is deranged, and produces severe pain in the stomach, with flatulency. The stomach swells, there are no dejections, no air escapes, and the person remains stupid, with his understanding impaired, and pain over the body.

In *Bidagdha Ajírna,* the bile is deranged, the person has sour eructations, complains of thirst, is giddy and often dozes. He has a free perspiration over the body, which feels hot.

कफसम्भवात्॥ समासमाग्नेरशिता मात्रा सम्यग्विपच्यते। स्वल्पापि
नैव मन्दाग्ने र्विषमाग्नेस्तु देहिनः॥ कदाचित् पच्यते सम्यक्
कदाचिच्च न पच्यते। मात्रातिमात्राप्यशिता सुखं यस्य विपच्यते।
तीक्ष्णाग्निरिति तं विद्यात् समाग्निः श्रेष्ठ उच्यते।

आमं विदग्धं विष्टब्धं कफपित्तानिलैस्त्रिभिः। अजीर्णं केचिदि
च्छन्ति चतुर्थं रसशेषतः॥ अजीर्णं पञ्चमं केचिन्निर्द्दोषं दिनपावि
च। वदन्ति षष्ठं चाजीर्णं प्राकृतं प्रतिवासरम्॥

अत्यम्बुपानाद्विषमाशनाच्च संधारणात् स्वप्नविपर्य्ययाच्च। काले
ऽपि सात्म्यं लघु चापि भुक्त मन्नं न पाकं भजते नरस्य॥ तत्रामे
गुरुतोत्क्लेदः शोथो गण्डाक्षिकूटगः। उद्गारश्च यथा भुक्त मवि
दग्धः प्रवर्त्तते॥ विष्टब्धे शूलमाध्मानं विविधा वातवेदना

When there is want of digestion, although the individual thinks the appetite good and eats, still it does not nourish the body, but acts as a poison in destroying the person. When the food is not taken in the usual quantities, digestion is not performed, and is often followed by disease. When a person eats like an animal, without consideration, he will be affected with indigestion, which is the cause of other diseases, as cholera, drum-belly, and constipation.

A'lasaka, (drum-belly.) The abdomen in this disease becomes enlarged and tight, with a rumbling noise, and the air passes upwards, followed by a constipation of fæces and air; with great thirst, eructations, and pain in the stomach.

Bilambika, or constipation, is somewhat different from drum-belly, as there is no swelling nor tightness of the abdomen; nor is the indigested food either rejected by vomiting nor by stool; but is retained in the abdomen causing much pain there, and likewise producing various diseases in different parts of the body. Constipation is always difficult to cure.

Dyspepsia, (*Agní Mándya.*)

This disease is supposed to be produced by derangements of the internal fire. It has four varieties.

मलवाताप्रवृत्तिश्च स्तम्भो मोहाङ्गपीड़नम् ॥ विदग्धे भ्रमतृण्मूर्च्छाः पित्ताच्च विविधा रुजः । उद्गारश्च सधुमाम्लः स्वेदो दाहश्च जायते ॥ रसशेषेऽन्नविद्वेषो हृदयाशुद्धिगौरवे ।

मूर्च्छा प्रलापो वमथुः प्रसेकः सदनं भ्रमम् । उपद्रवा भवन्तेऽग्रते मरणं वापग्रजीर्णतः । अनात्मवन्तः पशुवद्भुञ्जते येऽप्रमाणतः । रोगानीकस्य ते मूल मजीर्णं प्राप्नुवन्ति हि ॥

1st. When there is too little fire, it is called *Manda Agní* ; when food is not digested, or only imperfectly. In this form, the diseases of phlegm are often present.

2nd. When the fire is too strong, as when bile is deranged, it is called *Tikhna Agní*. In this case, little or even large quantities of food are digested; and the diseases of bile are liable to occur.

3rd. When the air is deranged the food is sometimes digested and sometimes not; from fire being sometimes in the natural state, and at other times it is deranged. In this case the disease is called *Bishama Agní*, when other diseases of air are present.

4th. *Bhasma Agní*, *(Bulimia,)* when pungent, sour and dry food are taken for some time; phlegm is diminished, and air is much increased; the internal fire, with the deranged air,

---

अथ विसूची-अलसक-विलम्बिका

निदानम् ।

अजीर्णमामं विष्टब्धं विदग्धञ्च यदीरितम्। विसूच्यलसकौ तस्माद्भवेच्चापि विलम्बिका ॥

सूचीभिरिव गात्राणि तुदन् सन्तिष्ठतेऽनिलः। यस्याजीर्णेन सा वैद्यैर्विसूचीति निगद्यते। न तां परिमिताहारा लभन्ते विदितागमाः। मूढास्तामजितात्मानो लभन्तेऽशनलोलुपाः मूर्च्छातिसारौ वमथुः, पिपासा शूलभ्रमोद्वेष्टनजृम्भदाहाः। वैवर्ण्यकम्पौ हृदये रुजश्च. भवन्ति तस्यां शिरसश्च भेदः।

कुक्षिरानह्यतेऽत्यर्थं प्रताम्यति परिकूजति। निरुद्धो मारुतश्चैव कुक्षावुपरि धावति ॥ वातवर्चोनिरोधश्च यस्यात्यर्थं भवेदपि तस्यलसकमाचष्टे तृष्णोद्गारौ च यस्य तु ॥

absorbs the liquid part of the body, and the food when taken is soon digested, or reduced to ashes, and the person is not satisfied. This disease is accompanied with great thirst, dry cough, fainting, giddiness, burning of the body and emaciation, with severe constipation, and much perspiration.

When there is no increase or diminution of the air, bile, and phlegm, in the same person; the fire remains in the natural state, and is called *Sama Agni.* This is not a disease, but is the most favourable state of digestion, and is the condition in which food is properly digested; when not taken in too small, or too large quantities. The divisions of the digestive organs into the parts in which the food are received, *Amasia*, (stomach;) *Agniaria*, (the duodenum;) and in which the digested food is removed *Pakasia*, (the small intestines,) is probably from the known structure of the intestines of the inferior animals.

This disease is produced by drinking much water, and eating at unusual hours, when very little food is taken, and the calls of nature are resisted; when the person is sleepy or

---

दुष्टन्तु भुक्तं कफमारुताभ्यां प्रवर्त्तते नोर्द्धमधश्च यस्य।
विलम्बिकां तां भृशदुश्चिकित्सा। माचक्षते शास्त्रविदः पुराणाः॥
यत्रस्थमाम् विरुजेत्तमेव देशं विशेषेण विकारजातैः।
दोषेण येनावततं शरीरं तल्लक्षणैरामसमुद्भवैश्च।
यः श्यावदन्तोष्ठनखोऽल्पसंज्ञो वम्यर्दितोऽभ्यन्तरयातनेत्रः।
क्षामस्वरः सर्व्वविमुक्तसन्धि र्यायान्नरः सोऽपुनरागमाय।
उद्गारशुद्धिरुत्साहो वेगोत्सर्गौ यथोचितः। लघुता क्षुत्-
पिपासा च जीर्णाहारस्य लक्षणम्॥

अथ क्रिमिनिदानम्।

क्रिमयश्च द्विधा प्रोक्ता वाह्याभ्यन्तरभेदतः। वहिर्मलकफा-
सृग्विट्-जन्मभेदाच्चतुर्व्विधाः॥ नामतो विंशतिविधा वाह्यास्तत्र

is in a passion, or is afraid, grieved, or fatigued at the time o eating; and when he dislikes the food during the time of eat ing. It is also produced, when the person sleeps during th day, instead of at night, or is irregular in the time of sleeping and when at the usual time of dinner, little is eaten. By such causes the food is not digested in the proper manner. When phlegm is deranged the food tastes sweet, and is indigested when bile, the taste is sour, and the food in the stomach pro duces eructations; and air when deranged causes the partiall digested food to be dried up, with pain in the stomach.

Bisuchika—(*Cholera.*)

The person first feels pain, as from indigestion, in the abdomen followed by frequent stools and vomiting, great thirst, and pain in the abdomen, fainting, giddiness, yawning, and cramps in the legs The colour of the body is altered, accompanied with shivering, pain in the chest, and head-ache. The unfavourable symptoms of choler are, the lips, teeth and nails become blackish, the person insen

---

मलोद्भवाः। तिलप्रमाणसंस्थानवर्णाः केशाम्बराश्रयाः॥ बहु पादाश्च सूक्ष्माश्च युका लिक्षाश्च नामतः। द्विधा ते कोठपिडक कण्डुगण्डान् प्रकुर्व्वते॥

अजीर्णभोजी मधुराम्लनित्यो द्रवप्रियः पिष्टगुड़ोपभोक्ता व्यायामवर्ज्जी च दिवाशयानो विरुद्धभुक् संलभते क्रिमींस्तु॥ मा पिष्टाम्ललवणगुड़शाकैः पुरीषजाः। मांसमत्स्यगुड़क्षीरदधि शुक्तैः कफोद्भवाः॥ विरुद्धाजीर्णशाकाद्यैः शोणितोत्था भवन्ति हि। ज्वरो विवर्णता शूलं हृद्रोगः सदनं भ्रमः॥ भक्तद्वेषोऽति सारश्च सञ्जातक्रिमिलक्षणम्। कफादामाशये जाता वृद्धाः सर्पन्ति सर्व्वतः॥ पृथुब्रध्ननिभाः केचित् केचिद्गण्डूपदोपमाः। रूढ़धा

ple, with freqnent vomiting. The eyes become sunken, voice feeble, nd the joints loose, with great debility. Such a person may be ken out to the burnt, as he will not recover. The most tal symptoms of cholera are, want of sleep, restlessness, tivering, no secretion of urine, and insensibility.

Worms,—(*Krimi.*)

There is an internal sort of worms, and another which pears upon the surface of the body. Others say that there are ır kinds ; one is external and produced by filth on the sur-ce ; others are internal and are produced by phlegm, by ood, and by the fæces. There are twenty varieties of worms, ch of which has a particular name. When produced exter-lly by filth, the insect is like a small Til-seed with many t, and is generally found in the hair and clothes. They are lled *juka* (lice). They produce small very itchy pimples, nd sometimes a large boil.

गण्डूराकारा स्तनुदीर्घा स्तथाणवः ॥ श्वेतास्ताम्रावभाषाश्च
मतः सप्तधा तु ते। अन्त्रादा उदरावेष्टा हृदयादा महागुदाः ॥
प्रवो दर्भकुसुमाः सुगन्धास्ते च कुर्व्वते। हृल्लासमास्यश्रवण मवि-
क्रमरोचकम्। मूर्च्छाच्छर्द्दिज्वरानाह कार्श्यक्षवथुपीनसान्॥
क्तवाहिशिराख्यान रक्तजा जन्तवोऽणवः। अपादा वृत्तताम्राश्च
ग्वात् केचिददर्शनाः॥ केशादा रोमविध्वंसा रोमद्वीपा उडुम्बराः।
ट् ते कुष्ठैककर्म्माणः सह सौरस मातरः। पक्वाशये पूरीषोत्था
यन्तेऽधो विसर्पिणः। वृद्धास्ते स्युर्भवेयुश्च ते यद्वामाशयोन्मुखाः।
दास्योद्गारनिश्वासविड्गन्धानुविधायिनः॥ पृथुवृत्ततनुस्थूलाः
नपीतश्वितासिताः। ते पञ्च नाम्ना क्रिमयः ककेरुकमकेरुकाः।

When *phlegm* produces the worms internally, it is deranged by indigestable food, particularly when taken at improper times, or with much sugar, or sweetmeats, or much liquids, as vinegar or sour food, curdled milk, vegetables, and unleavened flour when taken daily and frequently. A sedentary life, and sleeping during the day predisposes to worms.

When *blood* produces worms many diseases are the consequence. In this case it is caused by improper mixtures, or by indigestable food, or certain vegetables, &c. The worms are produced in the blood.

The general symptoms of internal worms are fever, paleness, and discoloration of the surface, severe pain, or *Sul*, especially in the breast, with languor, giddiness, loss of appetite, and diarrhœa. When produced by phlegm they are usually found in the stomach (*A'masiya*), and resemble earth-worms, and when very large they pass from one intestine to another. Some of the worms are like rice which has begun to germinate, some are long, others are short, and very small; some are white, or like nahogany, others are copper-coloured. There are seven varieties of worms found in the stomach. 1st, *Antrada*, or the gnawing

---

सौसुरादाः सशूलाख्या लेलिहा जनयन्ति हि॥ विड्भेदशूलविष्टम्भ-कार्श्यपारुष्यपाण्डुताः। रोमहर्षाग्निसदनं गुदकण्डुर्विमार्गगाः॥

अथ पाण्डुकामला-कुम्भकामला-हलीमक-निदानम्।

पाण्डुरोगाः स्मृताः पञ्च वातपित्तकफैस्त्रयः। चतुर्थः सन्निपातेन पञ्चमो भक्षणान्मृदः॥ व्यायाममम्लं लवणानि मद्यं, मृदं दिवास्वप्नमतीवतीक्ष्णम्। निषेव्यमाणस्य प्रदूष्य रक्तं दोषास्त्वचं पाण्डुरतां नयन्ति॥ त्वक्स्फोटन-ष्ठीवन-गात्रसाद-मृद्भक्षण-प्रेक्षण कूटशोथाः। विण्मूत्रपीतत्वमथाविपाको भविष्यतस्तस्य पुरःसराणि॥

kind; 2nd. *Udarábesta,* large form; 3rd. *Rhidayada,* produces a gnawing pain in the breast; 4th. *Mahágada,* with a large tail; 5th. *Chara,* like flattened rice; 6th. *Durbakusama,* like the flower of a certain grass, and 7th. *Sugandha,* which has a pleasant smell. These seven kinds of worms produce nausea, a copious discharge of saliva, indigestion, and want of appetite; fainting, dozing, vomiting and fever; constipation of urine and fæces, and weakness, sneezing, and a discharge of mucus from the nose.

The worms in the blood have no feet, some have a round figure and red colour (red globules of the blood), and they are so small that they cannot be distinctly seen. Their names are, 1. *Káysáda*: this form eats the roots of the hair of the head which drop out. 2. *Romabidhansa*: this form eats the roots of the hair over the body. 3. *Romadipa*: this variety produces elevations at the roots of the hair. 4. *Arambara,* are like the seeds of the wild fig; these worms may produce the (*kustha*), leprosy. 5. *Saurasa,* (father,) and 6. *Mátrí,* (mother.) These two pass quickly from one relation to another, or are hereditary.

त्वङ्मूत्रनयनादीनां रूक्षकृष्णारुणाभताः। वातपाण्डामये तोद कम्पानाह भ्रमादयः। पीतमूत्रशकृन्नेत्रो दाहतृष्णाज्वरान्वितः। भिन्नविट्कोऽतिपीताभः पित्तपाण्डामयी नरः। कफप्रसेकश्वयथु-तन्द्रालस्यातिगौरवैः। पाण्डुरोगी कफाच्छुक्लैस्त्वङ्मूत्रनयनाननैः। ज्वरारोचकहृल्लास-छर्द्दि-तृष्णाक्लमान्वितः॥ पाण्डुरोगी त्रिभिर्द्दोषै स्त्रग्राजग्रः क्षीणो हतेन्द्रियः। मृत्तिकादनशीलस्य कुप्यत्यन्यतमो मलः। कषाया मारुतं पित्तं उषरा मधुरा कफम्। कोपयेन्मृन्द्रसादींश्च रौक्ष्याद्भुक्तञ्च रूक्षयेत्। पूरयत्यविपक्वैव स्रोतांसि निरुणद्ध्यपि। इन्द्रियाणां बलं हत्वा तेजोवीर्यौजसी तथा। पाण्डुरोगं करोत्याशु बलवर्णाग्निनाशनम्।

Sushruta enumerates other kinds of worms generated in the blood; as, *Nakáda,* which destroys the nails.

Dantáda, which produces the caries of the teeth.

Kíkísa, which always accompanies leprosy.

When worms form in the small and large intestines they are called *Parisajya,* which are produced in the fæces, and are discharged by the anus. When these worms grow and ascend in the abdomen frequent eructations occur, which have the smell of the dejections. They are large, round, thick or thin, and are sometimes of a gray colour, or of a yellow white or dark colour. There are five kinds of such worms, 1. *Kakíraka*; 2. *Makíraka*; 3. *Sausuráda,* producing much pain; 4. *Sasulákiya*; 5. *Sailika,* which licks the intestines. These worms produce diarrhœa, pain in the stomach, dryness of the fæces, constipation, weakness, roughness, and dryness of the surface of the body, which is of a dirty yellow colour. There is loss of appetite with an itchiness towards the anus.

The thirteen first kinds of internal worms are curable, but the seven last are very difficult, or are incurable.

शूनाक्षिकूटगण्डभ्रूः शूनपान्नाभिमेहनः। क्रिमिकोऽष्ठोतिसार्य्येत मलं सासृक्कफान्वितम् ॥

पाण्डुरोगश्चिरोत्पन्नः खरीभूतो न सिध्यति। कालप्रकर्षाच्छूनानां यो वा पीतानि पश्यति। बद्धाल्पविट् सहरितं सकफं योऽतिसार्य्यते ॥ दीनः श्वेतादिदिग्धाङ्गश्छर्द्दिमूर्च्छातृड्र्दितः। स नास्त्र-सृक्क्षयाद् यश्च पाण्डुश्वेतत्वमाप्नुयात् ॥ पाण्डुदन्तनखो यस्तु पाण्डुनेत्रश्च यो भवेत्। पाण्डुसंघातदर्शी च पाण्डुरोगी विनश्यति। अन्तेषु शूनं परिहीनमध्यं, म्लानन्तथान्तेषु च मध्यशूनम्। गुदे च शेफस्यथ मुष्कयोश्च, शूनं प्रताम्यन्तमसंज्ञककल्पम्। विवर्ज्जयेत् पाण्डुकिनं यशोर्थी, तथातिसारज्वरपीड़ितञ्च ॥

Jaundice, (*Pándu.*)

This disease is produced by excesses in venery, eating earth, sour or salt food, or drinking much wine. It is likewise produced by sleeping during the day, and eating very hot things, which derange the air, bile, and phlegm.

There are five kinds of this disease produced by deranged air, bile, or phlegm; when these three are deranged together, and when produced by eating earth, especially chalk. When the air, bile, or phlegm are diseased, they derange the blood; and produce the pale or yellowish white colour of the skin. Before the disease appears the skin feels as if pinched, the sputa is red, the person cannot do any work, and has a desire to eat earth; his eyelids swell, the dejections and urine are yellow, and whatever is eaten is not digested

1. When *air* is deranged producing this disease, the skin, urine, and eyes, or other parts, are rough, dark-coloured, and brownish with shaking, pain over the body, and the dejections and urine are constipated, with giddiness.

2. When the *bile* is deranged, the urine, dejections, and eyes are of a yellow colour, the body is hot, with thirst, and

---

पाण्डुरोगी तु योऽत्यर्थं पित्तलानि निषेवते। तस्य पित्तमसृक्मांसं दग्ध्वा रोगाय कल्पते॥ हारिद्रनेत्रः स भृशं हारिद्रत्वङ्नखाननः। रक्तपीतशकृन्मूत्रो भेकवर्णो हतेन्द्रियः। दाहाविपाकदौर्ब्बल्यसदनारुचिकर्षितः। कामला बहुपित्तैषा कोष्ठशाखाश्रया मता॥ कालान्तरात् खरीभूता कृच्छ्रा स्यात् कुम्भकामला॥ कृष्णपीतशकृन्मूत्रो भृशं शूनश्च मानवः॥ स रक्ताक्षिमुखच्छर्दिविण्मूत्रो यश्च ताम्यति। दाहारुचितृड़ानाह तन्द्रामोहसमन्वितः। नष्टाग्निसंज्ञः क्षिप्रं हि कामलावान् विपद्यते। छर्द्यरोचकहृल्लास-ज्वरक्लमनिपीड़ितः। नश्यति श्वासकासार्त्तो विड्भेदी कुम्भकामली॥

fever, there are frequent dejections, and the surface of the body is very yellow.

3. *Phlegm.* In this form the phlegm proceeds from the mouth and nose, the person often dozes and complains of lassitude and heaviness of the body ; the skin, eyes, and face are of a whitish colour ; the urine is also pale.

4. When the *air, bile,* and *phlegm* are at the same time deranged, there is fever, no appetite, retching and vomiting, the person complains of thirst, and the body feels painful and tired. When such a person is very weak and insensible the person will die.

5. When produced by eating *earth* there are three kinds ; one deranging the *air*, another the *bile*, and a third the *phlegm.* Astringent earth (*kasáya mritiká*) also deranges *air* ; salt-earth (*usara*), deranges *bile* ; and sweet-earth (*madhura*), deranges the *phlegm.* When earth deranges the elements of the body, and whatever is eaten remains undigested, the blood which is formed stops the mouths of the vessels of the intestines that carry the chyle, blood, &c., and they derange the

---

यदा तु पाण्डोर्वर्णः स्याद्धरितः श्यावपीतकः। बलोत्साहक्षयस्तन्द्रा मन्दाग्नित्वं मृदुज्वरः॥ स्त्रीष्वहर्षोऽङ्गमर्दश्च दाहस्तृष्णारुचिभ्रमः। हलीमकं तदा तस्य विद्यादनिलपित्ततः॥

अथ रक्तपित्तनिदानम्।

घर्मव्यायामशोकाध्वव्यवायैरतिसेवितैः। तीक्ष्णोष्णक्षारलवणैरम्लैः कटुभिरेव च॥ पित्तं विदग्धं स्वगुणैर्विदहत्याशु शोणितम्। ततः प्रवर्त्तते रक्तमूर्द्ध्वञ्चाधो द्विधापि वा। ऊर्द्ध्वं नासाक्षिकर्णास्यैर्मेढ्रयोनिगुदैरधः। कूपितं रोमकूपैश्च समस्तैस्तत् प्रवर्त्तते। सदनं शीतकामित्वं कण्ठधूमायनं वमिः॥ लोहगन्धिश्च निश्वासो भवत्यस्मिन् भविष्यति॥

senses. The strength of the body is impaired, and the surface becomes pale and yellow, and it produces dyspepsia. In this form of *Jaundice* the person feels drowsiness, languor, cough, has difficulty in breathing, pain in the belly, and feels no appetite : his cheeks and eyelids swell, also the legs, umbilicus, and penis ; *diarrhœa* occurs, and the dejections are as if they consisted of a mixture of blood and phlegm, with worms.

Prognosis. When there is much fever with dyspepsia, nausia, vomiting, thirst, and languor occur ; when the person is very weak and insensible, or when caused by the derangement of the three humours, or when very chronic, with rough skin and swelling over the body the prognosis will be unfavourable. Should the patient see every thing yellow he will not soon get well. When constipated, when the dejections are yellow and mixed with bile, when accompanied with diarrhœa and much fever, restless and thirst, and when the eyes, teeth and nails become yellow, the prognosis must be unfavourable. In like manner, when the extremities are swollen, and the trunk is thin, or when the trunk is swollen and the extremities are small ; or when there is much swelling about the anus, penis

---

सान्द्रं सपाण्डु सस्नेहं पिच्छिलञ्च कफान्वितम्। श्यावारुणं सफेनञ्च तनुरूक्षञ्च वातिकम्॥ रक्तपित्तं कषायाभं कृष्णं गोमूत्रसन्निभम्। मेचकागारधूमाभमञ्जनाभञ्च पैत्तिकम्। संसृष्टलिङ्गं संसर्गात्त्रिलिङ्गं सान्निपातिकम्॥ ऊर्द्धगं कफसंसृष्टमधोगं पवनानुगम्। द्विमार्गं कफवाताभ्यामुभाभ्यामनुवर्त्तते। ऊर्द्ध्वं साध्यमधो याप्यमसाध्यं युगपद्गतम्। एकमार्गं बलवतो नातिवेगं नवोत्थितम॥ रक्तपित्तं सुखे काले साध्यं स्यान्निरुपद्रवम्। एकदोषानुगं साध्यं द्विदोषं याप्यमुच्यते॥ यत्त्रिदोषमसाध्यं स्यात् मन्दाग्नेरतिवेगवत्॥ व्याधिभिः क्षीणदेहस्य वृद्धस्यानश्नतश्च यत्॥

and scrotum, the prognosis must be guarded. When the patient suffers much, when senseless, or when attacked at the same time with dysentery and fever, such patients the physician should not treat.

A variety of Jaundice is named *kámalá*, which is produced by eating much sour, salt, and other indigestable articles of food after an attack of Jaundice. In this case the bile is much affected, and produces yellowness, particularly of the face, accompanied with drowsiness, loss of strength, and the other symptoms above stated.

If in *kámalá* there is swelling and pain in the joints, then it is called *kumbha-kámalá* (from *kumbha*, a water-pot, and *kámalá*, Jaundice). In this case the dejections and urine are of a dark or yellow colour ; the body is swelled, and the eyes and mouth are of a red colour. When vomiting takes place the matter vomited is of a red colour, as also the dejections and urine.

In some cases the patient is delirious, his body is hot, he has no appetite, is thirsty, and the dejections and urine become

---

दौर्ब्बल्य-श्वास-कास-ज्वर-वमथु-मदापाण्डुता-दाह-मूर्च्छा, भुक्ते घोरो विदाहस्त्वधृतिरपि सदा हृद्यतुल्या च पीड़ा। तृष्णा कोष्ठस्य भेदः शिरसि च तपनं पूतिनिष्ठीवनत्वम्॥ भक्तद्वेषा-विपाकौ विकृतिरपि भवेत् रक्तपित्तोपसर्गाः॥

मांसप्रक्षालनाभं क्वथितमिव च यत् कर्द्दमाम्भोनिभं वा, मेदः पूयास्रकल्पं यकृदिव यदि वा पक्वजम्बुफलाभम्। यत् कृष्णं यच्च नीलं भृशमतिकुणपं यत्र चोक्ता विकारा, स्तद्वर्ज्ज्यं रक्तपित्तं सुरपतिधनुषा यच्च तुल्यं विभाति॥ येन चोपहतो रक्तं रक्त-पित्तेन मानवः। पश्येद्दृश्यं वियच्चैव तच्चासाध्यमसंशयम्। लोहितं छर्द्दयेद् यस्तु बहुशो लोहितेक्षणः। लोहितोद्गारदर्शी च म्रियते रक्तपैत्तिकः॥

constipated : such cases are unfavourable. In other cases the person dozes, and the internal fire and the understanding, are much affected. Such persons will soon die ; as will be the case when there is vomiting with no appetite, fever, debility, noise in breathing, cough, and frequent dejections.

Another form of Jaundice is called *Halimaka* or *Lácorokaka*. This variety is produced by air and bile, and is characterized by fever, pain over the body, giddiness, languor, drowsiness, emaciation of the body, with the symptoms of the form of Jaundice produced by *air* and *bile*.

Hœmorrhagia, (*Raktapitta.*)

This order of disease is divided into those which occur from the mouth, nose, ears, eyes ; from the anus, urethra or vagina ; or from the skin.

Hœmorrhage is caused by anger, grief, fear, wrestling, and other severe exercises ; too much intercourse with women ; or

---

अथ राजयक्ष्म-शोष-क्षतक्षीण-निदानम् ।

वेगरोधात् क्षयाच्चैव साहसाद्विषमाशनात् । त्रिदोषो जायते यक्ष्मागदो हेतु चतुष्टयात् । कफप्रधानैर्दोषैस्तु रुद्धेषु रसवर्त्मसु । अतिव्यवायिनो वापि क्षीणे रेतस्यनन्तराः । क्षीयन्ते धातवः सर्व्वे ततः शुष्यति मानवः ॥

श्वासाङ्गमर्द्द-कफ-संस्रव-तालुशोष-वमथ्वग्निसाद-मदपीनस-कास-निद्राः । शोषे भविष्यति भवन्ति स चापि जन्तुः, शुक्लेक्षणो भवति मांसपरो रिरंसुः । स्वप्नेषु काकशुकशल्लकिनीलकण्ठा गृध्रास्तथैव कपयः कृकलासकाश्च । तं वाहयन्ति सनदीविजलाश्च पश्येच्छुष्कांस्तरून् पवनधुमदवार्द्दितांश्च ॥

too free use of hot things, as pepper and salt, or sour articles; when taken in considerable quantities. The improper mixtures of food, or exposure to the heat of the sun, or to fire. By these means the chyle is deranged, which irritates the bile, and this mixing with the blood produces *Rakta-pitta*. It may thus occur from above downwards, or from the surface of the body. This blood usually proceeds from the spleen or liver.

Immediately before the disease occurs the patient is languid, the body is weak, cold, and cool things are desired. His throat is burning hot, as if he had swallowed smoke, with vomiting. The breathing has the smell of quenched iron. When produced by deranged *air*, *bile*, and *phlegm*, it is known from the blood discharged being very thick, of a yellow colour, shining, and slippery, and mixed with phlegm of a grey colour, of a thick consistence, and with a yellow froth. In other cases it is thin. When bile is deranged in this disease, the blood has an astringent taste, and is of a dark colour, or of the colour of cow's urine, and as if mixed with different colours, as of the colour of smoke, or of a dark colour.

अंशपार्श्वाभितापश्च सन्तापः करपादयोः। ज्वरः सर्व्वाङ्गगश्चेति लक्षणं राजयक्ष्मणः॥ स्वरभेदोऽनिलाच्छूलं सङ्कोचश्चांसपार्श्वयोः। ज्वरो दाहोऽतिसारश्च पित्ताद्रक्तस्य चागमः॥ शिरसः परिपूर्णत्वमभक्तच्छन्द एवच। कासः कण्ठस्य चोध्वंसो विज्ञेयः कफकोपतः॥ एकादशभि रेभिर्व्वा षड्भिर्वापि समन्वितम्। जह्याच्छोषार्द्दितं जन्तु मिच्छन् सुविमलं यशः॥ कासातिसारपार्श्वार्त्तिस्वरभेदारुचिज्वरैः। त्रिभिर्व्वा पीड़ितं लिङ्गैः कासश्वासासृगामयैः॥ सर्व्वैरर्द्धैस्त्रिभिर्व्वापि लिङ्गैर्मांसवलक्षये। युक्तो वर्ज्यश्चिकित्स्यस्तु सर्व्वरूपोऽपरतोऽन्यथा॥ महाशनं क्षीयमानमतिसारनिपीड़ितम्॥ शूनमुष्कोदरञ्चैव यक्ष्मिणं परिवर्ज्जयेत्॥ उप-

The symptoms which terminate this order of diseases are weakness, difficult breathing, cough, fever, vomiting, and slight head-ache ; sometimes the patient faints, and his skin is yellow, hot, and after eating, the pit of the stomach burns. He is restless, and has severe pain in the chest, with hoarseness, head-ache, and the discharge of fecal matter from the mouth ; he has no appetite, is languid, and what is eaten is not digested.

The unfavourable symptoms in this disease are when the hœmorrhage is like the water in which flesh had been washed, or like a vegetable decoction ; is of a liver colour, or like water mixed with mud. When it resembles pus mixed with blood, when it is dark like the fruit of the *Jambu* tree (black-berry), or of a variegated colour, like the rain-bow, such cases are fatal.

When there is a frequent vomiting of blood ; when eructations have the taste of blood, when the eyes are red, and every thing appears the colour of blood, the case is hopeless.

When *phlegm* is deranged the blood is evacuated by the mouth; when *air* is deranged it is by the anus ; and when the two are

---

क्षामेदात्मवन्तं दीप्ताग्निमकृशं नरम्। शुक्लाक्षमन्नद्वेष्टारमूर्द्ध्वश्वास-
निपीड़ितम्। कृच्छ्रेण बहु मेहन्तं यक्ष्मा हन्तीह मानवम्॥

व्यवाय-शोकवार्द्धक्य-व्यायामाध्वप्रशोषितान्। व्रणोरःक्षतसंज्ञौ
च शोषिणौ लक्षणैः शृणु॥ व्यवायशोषी शुक्रस्य क्षय-
लिङ्गैरुपद्रुतः। पाण्डुदेहो यथापूर्व्वं क्षीयन्ते चास्य धातवः।
प्रध्यानशीलः स्रस्ताङ्गः शोकशोष्यपि तादृशः। जराशोषी कृशो
मन्द-वीर्यबुद्धिबलेन्द्रियः। कम्पनोऽरुचिमान् भिन्नकांस्यपात्रहतः
स्वरः॥ ष्ठीवति श्लेष्मणा हीनं गौरवारतिपीड़ितः॥ सम्प्रस्रुता-
स्यनासाक्षः शुष्करूक्षमलच्छविः॥ अध्वशोषी च स्रस्ताङ्गः संभृष्ट-
परुषच्छविः। प्रसुप्तगात्रावयवः शुष्कक्लोमगलाननः॥ व्यायाम-
शोषी भूयिष्ठमेभिरेव समन्वितः॥ लिङ्गैरुरःक्षतकृतैः संयुक्तश्च

deranged, the blood is evacuated above and below. When the blood passes above, the person may be cured; but not so when below. When evacuated both ways, it is incurable. When the person is strong, the disease recent, and not severe, and only occurs one way; and when the person in general feels well, with no other bad disease, it will be cured.

Phthisis Pulmonalis, (*Consumption.*)

Raj Jakshyá, (the prince of disease;) *Shosha, Kshyá, Khina*, (emaciation;) *Kshata*, (rapture or ulcer of the respiratory organs).

The mythological origin of this disease is that the moon married seven sisters, but attaching himself to one, the others complained to their father, who punished the moon, by declaring that he should be afflicted with consumption. This origin; and the precepts in the treatment, proclaim his frequent, and fatal nature. It is characterized by coughing accompanied with bloody expectoration.

क्षतं विना । रक्तक्षयाद्वेदनाभिस्तथैवाहारयन्त्रणात् । व्रणितस्य भवेच्छोषः स चासाध्यतमो मतः ॥

धनुषायास्यतोऽत्यर्थं भारमुद्वहतो गुरुम् । युध्यमानस्य बलिभिः पततो विषमोच्चतः ॥ वृषं हयं वा धावन्तं दम्यं वान्यं निगृह्णतः । शिलाकाष्ठाश्मनिर्घातान् क्षिपतो निघ्नतः परान् ॥ अधीयानस्य वात्युच्चैर्दूरं वा व्रजतो द्रुतम । महानदीर्वा तरतो हयैर्वा सह धावतः । सहसोत्पततो दूरं तूर्णं वापि प्रनृत्यतः ॥ तथान्यैः कर्म्मभिः क्रूरैर्भृशमभ्याहतस्य वा । विक्षते वक्षसि व्याधिर्बलवान् समुदीर्यते । स्त्रीषु चातिप्रसक्तस्य रूक्षाल्पप्रमिताशिनः ॥

It is produced by grief, by the evacuations being retained, when nature endeavours to expell them; by great loss of the humors of the body; by performing unusual and unnatural actions, as ineffectually endeavouring to raise heavy weights; and by running, swimming, or other violent exercise. Consumption is produced, by eating bad food, or at unusual times, and in unusual quantities, by fasting, by boils and sores in the chest, and by old age. Is also supposed to be produced by diminishing the mental and bodily strength, by blunting the senses, by producing difficulty in breathing, by altering the voice, by producing vomiting with expectoration, by a discharge from the eyes, nose, and mouth. In such cases the body dries, and the surface appears dirty.

When the air, phlegm, and bile, are deranged in the above disease; the chyle vessels are stopped by the humours, but particularly phlegm, and the other parts of the body are not nourished. Another form is produced by excessive venery,

---

उरो विरुज्यतेऽत्यर्थं भिद्यतेऽथ विभज्यते। प्रपीड्यते ततः पार्श्वे शुष्यत्यङ्गं प्रवेपते॥ क्रमाद्वीर्यं बलं वर्णो रुचिरग्निश्च हीयते। ज्वरो व्यथा मनोदैन्यं विड्भेदाग्निवधावपि॥ दुष्टः श्यावः दुर्गन्धः पीतो विग्रथितो बहुः। कासमानस्य चाभीक्ष्णं कफ सासृक् प्रवर्त्तते। स क्षतः क्षयतेऽत्यर्थं तथा शुक्रौजसो क्षयात्। अव्यक्तं लक्षणं तस्य पूर्व्वरूपमिति स्मृतम्॥

उरोरुक् शोणितच्छर्दिः कासो वैशेषिकः क्षते। क्षीणे सरक्तमूत्रत्वं पार्श्वपृष्ठकटीग्रहः॥ अल्पलिङ्गस्य दीप्ताग्नेः साध्यो बलवतो नवः॥ परिसंवत्सरो याप्यः सर्व्वलिङ्गन्तु वर्ज्जयेत॥

अथ कासनिदानम्।

धूमोपघाताद्रजसस्तथैव व्यायामरूक्षान्ननिषेवणाच्च। विमार्गगत्वाच्च हि भोजनस्य वेगावरोधात् क्षवथोस्तथैव॥ प्राणो

from the great discharge of semen, by which all the other elements are deranged. The disease commences by the person becoming emaciated and debilitated ; difficult breathing and pain over the body comes on, with cough, and a discharge of mucus, from the mouth and nose. The palate is dry, vomiting, and loss of appetite takes place, from the internal heat being diminished. There is also derangement of the mind, jaundice, cough with expectoration, and the loss of taste, and smell. The patient sleeps continually, and the eyes become of a pearl white colour. The person is fond of animal food, and is desirous of intercourse with women. The following symptoms indicate the presence of this disease ; when the patient's voice changes, he sees in his dream crows, parrots, porcupines, peacocks, vultures, monkeys, and lizards ; and he supposes he is mounted upon these animals. He sees also dry beds of rivers, dry trees, as if destroyed by storms, and by fire.

The characteristic symptoms are pain in the shoulders, and sides of the chest. A burning feverish feel of the palms of the hands and soles of the feet, which extends over the body.

छ्यदानानुगतः प्रदुष्टः संभिन्नकांस्यस्वन-तुल्यघोषः। निरेति वक्त्रात् सहसो सदोषो मनीषिभिः कास इति प्रदिष्टः॥ पञ्च कासाः स्मृता वातपित्तश्लेष्मक्षतक्षयैः। क्षयायोपेक्षिताः सर्व्वे बलिनश्चोत्तरोत्तरम्। पूर्व्वरूपं भवेत्तेषां शूकपूर्णगलास्यता॥ कण्ठे कण्डुश्च भोज्यानामवरोधश्च जायते॥

हृच्छङ्खमूर्द्धोदरपार्श्वशूली क्षामाननः क्षीणबलस्वरौजाः। प्रसक्तवेगस्तु समीरणेन भिन्नस्वरः कासति शुष्कमेव। उरोविदाह ज्वरवक्त्रशोषै रभ्यर्द्दितस्तिक्तमुखस्तृषार्त्तः। पित्तेन पीतानि वमेत् कटूनि कासेत् सपाण्डुः परिदह्यमानः॥ प्रलिप्यमानेन मुखेन सीदन् शिरोरुजार्त्तः कफपूर्णदेहः। अभक्तरुग् गौरवस्वादयुक्तः कासेद्भृशं सान्द्रकफः कफेन॥

The characteristic symptoms are pain in the shoulders, and sides of the chest. A burning feverish feel of the palms of the hands and soles of the feet is felt, which extends over the body.

Consumption is sometimes produced by derangements of one of the three humours. The symptoms produced by derangement of the air are hoarseness ; pain, particularly in the shoulders and sides of the chest, and a bent form of the body. The symptoms of bile are fever, the body burning, diarrhœa, and hemoptisis. The symptoms of phlegm are a fulness and heaviness of the head, no appetite, cough, and the wind-pipe is painful as if bruised, with a change in the voice. When all the above symptoms are present at the same time, and in the same person ; or when there is cough, diarrhœa, pain of the chest and sides, hoarseness, loss of appetite and fever, or when cough, asthma, and the discharge of blood is present, with imaciation, the person will die. When these bad symptoms are absent the physician may attend the person, but when the person has a strong appetite, the food does not produce strength, flesh, or diarrhœa ; or when the testicles or

---

अतिव्यवायभाराध्व-युद्धाश्वगजविग्रहैः । रूक्षस्योरःक्षतं वायुर्गृहीत्वा कासमाचरेत् । स पूर्व्वं कासते शुष्कं ततः ष्ठीवेत् सशोणितम् ॥ कण्ठेन रुजतात्यर्थं विरुग्णेनेव चोरसा । सूचीभिरिव तीक्ष्णाभिस्तुद्यमानेन शूलिना ॥ दुःखस्पर्शेन शूलेन भेदपीडाभितापिना । पर्व्वभेद-ज्वरश्वास-तृष्णावैस्वर्य्यपीड़ितः ॥ पारावत इवाकूजन् कासवेगात् क्षतोद्भवात् ॥

विषमासात्म्यभोज्याति व्यवायाद्वेगनिग्रहात् । घृणिनां शोचतां नृणां व्यापन्नेऽग्नौ त्रयो मलाः ॥ कुपिताः क्षयजं कासं कुर्य्युर्द्देहक्षयप्रदम् ॥ सगात्रशूल-ज्वर-दाहमोहान् प्राणक्षयञ्चोपलभेत कासी । शुष्यन् विनिष्ठीवति दुर्व्वलस्तु प्रक्षीणमांसो रुधिरं सपूयम् ॥

7

stomach swell, the person will not recover. When the person is strong, the disease recent, and he has slight fever ; when he can work, has a good appetite, is equal to the treatment, and follows the judicious instructions of the physician, such a person may recover.

When the eye is white, when there is no appetite, with great derangement of breathing ; when there is a great secretion of urine, with pain, the person will not recover. The other form of consumption is produced by excessive venery, grief, old age, great fatigue, by taking long journies on foot, by the debility produced by old ulcers, and by the rupture o' the organs of respiration, by which the body will become thin, and the disease declare itself. By excessive venery the body becomes emaciated, debilitated, with the other symptoms of diminished semen, such as pain in the scrotum and penis, impotency, or a slight discharge of semen, mixed with blood, when the body becomes yellow, and the other humours are diminished.

When consumption is produced by *grief* the person remains complaining, with the other symptoms of the last

---

तं सर्व्वलिङ्गं भृशदुश्चिकित्स्यं चिकित्सितज्ञाः क्षयजं वदन्ति ॥ इतेयष क्षयजः कासः क्षीणानां देहनाशनं। साध्यो बलवतां वा स्याद् याप्यस्त्वेवं क्षतोत्थितः। नवौ कदाचित् सिध्येतामपि पादगुणान्वितौ। स्थविराणां जरा कासः सर्व्वो याप्यः प्रकीर्त्तितः। त्रीन् पूर्व्वान् साधयेत् साध्यान् पथ्यैर्याप्यांस्तु यापयेत् ॥

अथ हिक्कानिदानम्।

विदाहि गुरु विष्टम्भि रूक्षाभिष्यन्दि भोजनैः। शीतपानाशनस्थान-रजो-धूमातपानिलैः। व्यायामकर्म्म-भाराध्व-वेगाघातापतर्पणैः ॥ हिक्का श्वासश्च कासश्च नृणां समुपजायते। मुहुर्मुहुर्वायुरुदेति सस्वनो यकृतप्लिहान्त्राणि मुखादि वा क्षिपन्। सघोष

form; but without the evacuation and the symptoms of deranged semen. When the disease is produced by old age the body becomes very thin, the person cannot labour, his organs of sense and strength are diminished, his body shakes, he has no appetite, and his voice is like a broken pewter-plate when struck. There is always a flow of saliva from the mouth, weakness, and heaviness; and his eyes, nose, and mouth discharge mucus. The dejections, and surface of the body are in these patients dry and rough. When the body is thin from great fatigue, or walking; the person cannot get up, his body changes in colour, is painful and some parts lose their sensibility. The palate, throat, and mouth are dry. When produced by other kinds of violent exercise or by a rupture of the lungs, the symptoms are the same as above.

When old ulcers debilitate the body, by the great loss of blood, when there is much pain, and there is little nourishment in the food which is taken, the disease is incurable. When consumption is produced by a rupture of the respiratory organs, as by the frequent use of the bow and arrow, by carrying great weights, when a weak person fights with a strong man,

---

वानाशु ह्निनस्तग्रसून् यतस्ततस्तु ह्निक्केतग्रभिधीयते बुधैः ॥ अन्नजां यमलां क्षुद्रां गम्भीरां महतीं तथा ॥ वायुः कफेनानुगतः पञ्च-ह्निक्काः करोति ह्नि। कण्ठोरसोर्गुरुत्वञ्च वदनस्य कषायता। ह्निक्कानां पूर्व्वरूपानि कुक्षेराटोप एव च ॥

पानान्नैरतिसंयुक्तैः सहसा पीड़ितो निलः। ह्निक्कयतूर्ग्रर्द्धगो भूत्वा तां विद्यादन्नजां भिषक् ॥ चिरेण यमलैर्व्वेगैर्या ह्निक्का सम्प्रवर्त्तते। कम्पयन्ती शिरो ग्रीवां यमलां तां विनिर्द्दिशेत्। विकृष्टकालैर्या वेगैर्म्मन्दैः समभिवर्त्तते। क्षुद्रिका नाम सा ह्निक्का जत्रुमूलात् प्रधाविता ॥ नाभिप्रवृत्तः या ह्निक्का घोरा गम्भीर-नादिनी। अनेकोपद्रववती गम्भीरा नाम सा स्मृता ॥ मर्म्मघ्नग्रत्-

when jumping from a great height, or when a person attempts to run after and seize an ox, a horse, or a dacoit, or pull at a bow, or throw pieces of wood or stone, the disease is dangerous. In like manner, loud reading, walking quickly and to a great distance, or swimming much, much horse exercise, or running up a height or to a great distance, dancing quickly, or other bad customs, eating very dry articles, or very little food, or only one kind of food, will produce the disease. When this disease is present there is great pain in the breast as if it was wounded, pain in the sides, and the body dries up, and shakes. By degrees the spirit and strength fail, and the colour of the skin is diminished or unnatural, there is no appetite, with fever, pain, dejection of mind, diarrhœa and loss of appetite. The sputa is of a light blue or yellow colour, with a bad smell, and like the knot of a piece of rope, being unequal. At other times the sputa is mixed with blood. These symptoms increase daily, with pain in the chest, more blood is vomited, and the cough becomes more severe. When the body is much emaciated from the drying up of the juices, indicated by the parched dry mouth, &c., the urine has the colour of blood, and the sides, back and thighs are painful.

पीड़यन्तीव सततं या प्रवर्त्तते। महाहिक्केति सा ज्ञेया सर्व्वगात्रविकम्पिनी ॥

आयम्यते हिक्कतो यस्य देहो दृष्टिश्चोर्द्ध्वं नाम्यते यस्य नितराम्। क्षीणोऽन्नद्विट् क्षौति यश्चातिमात्रं तौ द्वौ चान्त्यौ वर्ज्जयेद्धिक्कमानौ। अतिसञ्चितदोषस्य भक्ताच्छेदकृशस्य च॥ व्याधिभिः क्षीणदेहस्य वृद्धस्यातिव्यवायिनः। आसां या सा समुत्पन्ना हिक्का हन्त्याशु जीवितम्। यमिका च प्रलापार्त्ति मोह तृष्णासमन्विता। अक्षीणश्चाप्यदीनश्च स्थिरधात्विन्द्रियश्च यः। तस्य साधयितुं शक्या यमिका हन्त्यतोऽन्यथा ॥

Consumption often occurs in the progress of other diseases, and is always accompanied with danger, being cured with much difficulty. When the internal heat is natural, and the symptoms not severe, and remain but a few days, the person will be cured. If it continues one year the cure will not be accomplished, and when the severe symptoms above enumerated are present the person will die.

Cough, (*Kása.*)

This disease is produced, by smoke or dust entering the mouth and nostrils, by fighting, by great fatigue, by dry food, by articles of food entering the air passages, by sneezing, or by resisting the calls of nature. These causes derange the vital air *(Prán-báyu)* in the chest, and the *Udán-báyu* which is situated in the trachea, by which the air which passes through the air passages to the mouth, produces a peculiar noise, like a broken metallic vessel.

अथ श्वासनिदानम्।

महोर्द्धच्छिन्नतमकक्षुद्रभेदैस्तु पञ्चधा। भिद्यते स महाव्याधिः श्वास एको विशेषतः। वाताधिको भवेत् क्षुद्र स्तमकस्तु कफोद्भवः। कफ वाताधिक स्त्वेव संसृष्टः छिन्नसंज्ञकः॥ श्वासो मारुतसंसृष्टो महानूर्द्ध स्ततो मतः। प्राग्रूपं तस्य हृत्पीड़ा शूलमाधानमेव च॥ आनाहो वक्त्रवैरस्यं शङ्खनिस्तोद एव च॥

यदा स्रोतांसि संरुध्य मारुतः कफपूर्व्वकः। विष्वग्व्रजति संरुद्धस्तदा श्वासान् करोति सः॥ उद्धूयमानवातो यः शब्दवद्दुःखितो नरः। उच्चैः श्वसिति संरुद्धो मत्तर्षभ इवानिशम्॥ प्रनष्टज्ञानविज्ञानस्तथा विभ्रान्तलोचनः। विवृताक्ष्याननो बद्धमूत्र-

The disease may likewise be produced by air, bile, and phlegm, by ruptures of the respiratory organs, or by the loss of particular humours. All these varieties of cough, pass to consumption if neglected. The disease commences with a feeling in the mouth and throat as if it was covered with some irritating substance. It feels itchy, or there is a stinging which prevents the passage of the food into the stomach.

The symptoms of cough are produced by deranged *air*, the change of voice, the dry and frequent cough, distresses the patient, with pain in the temples, head, stomach, and chest. The face becomes sallow, and the person becomes weak.

When *bile* is deranged the mouth is dry and bitter, and the breath is hot with fever ; the person complains of thirst, and severe pain over the body ; the expectoration is sour, and of a yellowish colour, and the skin becomes yellow and hot.

When *phlegm* is deranged, the mouth is full of mucus with head-ache, loss of appetite, languor, frequent cough, with thick mucus expectoration. The person cannot labour, has frequent fits of coughing, the body is heavy and weak,

---

वर्च्चा विशीर्णवाक् । दीनः प्रश्वसितश्चास्य दूराद्विज्ञायते भृशम् । महाश्वासोपसृष्टस्तु क्षिप्रमेव विपद्यते । ऊर्द्ध्वं श्वसिति यो दीर्घं न च प्रत्याहरत्यधः ॥ श्लेष्मावृतमुखस्रोता क्रुद्धगन्धवहार्द्दितः ॥ ऊर्द्ध्वदृष्टिर्विपश्यंस्तु विभ्रान्ताक्ष इतस्ततः । प्रमुह्यन् वेदनार्त्तश्च शुष्कास्योऽरतिपीड़ितः । ऊर्द्ध्वश्वासे प्रकुपिते ह्यधःश्वासो निरुध्यते ॥ मुह्यत स्ताम्यतश्चोर्द्ध्वं श्वास स्तस्यैव हन्त्यसून् । यस्तु श्वसिति विच्छिन्नं सर्व्वप्राणेन पीड़ितः । न वा श्वसिति दुःखार्त्तो मर्म्मच्छेदरुगर्द्दितः ॥ आनाह स्वेद-मूर्च्छार्त्तो दह्यमानेन वस्तिना । विप्लुताक्षः परीक्षिणः श्वसन् रक्तैकलोचनः ॥ विचेताः परिशुष्कास्यो विवर्णः प्रलपन्नरः । छिन्नश्वासेन विच्छिन्नः स शीघ्रं विजहात्यसून् ।

he has no appetite, the frequency of coughing increases, and much phlegm is expectorated.

Katazoá Kása is caused by excessive venery, fatigue, carrying heavy weights, going great distances when unaccustomed, and violent exercise upon horseback or elephants. By these causes the air passages are injured or ulcerated, when the patient is first affected with dry cough followed by spitting of blood, much pain in the throat and chest, which is increased by pressure. The joints and other parts of the body are painful, as if pins were penetrating it ; pain in the muscles, fever, difficulty of breathing, thirst, hoarseness, and change in the voice, so that it resembles that of wild pigeon.

Khyá Kása (Pneumonia) This form of the disease is produced by taking improper food, at improper, or unusual times ; excessive venery, and neglect of the calls of nature. In other cases the disease is produced by grief, by food which has a bad taste, or produces disgust by which the internal heat is diminished and deranged, with the air, bile, and phlegm. This disease is characterized by the person being affected with severe pain and emaciation of the body, fever, and a burning sensation of the body. His intellect becomes affected, and

---

प्रतिलोमं यदा वायुः स्रोतांसि प्रतिपद्यते। ग्रीवां शिरश्च संगृह्य श्लेष्माणं समुदीर्य च॥ करोति पीनसं तेन रुद्धोघुर्घुरकं तथा। अतीवतीव्रवेगञ्च श्वासं प्राणप्रपीड़कम्॥ प्रताम्यति स वेगेन तृष्यते सन्निरुध्यते। प्रमोहं कासमानश्च स गच्छति मुहुर्मुहुः। श्लेष्मण्यमुच्यमाने तु भृशं भवति दुःखितः॥ तस्यैव च विमोक्षान्ते मुहूर्त्तं लभते सुखम्। तथास्योध्वंसते कण्ठः कृच्छ्राच्छक्नोति भाषितम्। न चापि लभते निद्रां शयानः श्वासपीड़ितः॥ पार्श्वे तस्यावगृह्णाति शयानस्य समीरणः। आसीनो लभते सौख्यमुष्णञ्चैवाभिनन्दति॥ उच्छ्रिताक्षो ललाटेन स्विद्यता

the person loses his strength. The cough is at first dry, is accompanied with vomiting, and is followed by purulent and bloody expectoration. When these symptoms are present they are rarely cured; and in weak persons the disease is generally fatal, unless when recent. In old age the cough *(Jará Kása)* will remain, and not be removed.

When *Kátazoa* and *Khyá Kása* are recent, with the assistance of a good physician, and proper remedies, a cure may be obtained. When air, bile and phlegm produce these diseases separately, it may be cured

---

Hiccup, (*Hikka.*)

This disease is produced by nearly the same causes as *Swása* (asthma), and *Kása* (cough). Such as heavy and indigestable food, or roasted, hot, and dry food; or much food, or an improper mixture of food, or articles that increase cough, &c., so as to produce constipation. In other cases very dry things,

---

भृशमर्त्तिमान् विशुष्कास्यो मुहुःश्वासो मुहुश्चैवावधम्यते। मेघाम्बुशीतप्राग्वातैः श्लेष्मलैश्च विवर्द्धते। स याप्यस्तमक श्वासः साध्योवास्यान्नवोत्थितः॥ ज्वरमूर्च्छापरीतस्य विद्यात् प्रतमकन्तु तम्। उदावर्त्तरजोजीर्णक्लिन्नकायनिरोधजः॥ तमसा वर्द्धतेऽत्यर्थं शीतैश्चाशु प्रशाम्यति॥ मज्जतस्तमसीवास्य विद्यात् सन्तमकन्तु तम्॥

रूक्षायासोद्भवः कोष्ठे क्षुद्रो वात उदीरयन्। क्षुद्रश्वासो न सोऽत्यर्थं दुःखेनाङ्ग प्रबाधकः॥ हिनस्ति न स गात्राणि नच दुःखो यथेतरे। नच भोजनपानानां निरुणद्ध्युचितां गतिम्॥ नेन्द्रियाणां व्यथां नापि काञ्चिदापादयेद्रुजम्। स साध्य उक्तो बलिनः

cold things, or situations, exposure to dust, smoke entering the mouth or nostrils; or much heat, as exposure to the sun, and hot air. Violent exercise, as shooting arrows, carrying heavy loads, walking great distances, not attending to the calls of nature, or long fasting produce this disease. It is called *hikka*, because the air comes to the mouth frequently, with a peculiar noise, and the spleen, liver, and intestines seem to be coming up to the mouth. This disease quickly debilitates, and destroys the *prána* (life).

The precursory symptoms are a heaviness of the throat and chest, an astringent taste in the mouth, and a rumbling noise in the belly. There are five kinds of hiccup, in all of which air and phlegm are deranged.

1. *Unnugá.* This form is produced by taking too much food and drink, which deranges the air, and produces the disease.

2. *Jumulá.* In this form the passage of air proceeds, after a considerable time, with eructations of air, and the head and neck shake at the moment; hence the name.

सर्व्वं चाव्यक्तलक्षणाः। क्षुद्रःसाध्यमतस्तेषां तमकः कृच्छ्र उच्यते। त्रयः श्वासा न सिद्ध्यन्ति तमको दुर्व्वलस्य च। कामं प्राणहरा रोगा बह्वो नतु ते तथा। यथा श्वासश्च हिक्का च हरतः प्राण माशु च।

अथ स्वरभेद-निदानम्।

अत्युच्चभाषण-विषाध्ययनाभिघात-संदूषणैः प्रकुपिताः पवनादयस्तु। स्रोतःसु ते स्वरवहेषु गताः प्रतिष्ठां, हन्युः स्वयं भवति वापि हि षड्विधः सः। वातादिभिः पृथक् सर्व्वैर्मेदसा च क्षयेण च। वातेन कृष्णनयनानन्-मूत्रवर्च्चा भिन्नं शनै र्वदति गर्द्दभवत् स्वरञ्च। पित्तेन पीतनयनानन-मूत्रवर्च्चा ब्रूयाद्गलेन स च दाह-समन्वितेन। ब्रूयात् कफेन सततं कफरुद्धकण्ठः स्वल्पं शनै-

3. *Khudrá.* (hiccup) takes place slowly, is not strong, and proceeds from the scrobiculus cordis.

4. *Gambirá.* In this form the hiccup commences from the navel, is strong, and very noisy, and is always accompanied with other severe or fatal symptoms.

5. *Mahatí.* There is frequent hiccup, which produces pain in the vital parts, and shakes the whole body. The unfavourable symptoms are when hiccup is accompanied with fixed eyes, as if drawn up by some one; when there is great weakness, and the patient's arms and legs are thrown out, with frequent sneezing. When the person is very weak, and old, or becomes weak after excessive venery, with no appetite, and a cough, it will soon prove fatal. When combined with other diseases, as delirium, fainting, great thirst, &c., it will be fatal. When the person is strong, has a good constitution, hiccup may be cured. Thus when the patient is not thin, when his memory is good, his tissues and senses are healthy, the person will recover.

Asthma, (*Swása*).

This disease is produced by the same causes as produce hiccough. It is by the *Prán-báyu* changing its place, and being

---

र्वदति चापि दिवा विशेषात्। सर्व्वात्मके भवति सर्व्वविकार-सम्पत् तञ्चापसाध्यमृषयः स्वरभेदमाहुः॥ धूमेरत वाक् चय-कृते चयमाप्नुयाच्च वागेष चापि हतवाक् परिवर्ज्जनीयः। अन्तर्गतं स्वरमलच्यपदं चिरेण मेदोऽन्वयाद्दति दिग्धगलस्तृषार्त्तः। चीणस्य वृद्धस्य कृशस्य वापि चिरोत्थितो यश्च सहोपजातः। मेद-स्विनः सर्व्वसमुद्भवश्च स्वरामयो यो न स सिद्धिमेति॥

confined in its passage by phlegm, which produces the difficulty in breathing. There are the following five varieties of asthma :—

1. *Swása* is a severe disease, and has only slight varieties. It is ushered in with pain in the chest and sides, loss of appetite, restlessness, tightness of the abdomen, a bad taste in the mouth, and a constipation of the bowels and bladder.

2. *Mahá-swása.* The air is confined in the air passages by the phlegm, and thus produces Asthma. The patient respires with difficulty, and with a noise like that of a wild bullock. He becomes low-spirited, his eyes are always moving about; his mouth open, with constipation of urine and fæces; he speaks with difficulty, and his distress may be observed from a distance.

3. *Urdha-swása.* The patient in this disease respires with difficulty and with an effort; the air passages being closed by phlegm, and the air trying to escape gives much pain. His eyes are directed upwards, he cannot see, and different objects appear before the eyes; sometimes he faints, his mouth re-

---

अथारोचक-निदानम् ।

वातादिभिः शोकभयातिलोभ-क्रोधैर्मनोघ्नानाशनरूपगन्धैः । अरोचकाः स्युः परिहृष्टदन्तः कषायवक्त्रश्च मतोऽनिलेन । कटूष्ण-मुष्णं विरसञ्च पूति पित्तेन विद्याल्लवणञ्च वक्त्रम् । माधुर्यपैच्छिल्यगुरुत्वशैत्य-विबद्धसंबद्धयुतं कफेन ॥ अरोचके शोक-भयातिलोभ क्रोधाद्यहृद्याशुचिगन्धजे स्यात् । स्वाभाविकञ्चास्यमथारुचिश्च त्रिदोषजे नैकरसं भवेत्तु ॥ हृच्छूलपीड़नयुतं पवनेन पित्तात् तृड़्दाहचोषबहुलं सकफप्रसेकम् । श्लेष्मात्मकं बहुरुजं बहुभिश्च विद्याद्वैगुण्यमोहजड़ताभिरथापरञ्च ॥

mains dry with restlessness and severe pain over the body. The respiration becomes more difficult, and he dies.

4. *China-swása.* This form occurs in fits at irregular intervals. In these cases he is sometimes still, and cannot breathe. The vital parts are much affected, and very painful. He is constipated in his bowels, with much perspiration and drowsiness. He complains of much pain in the bladder, which is very hot, his eyes are always rolling about, and red; great debility, low spirits, mouth dry, bad colour of the skin, and delirium. Such persons quickly die.

5. *Tamaka-swása.* In this variety the air passes in, but is not discharged easily. The vessels of the neck and air passages are affected, with a collection of mucus in the air passages. Catarrh is produced, as indicated by yellow sputa from the mouth, and snoring, with great uneasiness and difficulty in breathing. When he coughs he often faints, but on mucus being discharged he feels easier. At times he cannot speak, does not sleep, and when he does he complains of much pain in the sides and chest. He is easiest in the sitting posi-

---

अथ छर्द्दिनिदानम् ।

दुष्टैर्दोषैः पृथक् सर्व्वैर्वीभत्सालोचनादिभिः । छर्द्दयः पञ्च विज्ञेया स्तासां लक्षणमुच्यते ॥ अतिद्रवैरतिस्निग्धैरहृद्यैर्लवणैरति । अकाले चातिमात्रैश्च तथासात्म्यैश्च भोजनैः ॥ श्रमाद्भया-त्तथोद्वेगादजीर्णात् क्रिमिदोषतः । नार्य्याश्चापन्नसत्वायास्तथाति-द्रुतमश्नतः ॥ वीभत्सैर्हेतुभिश्चान्नैर्द्रुतमुत्क्लेशितो बलात् ॥ छादयन्नाननं वेगैरर्द्दयन्नङ्गभञ्जनैः । निरुच्यते छर्द्दिरिति दोषो वक्त्रं प्रधावितः ॥

हृल्लासोद्गाररोधौ च प्रसेको लवणस्तनुः । द्वेषोऽन्नपाने च भृशं वमीनां पूर्व्वलक्षणम् ॥

tion, and likes hot things. His eyes are turned upwards, he perspires much in the forehead, his mouth is dry, and the body swings about as if he was riding upon an elephant. From time to time his breathing is difficult. This disease is increased in cloudy, rainy, and cold weather ; especially during the prevalence of easterly winds. Whatever increases phlegm, is liable to increase the disease. This form of disease may be cured if recent, but in the old, or when it has continued for some time, it is not curable. When this form is combined with fever, and dozing, it forms *Pratamaka*. When produced or increased by *Udabarta*, (constipation,) *Ajirna*, (dyspepsia,) *Rajah*, (or dust) and darkness. In this form cold things give relief, and the person sees imperfectly like one in darkness. This is called *Sangtamaka*.

6. *Khudra-swása*. It is produced by dry food and exercise. In this form there is less difficulty in breathing, and there is no pain or uneasiness. It does not prevent deglutition, nor the action of the senses, and only produces difficulty

---

हृत्पार्श्वपीड़ा मुखशोष-शीर्ष-नाभ्यर्त्ति-कास-स्वरभेदतोदैः उद्गारशब्दं प्रबलं सफेनं विच्छिन्नमुष्णां तनुकं कषायम् ॥ कृच्छ्रेण चाल्पं महता च वेगेनार्त्तोऽनिलाच्छर्द्दयतीह दुःखम् । मूर्च्छा पिपासा मुखशोषमूर्द्ध तालुच्चिसन्तापतमो भ्रमार्त्तः ॥ पीतं भृशोष्णं हरितं सतिक्तं धूम्रञ्च पित्तेन वमेत् सदाहम् । तन्द्रास्य-माधुर्य्य-कफप्रसेक-सन्तोषनिद्रारुचिगौरवार्त्तः ॥ स्निग्धं घनं स्वादु कफाद्विशुद्धं सरोमहोर्षोऽल्परुजं वमेत्तु । शूलाविपाकारुचिदाह-तृष्णा श्वासप्रमेहप्रबला प्रसक्ताम् ॥ छर्द्दिस्त्रिदोषाल्पवर्णाम्ल-नील सान्द्रोष्णारक्तं वमतां नृणां स्यात् ॥

विट्स्वेदमूत्राम्बु-वहानि वायुः स्रोतांसि संरुद्ध्य यदोर्द्धमेति । उत्सन्नदोषस्य समाचितं तं दोषं समुद्धूय नरस्य कोष्ठात् ॥ विमू-

in breathing on running, &c. No other disease is produced by this one, and it is curable unless when combined with some other disease.

Hoarseness, (*Swarabheda.*)

The causes of this disease are loud speaking, poison, long continued reading, external injuries, exposure to cold, &c. When air, bile and phlegm are deranged in the air-passages they produce the six varieties of hoarseness. One is produced by derangements of the air, bile, or phlegm ; by the combination of the three ; by fatness ; and by weakness.

1st. *Air* when deranged produces this disease, when the person's eyes, mouth, urine, and dejections become black, and his tone of speaking is slow, and like an ass braying.

2nd. When *bile* is deranged, the eyes, mouth, urine, and dejections are of a yellowish colour, and the patient speaking from the throat, with a sense of burning pain in the part.

क्षयो तत्समगन्धवर्णं तृट्-श्वासहिक्कार्त्तियुतं प्रसक्तम् ॥ प्रच्छर्दयेद्दुष्टमिहातिवेगात्तयर्द्दितश्चाशु विनाशमेति ॥

वीभत्सजा दौर्हृदजामजा च असात्म्यजा च क्रिमिजा च या हि। सा पञ्चमी तां च विभावयेच्च, दोषोच्छ्रयेणैव यथोक्तमादौ शूलहृल्लासबहुला क्रिमिजा च विशेषतः॥ क्रिमिहृद्रोगतुल्येन लक्षणेन च लक्षिता॥ क्षीणस्य या छर्द्दिरतिप्रसक्ता सोपद्रवा। शोणितपूययुक्ता। सचन्द्रिकां तां प्रवदेदसाध्यां साध्यां चिकित्सेन्निरुपद्रवां च॥

तृष्णानिदानम्।

भयश्रमाभ्यां बलसंक्षयाद्वा ऊर्द्ध्वञ्चितं पित्तविवर्द्धनैश्च। पित्तं सवातं कुपितं नराणां तालुप्रपन्नं जनयेत् पिपासाम्। स्रोतः-

3rd. *Phlegm* when deranged, the throat is filled with mucus, and the person speaks little and that slowly and with difficulty, particularly at night.

When air, bile, and phlegm are deranged, the combined symptoms of the three varieties are present; and the patient speaks so indistinctly that he cannot be understood. This form is incurable.

4th. When weakness or diminution of the essential parts (*dhátu*) produce the disease, the patient cannot speak, and when he tries, smoke appears to proceed from the mouth, with pain. He speaks very little. This form is also incurable.

5th. When it is produced by *fatness* the person's speaking is indistinct, and he thinks his throat and palate are covered with something. Such disease will not be cured when the person is weak, old, thin; when it has been of long continuance, and is congenital. In fat people, and when produced by the combination of the three humours it is also incurable.

स्वपां वाहिषु दूषितेषु दोषैश्च तृट् संभवतीह जन्तोः। तिस्रः
स्मृतास्ताः क्षतजा चतुर्थी क्षयात्तथाद्यामसमुद्भवा च। भक्तोद्भवा
सप्तमिकेति तासां निबोध लिङ्गान्यनुपूर्व्वशस्तु। क्षामास्यतामारु-
तसम्भवायां तोदस्तथा शङ्ख शिरःसु चापि॥ स्रोतोनिरोधो विर-
सश्च वक्त्रं शीताभिरद्भिश्च विवृद्धिमेति। मूर्च्छान्नविद्वेष विलाप-
दाहा रक्तेक्षणत्वं प्रततश्च शोषः॥ शीताभिनन्दा मुखतिक्तता
च पित्तात्मिकायां परिदूयनञ्च। वाष्पावरोधात् कफसंवृतेऽग्नौ,
तृष्णा बलासेन भवेत्तथा तु॥ निद्रा गुरुत्वं मधुरास्यता च तृष्णा-
र्दितः शुष्यति चातिमात्रम्॥ क्षतस्य रुक्शोणितनिर्गमाभ्यां
तृष्णा चतुर्थी क्षतजा मता तु॥ रसक्षयाद्याक्षयसम्भवा सा तया-
भिभूतश्च निशादिनेषु। पेपीयतेऽम्भः ससुखं न याति तां सन्नि-
पातादिति केचिदाहुः॥

Chardi, *or Vomiting.*

Deranged air, bile, and phlegm, produce this disease; as also when the three humours are deranged, or when the person takes too much fluid, or bad articles of food. When disgusting objects are seen, smelt, or eaten, it may produce this disease. In other persons it is produced by eating food too fast, or at unusual times, and by great fatigue, grief, indigestion, and worms. The state of pregnancy likewise produces vomiting.

Before vomiting occurs, the person complains of nausea, a cessation of belching, a watery and saltish discharge from the mouth, he dislikes food, becomes weak and unsteady in walking, which is followed by vomiting.

When produced by air the vomiting is frothy and scanty, much pain is felt in the back, and sides of the abdomen; great exhaustion, and vomiting occurs, with a loud noise, and an astringent taste in the mouth. When *bile* produces vomi-

---

रसक्षयोक्तानि च लक्षणानि, तस्यामशेषेण भिषग्व्यवस्येत् । त्रिदोषलिङ्गामसमुद्भवा च हृच्छूलनिष्ठीवन सादकर्त्री । स्निग्धं तथाम्ल लवणाच्च भुक्तं गुर्व्वन्नमेवाशु तृषां करोति ॥ दीनस्वरः प्रताम्यन् दीनः संशुष्ककण्ठगलतालुः ॥ भवति खलु योपसर्गात् तृष्णा सा शोषिणी कष्टा ॥ ज्वर मोहक्षयकासश्वासाद्युपसृष्टदेहानां सर्व्वस्त्वतिप्रसक्ता रोगकृशानां वमिप्रयुक्तानाम् ॥ घोरोपद्रवसंयुक्ता तृष्णा मरणाय विज्ञेया ।

अथ मूर्च्छाभ्रमनिद्रासंन्यासनिदानम् ।

क्षीणस्य बहुदोषस्य विरुद्धाहारसेविनः । वेगाघातादभीघाताद्धीनसत्वस्य वा पुनः ॥ करणायतनेषूग्रा बाह्येष्वभ्यन्तरेषु च । निविशन्ते यदा दोषास्तदा मूर्च्छन्ति मानवाः ॥ संज्ञावहासु नाड़ीषु पिहितास्वनिलादिभिः । तमोऽभ्युपैति सहसा सुखदुःख-

ing, the person feels faint, thirsty, the mouth is dry and the head, palate, and eyes hot. He sees indistinctly as if he was in darkness, his body turns round, and he vomits a bitter matter of a yellow, hot, green, or sour nature. When phlegm is the cause the patient is heavy and dozes, his mouth is sweet, phlegm is discharged, thick, white, and copiously mixed with mucus, and a horripilation is felt. The person has no appetite, and the fluid vomited is neither salt, sour, nor bitter. When air, bile, and phlegm are deranged, all the above symptoms are present. When produced by the sight of disagreeable objects, pregnancy or worms, the humours will be deranged, and the variety of the disease will be distinguished by their peculiar symptoms. When produced by worms, there is frequent eructations, and much pain, accompanied with the symptoms of those diseases of the chest which are produced by worms.

The unfavourable symptoms are great debility, and the matter vomited being mixed with blood and pus, or resembles the variegated colour of the peacock's tail. There is also frequent vomiting in other dangerous diseases. All the varieties of vomiting are produced by disorders of the stomach.

व्यपोहकृत्। सुखदुःखव्यपोहाच्च नरः पतति काष्ठवत्॥ मोहो मूर्च्छेति तामाहुः षड्विधा सा प्रकीर्त्तिता। वातादिभिः शोणितेन मद्येन च विषेण च॥ षट्स्वप्येतासु पित्तन्तु प्रभुत्वेनावतिष्ठते॥

हृत्पीड़ा जृम्भणं ग्लानिः संज्ञा दौर्व्वल्यमेव च। सर्व्वासां पूर्व्वरूपाणि यथास्वञ्च विभावयेत्॥ नीलं वा यदि वा कृष्णमाकाशमथवारुणम्। पश्यंस्तमः प्रविशति शीघ्रञ्च प्रतिबुध्यते॥ वेपथुश्चाङ्गमर्द्दश्च प्रपीड़ा हृदयस्य च। कार्श्यं श्यावारुणा च्छाया मूर्च्छायां वातसम्भवे॥ रक्तं हरितवर्णं वा वियत् पीतमथापि वा। पश्यंस्तमः प्रविशति सस्वेदश्च प्रबुध्यते॥ सपिपासः ससन्तापः

9

Swooning, (*Murchhá.*)

When the person is weak, or when the *air*, *bile* and *phlegm* are very much deranged, by eating improper mixtures of food, such as milk and fish, or flesh, &c., by constipation, &c., this disease is produced; in which the organs of sense, both external and internal are deranged, with faintness.

When the derangements of *air*, *bile* and *phlegm* close the passages of the vessels, the person connot see, and falls down as a piece of wood: this disease is called *Múrchhá* or *moha.*

There are six varieties of this disease, but in all the bile is deranged. The six are produced by derangements of *air*, *bile* or *phlegm*, by blood, by drinking spirits, and by poison.

The approach of this disease is known by pain in the breast, gaping, languor, loss of sense, and strength. These symptoms are the same in all the varieties.

When produced by derangements of *air*, every thing appears of a dark-blue or red colour, or like the sky. The person cannot see, and faints, but the senses soon return. There is

---

रक्तपीतारुणेक्षणः। संभिन्नवर्च्चाः पीताभो मूर्च्छायां पित्तसम्भवे। मेघसङ्काशमाकाशमावृतं वा तमोघनैः। पश्यंस्तमः प्रविशति चिराच्च प्रतिबुध्यते॥ गुरुभिः प्रावृतैरङ्गैर्यथैवार्द्रेण चर्म्मणा॥ सप्रसेकः सहृल्लासो मूर्च्छायां कफसम्भवे॥

सर्व्वाकृतिः सन्निपातादपस्मार इवागतः। स जन्तुं पाययत्याशु विना वीभत्सचेष्टितैः॥

पृथिव्यापस्तमोरूपं रक्तगन्धस्तदन्वयः। तस्माद्रक्तस्य गन्धेन मूर्च्छन्ति भुवि मानवाः॥ द्रव्यस्वभाव इत्येके दृष्ट्वा यदभिमुह्यति गुणास्तीव्रतरत्वेन स्थितास्तु विषमद्ययोः। तएव तस्मात्ताभ्यान्तु मोहौ स्यातां यथेरितौ। स्तव्धाङ्गदृष्टिस्त्वसृजा गूढोच्छ्वासश्च मूर्च्छितः॥ मद्येन विलपन् शेते नष्टविभ्रान्तमानवः। गात्राणि

shivering, pain of the body and breast, weakness, and the skin becomes dirty, and of a reddish or green colour.

Bile. The person sees every thing of a yellow, or green colour; he cannot see, and faints. He is soon restored to his senses, with perspiration. When he recovers, the skin becomes yellow, the body becomes hot, eyes red, and dejections yellow.

Phlegm. He sees every thing of the colour of clouds; the sky appears misty and dark, followed by fainting, in which sensation remains long absent. The body feels like as if a piece of soaked leather had been put upon it: and phlegm is discharged from the mouth and nose, followed by nausea and vomiting.

When these three humours are deranged at the same time, they produce all the symptoms of the three separate diseases; but without the symptoms of Epilepsy. When these diseases occur, and the person does not feel when needles are thrust into his flesh, red hot irons put upon the surface, or hot substances put into his mouth, the person will soon die.

विक्षिपन् भूमौ जरां यावन्न याति तत्। वेपथुस्वप्नतृष्णाः स्युस्त-मश्च विषमूर्च्छिते। वेदितव्यञ्च तीव्रतरं यथास्वं विषलक्षणम्॥

मूर्च्छा पित्ततमःप्राया, रजःपित्तानिलाद्भ्रमः। चक्रवद् भ्रमतो गात्रं भूमौ पतति सर्व्वदा॥ भ्रमरोग इति ज्ञेयो रजपित्ता-निलात्मकः। तमोवातकफात्तन्द्रा निद्रा श्लेष्मतमोभवा॥ इन्द्रि-यार्थेष्वसंवित्ति गौरवं जृम्भणं क्लमः। निद्रार्त्तस्येव यस्येहा तस्य तन्द्रां विनिर्द्दिशेत्॥ दोषेषु मदमूर्च्छाया हृतवेगेषु देहिनाम्। स्वयमेवोपशामयन्ति संन्यासो नौषधैर्व्विना॥

वाग्देहमनसां चेष्टामाक्षिप्यातिबला मलाः। सन्यस्यन्त्यबलं जन्तुं प्राणायतनमाश्रिताः॥ स ना सन्याससन्यस्तः काष्ठीभूतो-मृतोपमः। प्राणै र्व्विमुच्यते शीघ्रं मुक्ता सद्यःफलां क्रियाम्॥

Seeing *blood* often produces swooning from its containing earth and water, which possess the properties of *tamoguna,* the cause of darkness. In this manner the occurrence of fainting, on seeing blood, by the quality of darkness which it possesses.

When swooning is produced by *poison* there is shivering, drowsiness, thirst, followed by weakness and insensibility. There are various kinds of this variety, but all produce these symptoms. Fainting is generally produced by deranged bile, when mixed with *tamoguna,* or darkness. When bile and air are mixed with *rajoguna,* it produces swooning, and drowsiness; coma is produced when air and phlegm are mixed with *tamoguna*; and phlegm and *tamoguna* when mixed together produce sleep. Drinking spirits derange the *air, bile* and *phlegm,* and produce swooning, which continues until the effects of the spirits cease.

Another form of this disease is called *sangnyása* (apoplexy). It is produced by the deranged air, bile and phlegm, which

---

अथ पानात्ययपरमदपानाजीर्णपान-
विभ्रमनिदानम्।

ये विषस्य गुणाः प्रोक्तास्तेऽपि मद्ये प्रतिष्ठिताः। तेन मिथ्योपचारेन भवत्युग्रो मदात्ययः॥ किन्तु मद्यं स्वभावेन यथैवान्नं तथा स्मृतम्। अयुक्तियुक्तं रोगाय युक्तियुक्तं यथामृतम्॥ प्राणाः प्राणभृतामन्नं तदयुक्त्या निहन्त्यसून्। विषं प्राणहरं तच्च युक्तियुक्तं रसायनम्॥ विधिना मात्रया काले हितैरन्नैर्यथाबलम्। प्रहृष्टो यः पिबेन्मद्यं तस्य स्यादमृतोपमम्॥ स्निग्धैस्तदन्नैर्म्मांसैश्च भक्ष्यैश्च सह सेवितम्। भवेदायुःप्रकर्षाय बलायोपचयाय च॥ कामता मनसस्तुष्टि स्तेजो विक्रम एव च। विधिवत् सेव्यमाने तु मद्ये सन्निहिता गुणाः॥

pass to the place in which life is retained, and overpowers all the functions of both mind and body, and the person suddenly falls down, and remains as if dead, or like a piece of wood. If not immediately, and properly treated, such a person will die.

Burning of the body, (*Dáha.*)

This is generally a symptomatic disease attended with fever The blood of the whole body is affected in this disease, the body becomes hot, and the patient complains of a burning sensation over the body, as if hot charcoal was applied to the surface which becomes of a red colour like copper. The eyes of such a person are red, and his breath is like hot iron.

There are seven forms of this disease, one being produced by bile, another by blood, the third by external injury of the trunk, the fourth by not quenching thirst, the fifth by the

---

बुद्धि-स्मृति-प्रीतिकरः सुखश्च पानान्न-निद्रा-रति-वर्द्धनश्च। संपाठ गीतस्वरवर्द्धनश्च प्रोक्तोऽतिरम्यः प्रथमो मदो हि॥ अव्यक्त-बुद्धिस्मृतिवाग्विचेष्टः सोन्मत्तलीलाकृतिरप्रशान्तः। आलस्यनिद्रा-भिहतो मुहुश्च मध्येन मत्तः पुरुषो मदेन॥ गच्छेदगम्यां न गुरूंश्च मन्येत् खादेदभक्ष्याणि च नष्टसंज्ञः॥ ब्रूयाच्च गुह्यानि हृदि स्थितानि मदे तृतीये पुरुषोऽस्वतन्त्रः॥ चतुर्थे तु मदे मूढ़ो भग्नदार्व्विव निष्क्रियः। कार्य्याकार्य्यविभागज्ञो मृता-दप्यवरो मतः। को मदं तादृशं गच्छेदुन्मादमिव चापरम्। बहुदोषमिवामूढ़ः कान्तारं स्ववशः कृती।

निर्भक्तमेकान्तत एव मद्यं निषेव्यमानं मनुजेन नित्यम्। आपा-दयेत् कष्टतमान् विकारानापादयेच्चापि शरीरभेदम्॥ क्रुद्धेन

injury of vital parts, the sixth by excess in drinking, and the seventh by the loss of the essential parts of the body, as chyle, blood, &c.

1st and 2nd. When produced by *bile*, it is accompanied with fever. When *blood* is affected the body, eyes, &c., become red, and he complains of a burning sensation over the body.

3rd. When any viscus is injured, and is filled up with blood, and affects a *dáha* which is difficult to cure.

4th. When produced by excessive drinking the internal heat comes out externally, and is increased by the derangement of bile and blood. It then produces great burning of the body.

5th. If a foolish person does not drink water, when he is very thirsty, the watery part of the body is diminished ; and the internal heat is increased, producing a burning of the external and internal parts of the body ; his throat, palate, tongue and lips, become dry, and the tongue protrudes, with shaking of the body.

भीतेन पिपासितेन शोकाभितप्तेन क्षुधितेन। व्यायामभाराध्वप्रक्षितेन वेगावरोधाभिहतेन चापि॥ अत्यम्लभक्षावततोदरेण साजीर्णभुक्तेन तथाबलेन। उष्णाभितप्तेन च सेव्यमानं करोति मद्यं विविधान् विकारान्॥ पानात्ययं परमदं पानाजीर्णमथापि वा। पानविभ्रममुग्रञ्च तेषां वक्ष्यामि लक्षणम्॥ हिक्का श्वासशिरःकम्प पार्श्वशूलप्रजागरैः। विद्याद्बहुप्रलापस्य वातप्रायं मदात्ययम्। तृष्णादाहज्वरस्वेद-मोहातिसारविभ्रमैः॥ विद्याद्धरितवर्णस्य पित्तप्रायं मदात्ययम्॥ छर्द्यरोचकहृल्लास-तन्द्रा-स्तैमित्यगौरवैः। विद्याच्छीतपरीतस्य कफप्रायं मदात्ययम्॥ ज्ञेयस्त्रिदोषजश्चापि सर्वलिङ्गै र्मदात्ययः। श्लेष्मोच्छ्रयोऽङ्गगुरुता विरसास्यता च विण्मूत्रसक्तिरथ तन्द्रिररोचकश्च॥ लिङ्गं परस्य च मदस्य वदन्ति तज्ज्ञा स्तृष्णा रुजा शिरसि सन्धिषु चापि भेदः।

6th. When the essential fluids of the body are diminished by any cause, as an excess in venery, too much exercise, copious evacuation of any of the fluids, the body feels very hot, and the patient faints, has much thirst, his voice becomes low and altered, he cannot move his body, and soon dies.

7th. When any vital part is injured, as the bladder, heart, or brain, it produces a burning sensation over the body which is incurable.

When the body feels cold to another while the patient is suffering from an internal burning, it is always a very unfavourable symptom in this kind of disease.

Burning of the feet (Páda-dáha) is a variety of this order; and is a peculiar, severe and very untractable disease.

Madness, (*Unmáda.*)

The causes producing this disease are improper food, endeavouring to perform impossibilities, strong passions of the

---

आध्मानमुग्रमथ चोद्गिरणं विदाहः पाने जरां समुपगच्छति लक्षणानि। हृद्गात्रतोदकफसंस्रवकण्ठधूमा, मूर्च्छावमि ज्वर-शिरोरुजनप्रदाहाः। द्वेषः सुरान्नविकृतेष्वपि तेषु तेषु तं पान-विभ्रम मुशन्त्यखिलेन धीराः। हीनत्तरौष्ठमतिशीतममन्ददाहं तैलप्रभास्यमपि पानहतं त्यजेत्तु॥ जिह्वौष्ठदन्तमसितस्त्वथ वापि नीलं पीतञ्च यस्य नयने रुधिरप्रभे वा। हिक्काज्वरौ वमथु-वेपथु-पार्श्वशूलाः कासभ्रमावपि च पानहतं भजन्ते॥

अथ दाहनिदानम्।

त्वचं प्राप्तः स पानोष्मा पित्तरक्ताभिमूर्च्छितः। दाहं प्रकुरुते घोरं पित्तवत्तत्र भेषजम्॥ कृत्स्नदेहानुगं रक्तमुद्रिक्तं

mind, cursing the gods, bráhmans, and spiritual guides ; eating poison, &c.

The *air, bile* and *phlegm* are affected by the above causes, which deranged knowledge (*satwagun*), affects the seat of understanding and the heart, and pass through the vessels conveying sense (*mana*) when the person becomes mad, speaks foolishly, is restless, and his eyes are continually moving about.

There are six kinds of madness. Three being produced by derangements of air, bile and phlegm ; one by the combination of these ; another by the violent actions of the passions ; and the last by poison.

Air is deranged and the mind is thus affected by the use of dry, cooling, articles of food ; by food in small quantities ; by strong purgatives ; by the causes diminishing the humours (*dhátu*), or by fasting. By these causes the air is deranged, producing madness ; in which the man laughs, dances, and sings unreasonably, and moves his limbs about. At other times he cries without cause ; the skin of his body becomes dry, rough, and of a dark-red colour. These symptoms are more violent after the digestion of food ; and the patient becomes greatly emaciated.

दहति ध्रुवम्। स उष्यते तृष्यते वा ताम्राभस्ताम्रलोचनः लोहगन्धाङ्गवदनो वह्निनेवावकीर्य्यते। पित्तज्वरसमः पित्तात् स चाप्यस्य विधिः स्मृतः॥ तृष्णानिरोधादब्धातौ क्षीणे तेजः समुद्धतम्। सबाह्याभ्यन्तरं देहं प्रदहेन्मन्दचेतसः॥ संशुष्कगलताल्वोष्ठो जिह्वां निष्कृष्य वेपते। असृजः पूर्णकोष्ठस्य दाहोऽन्यः स्यात् सुदुस्तरः। धातुक्षयोक्तो यो दाहस्तेन मूर्च्छातृड़र्द्दितः॥ क्षामस्वरः क्रियाहीनः स सीदेद्भृशपीड़ितः॥ मर्म्माभिघातजोऽप्यस्ति सोऽसाध्यः सप्तमो मतः। सर्व्व एव च वर्ज्याः स्युः शीतगात्रेषु देहिनः॥

When *bile* is generally deranged by the use of indigestible food, and the use of pungent and heating substances, the symptoms it produces are impatience of control, and anger; the person wishes to use violence to others; he remains naked, prefers cooling food, and wishes to live under the shade, or in water. The body is yellow and hot.

When *phlegm* is deranged by the usual causes, as a too sedentary life, and taking too much nourishing food; by which the phlegm is deranged, affecting the functions of the heart, and producing the following symptoms: A love of solitude, taciturnity, and loss of appetite; the person has a desire for women, enjoys deep sleep, and has vomiting, or expectoration. After eating any thing the symptoms are very violent, and the body as well as the nails and countenance are whitish.

When *air, bile,* and *phlegm* are deranged together, all the separate symptoms are produced, and the disease becomes of very difficult cure.

When the disease is produced by the passions; as when frightened by a robber, a tyrannical official, &c.; by the

---

अथ उन्माद-भूतोन्मादनिदानम्।

मदयन्त्युद्धता दोषा यस्मादुन्मार्गमागताः। मानसोऽयमतो व्याधिरुन्माद इति कीर्त्तितः॥ एकैकशः सर्व्वशश्च दोषैरत्यर्थमूर्च्छितैः॥ मानसेन च दुःखेन स च पञ्चविधो मतः। विषाद्भवति षष्ठश्च यथास्वं तत्र भेषजम्॥ स चाप्रवृद्धस्तरुणो मदसंज्ञां बिभर्त्ति च॥ विरुद्धदुष्टाशुचिभोजनानि प्रधर्षणं देवगुरुद्विजानाम्। उन्मादहेतुर्भयहर्षपूर्व्वो मनोऽभिघातो विषमाश्च चेष्टाः। तैरल्पसत्वस्य मलाः प्रदुष्टा बुद्धेर्निवासं हृदयं प्रदुष्य॥ स्रोतांस्यधिष्ठाय मनोवहानि प्रमोहयन्त्याशु नरस्य चेतः॥

धीविभ्रमः सत्वपरिप्लवश्च पर्य्याकुला दृष्टिरधीरता च। अबद्धवाक्त्वं हृदयञ्च शून्यं सामान्यमुन्मादगदस्य लिङ्गम्॥ रुक्षाल्प-

loss of wealth, and friends, or by the love of particular women, the symptoms are characterized by talking, laughing, singing, and sometimes crying. This variety terminates in idiocy.

When madness is produced by poison, the person becomes faint, from the sudden loss of strength; his eyes become red, and the countenance and the body become yellow or blue. The unfavourable symptoms are when the person is weak and emaciated, remains in one position, and is always looking downwards, or upwards. When the patient has no sleep, and is so courageous that he will throw himself from a height, the disease will be fatal.

Possessed persons, or Devil-Madness, (*Bhutonmáda*).

There are two kinds of spiritual beings, a good and a bad spirit, which are supposed to enter the body, and to produce disease. These are called *Bhútonmáda, (Devil-Madness)*; and *Debonmáda,* (madness produced by good spirits).

शीतान्नविरेक-धातुक्षयोपवासैरनिलोऽतिवृद्धः ॥ चिन्तादिदुष्टं हृदयं प्रदुष्य बुद्धिं स्मृतिञ्चाप्युपहन्ति शीघ्रम्। अस्थानहासस्मित नृत्यगीत-वागङ्गविक्षेपण-रोदनानि ॥ पारुष्यकार्श्यारुणवर्णता च, जीर्णे बलञ्चानिलजस्य रूपम्। अजीर्णकट्वम्लविदाहशीतै र्भोज्यैश्चितं पित्तमुदीर्णवेगम् ॥ उन्मादमत्युग्रमनात्मकस्य हृदि स्थितं पूर्ब्बवदाशु कुर्य्यात्। अमर्षसंरम्भविमग्नभावाः सन्तर्ज्ज-नातिद्रवणौष्ण्यरोषाः। प्रच्छाय शीतान्नजलाभिलाषाः पीता च भा पित्तकृतस्य लिङ्गम् ॥ सम्पूरणै र्मन्दविचेष्टितस्य, सोष्मा कफो मर्म्मनि सम्प्रदुष्टः। बुद्धिं स्मृतिञ्चाप्युपहत्य चित्तं प्रमोहयन् संज-नयेद्विकारान् ॥ वाक्चेष्टितं मन्दमरोचकश्च नारी विविक्तप्रियता च निद्रा। छर्द्दिश्च लाला च बलञ्च भुङ्क्ते नखादिशौक्ल्यञ्च कफा

When produced by attack of devils, the person shews his aversion to every thing divine, is very strong, and has much knowledge ; and when from the entrance of good spirit or (*Debtá*) the person has a pleasure in flowers and good smells, becomes pure and holy, and is inclined to speak Sanskrit. He obeys *bráhmans* with strictness, and looks courageous. There are no intermissions in these forms of madness.

Devils know the present, the future, and what is hid or unknown. They are never at rest ; and they are employed in different kinds of business. An unclean or wounded person, or those who do not perform their ceremonies, may be injured by devils. They are very numerous and powerful, and are usually considered as the attendants, or servants of *Shiva.* This explains how the energy, and work of the affected person, is much beyond that of man ; his mind is now powerful, his knowledge extensive, and he understands the *shástras.* Sometimes the person appears sane, and at another time is mad, Such madness is produced by a devil, which is known by the unnatural motion of the person's eyelids.

There are eight principal devils that torment the human species.

त्वके स्यात् ॥ यः सन्निपातप्रभवोऽतिघोरः सर्व्वैः समस्तैः स च हेतुभिः स्यात् ॥ सर्व्वाणि रूपाणि विभर्त्ति तादृग्विरुद्धभेषज्य विधि र्विवर्ज्यः ।

चोरैर्नरेन्द्रपुरुषैररिभिस्तथान्यै र्वित्रासितस्य धनवान्धवसंक्षयाद्वा । गाढ़ं क्षते मनसि च प्रियया रिरंसो र्जायेत चोत्कटतरो मनसो विकारः ॥ चित्रं ब्रवीति च मनोऽनुगतं विसंज्ञो गायत्यथो हसति रोदिति चापि मूढ़ः । रक्तेक्षणो हतबलेन्द्रियभाः सुदीनः श्यावाननो विषकृतेऽथ भवेद्विसंज्ञः । अवाञ्ची वाप्युदञ्ची वा क्षीणमांसबलो नरः । जागरूको ह्यसन्देहमुन्मादेन विनश्यति ॥

1. When *Debagraha*, or good spirit, enters a body, the person is always happy and contented, remains clean in his person, and wears garlands of the sacred flowers, &c.; his person has a pleasant smell, and he has no sleep. He speaks Sanskrit correctly The person is strong, his eyes remain fixed, and he blesses those who approach him. He has a great love for *bráhmans*, and performs the prescribed ceremonies, and attends to old customs of his ancestry.

2. *Asuragraha*. They are the enemies of the *Debtás*. When the person is possessed with them, he perspires much, speaks of the bad conduct of *bráhmans*, and the *Debtás*. His eyes are turned and fixed, he has no fear, and is always performing bad actions. He is a glutton, is not pleased with his food and drink, and is always mischievous.

3. *Gandarbagraha*. The person possessed with this devil is always happy, prefers living in an island, near the bank of a river, or in the jungle; and his conduct is good. He is fond of singing, of sweet smells, and of looking at flowers. He is fond of dancing, and laughing. Those are the choristers of heaven (demigods) who wear sacred flowers, put marks on

---

अमर्त्यवाग्विक्रमवीर्य्यचेष्टो ज्ञानादि-विज्ञान-बलादिभि र्यः।
उन्मादकालोऽनियतश्च यस्य भूतोत्थमुन्मादमुदाहरेत्तम् ॥

सन्तुष्टः शुचिरतिदिव्यमाल्यगन्धो निस्तन्द्री रवितथ-संस्कृत प्रभाषी। तेतस्वी स्थिरनयनो वरप्रदाता ब्रह्मण्यो भवति नरः स देवजुष्टः ॥ संस्वेदी द्विज गुरुदेवदोषवक्ता जिह्माक्षो विगत-भयो विमार्गदृष्टिः। सन्तुष्टो न भवति चान्नपानजातैर्दुष्टात्मा भवति स देवशत्रुजुष्टः ॥ हृष्टात्मा पुलिनवनान्तरोपसेवी स्वाचारः प्रियपरिगीतगन्धमाल्यः। नृत्यन् वै प्रहसति चारु चाल्पशब्दं गन्धर्व्व ग्रहपरिपीड़ितो मनुष्यः। ताम्राक्षः प्रियतनु-रक्तवस्त्र-धारी गम्भोरो द्रुतगतिरल्पवाक् सहिष्णुः। तेजस्वी वदति च

their person, and have a great love for adorning their persons. They speak little but properly, and agreeably.

4. *Jakshyagraha.* This class of demigods are fabled to superintend the treasures, and gardens of heaven. When he enters the body, the person's eyes become yellowish red like copper. They wear thin red clothes, talk little, but are profoundly intelligent, and have much patience; such a person walks fast, is never revengeful, though very strong, and is always wanting to bestow his means upon others.

5. *Pitrigraha.* These are spirits which are separated after death from the bodies of mankind. When an ancestor thus enters the body, the person is always preparing prayers for them, and performing the different ceremonies *(shráddha)* for ancestors. Such a patient is quiet and peaceable, and is fond of animal food, and sweetmeats.

6. *Sarpagraha.* When the serpent-devil enters the body, the person walks irregularly, or from one side to another, like a serpent; his tongue is thrust from one side of the mouth to the other; and he is passionate, and is fond of treacle, honey, and sweetmeats.

किं ददामि कस्मै यो यक्षग्रहपरिपीड़ितो मनुष्यः ॥ प्रेतानां स क्षिपति संस्तरेषु पिण्डान् शान्तात्मा जलमपि चापसव्यवस्त्रः । मांसेप्सुस्तिलगुड़पायसाभिकामः स्तद्भक्तो भवति पितृग्रहाभिजुष्टः ॥ यस्तुर्वीं प्रसरति सर्पवत् कदाचित् सृक्किण्यौ विलिह्यति जिह्वया तथैव ॥ क्रोधालु गुड़मधुदुग्धपायसेप्सु ज्ञातव्यो भवति भुजङ्गमेन जुष्टः । मांसासृग्विविधसुराविकारलिप्सु निर्लज्जो भृशमतिनिष्ठुरोऽतिशूरः ॥ क्रोधालु विपुलबलो निशाविहारी शौचद्विड् भवति स राक्षसै र्गृहीतः । उद्धस्तः कृशपरुषोऽचिरप्रलापी दुर्गन्धो भृशमशुचि स्तथातिलोलः ॥ बह्वाशी विजनवनान्तरोपसेवी व्याचेष्टन् भ्रमति रुदन् पिशाचजुष्टः ॥ स्थूलाक्षो द्रुतम-

7. *Rákshyasagraha*, or cannibal-devil. When one of these devils enters the body of a person, he is fond of eating flesh, blood, and wine. He has no shame, his appearance is disagreeable, and he is very strong, and passionate. Such a person walks about at night, is unclean, and is always performing bad actions.

8. *Pishácha*, or fiend, is known to have entered the body, by the person always stretching out his hands. His body is thin, and is disagreeable to look upon, and he speaks fast, and without meaning. His body has a disagreeable smell, and he is unclean, restless, and covetous. Such a person eats much, prefers living in jungles, and retired places; he walks with an unnatural motion of the limbs and is sorrowful, and frequently cries.

The unfavourable symptoms of such persons possessed with devils are; his eyes are swollen, he walks fast, and his tongue is passed rapidly, and continually, from one side of the mouth

---

टनः स फेनलेही निद्रालुः पतति कम्पते च यो हि। यश्चाद्रि-
द्विरदनगादिविच्युतः स्यात् सोऽसाध्यो भवति तथा त्रयोदशाब्दैः॥

देवग्रहाः पौर्णमास्यामसुराः सन्ध्ययोरपि। गन्धर्वाः प्राय-
शोऽष्टम्यां यक्षाश्च प्रतिपद्यत॥ पितरः कृष्णक्षये हिंस्राः पञ्च-
म्यामपि चोरगाः। रक्षांसि रात्रौ पिशाचाश्चतुर्द्दश्यां विशन्ति हि।
दर्पणादीन् यथा छाया शीतोष्णं प्राणिनो यथा। स्वमणिं
भास्करार्चिश्च यथा देहञ्च देहधृक्। विशन्ति च न दृश्यन्ते
ग्रहास्तद्वच्छरीरिणः॥

अथापस्मारनिदानम्।

तमःप्रवेशः संरम्भो दोषोद्रेकहतस्मृतेः। अपस्मार इति ज्ञेय
गदो घोरश्चतुर्व्विधः। हृत्कम्पः शून्यता स्वेदो ध्यानं मूर्च्छा
प्रमूढ़ता। निद्रानाशश्च तस्मिंश्च भविष्यति भवत्यथ।

to the other; he is always sleepy and sometimes falls down; and at other times he is affected with severe shivering. When the madness is produced by falls from high places, such as from elephants, or trees, they are more difficult to cure. It is also dangerous in old age, and when hereditary. When the disease has continued 13 years it will not be cured.

The devils invade the body of persons on different days according to the species. *Debtá* invade at full moon, and devils (*Asur*), enter in the morning and evening. The *Gandarba* enters on the eighth, and *Jakshya* on the first day of the moon. *Sarpagraha*, or serpent-devils, enter on the fifth day after new and full moon. *Rákshyasa* enter at night. *Pishácha* enter on the 15th day after new and full moon. We cannot see when a spirit enters the body, in the same manner as the soul enters, and leaves the body without being seen; as light enters the water in a glass, or as heat or cold enters a body, without our being aware how it takes place. *Unmáda*, and *Bhútonmada*, are said to be cured when the functions of the sense, judgment, and heart, are restored to a perfect state, and the tissues are natural.

कम्पते प्रदशेद्दन्तान् फेनोद्वामी श्वसित्यपि। परुषारुण-
कृष्णानि पश्येद्रूपाणि चानिलात्॥ पीतफेनाङ्गवक्त्राक्षः पीता-
सृग्रूपदर्शकः॥ सतृष्णोष्णानलव्याप्तलोकदर्शी च पैत्तिकः। शुक्ल-
फेनाङ्गवक्त्राक्षः शीतहृष्टाङ्गजो गुरुः॥ पश्यन् शुक्लानि रूपाणि
श्लैष्मिको मुच्यते चिरात्। सर्व्वैरेतैः समस्तैश्च लिङ्गैर्ज्ञेयस्त्रिदो-
षजः॥ अपस्मारः स चासाध्यो यः क्षीणस्यानवश्च यः। प्रस्फु-
रन्तं सुबहुशः क्षीणं प्रचलितभ्रुवम्। नेत्राभ्यां च विकुर्व्वाण-
मपस्मारो विनाशयेत्॥

पक्षाद्वा द्वादशाहाद्वा मासाद्वा कुपिता मलाः। अपस्माराय
कुर्व्वन्ति वेगं किञ्चिदथान्तरम्॥ देवे वर्षत्यपि यथा भूमौ
बीजानि कानिचित्। शरदि प्रतिरोहन्ति तथा व्याधिसमुच्छ्रयाः॥

Persons not liable to be afflicted by devils are, prophets, charitable persons, those who speak the truth, and those who attend to the orders of the *shástras*, and perform particular duties, and employ proper terms in addressing holy men. Those who have the eight qualities of the body, are always pure, humble, and wise, visit holy places, always govern their passions, and speak the truth ; and those who pray, and attend to the prescribed ceremonies and are charitable, over such persons devils have no power. Devils only go about at night, and they live, under their eight chiefs, on blood, fat, flesh, and disgusting animals.

Epilepsy, (*Apasmara or Mrigi*).

Generic character. Sudden loss of sense, loss of sight, and the person falls down with convulsions. These symptoms are preceded by palpitation of the heart, lightness and hollowness of the chest and body, perspiration, inaccurate thinking, dullness of sense, and loss of sleep.

अथ वातव्याधिनिदानम् ।

रूक्षशीताल्पलघ्वन्न-व्यवायातिप्रजागरैः । विषमादुपचाराच्च दोषासृक् स्रवणादपि ॥ लङ्घनप्लवनात्यध्व-व्यायामादिविचेष्टितैः । धातुनां संक्षयाच्चिन्ताशोकरोगातिकर्षणात् ॥ वेगसन्धारणादामादभिघातादभोजनात् । मर्म्माबाधाद्गजोष्ट्राश्व-शीघ्रयानापतंसनात् । देहे स्रोतांसि रिक्तानि पूरयित्वानिलो बली ॥ करोति विविधान् व्याधीन् सर्व्वाङ्गैकाङ्गसंश्रयान् । अव्यक्तलक्षणं तेषां पूर्व्वरूपमिति स्मृतम् । आत्मरूपन्तु यद्व्यक्तमपायो लघुता पुनः ॥

सङ्कोचः पर्व्वणां स्तम्भो भङ्गोऽस्थ्नां पर्व्वणामपि । रोमहर्षः प्रलापश्च पाणिपृष्ठशिरोग्रहः ॥ खाञ्जपाङ्गुल्यकुब्जत्वं शोषोऽङ्गा-

When air, bile, and phlegm are deranged by grief, sorrow, or the like, they pass into the vessels immediately communicating with the heart, and produce this disease, with the loss of sense and memory.

Exciting causes. This disease is produced by the improper use and indulgence of the senses ; as too much, or too little listening, seeing, tasting, smelling, &c. ; the improper mixtures of food, or putrified articles of food ; the neglect of the calls of nature, connection with women during the flow of the menses, and by such passions, as sorrow, grief, and anger. By these causes the mind is so effected as to produce epilepsy.

There are four kinds of disease, one being produced by the derangement of each of the three humours, and the fourth by the combination of the three.

When *air* is deranged, the symptoms of epilepsy are followed by shivering, grinding of the teeth, foaming at the mouth, hurried respiration, and to the patient every object appears obscured, red, and confused.

When *bile* is deranged the symptoms are accompanied with a yellowness of the body and countenance. To the patient

---

नामनिद्रता । गर्भशुक्ररजोनाशः स्पन्दनं गात्रसुप्तता ॥ शिरो-नासाक्षिजत्रूणां ग्रीवायाश्चापि हुण्डनम् । भेदस्तोदोऽर्त्तिराक्षेपो मुहुश्चायास एव च ॥ एवंविधानि रूपाणि करोति कुपितोऽनिलः । हेतुस्थानविशेषाच्च भवेद्रोगविशेषकृत् ॥

तत्र कोष्ठाश्रिते दुष्टे निग्रहो मूत्रवर्च्चसोः । व्रध्नहृद्रोग-गुल्मार्श-पार्श्वशूलञ्च मारुते ॥ सर्व्वाङ्गकुपिते वाते गात्रस्फुरणभञ्जनम् ॥ वेदनाभिः परीतश्च स्फुटन्ति वास्य सन्धयः । ग्रहो विण्मूत्रवातानां शूलाध्मानाश्मशर्कराः ॥ जङ्घोरु-त्रिक-पात् पृष्ठरोगशोषौ गुदे स्थिते । रुक् पार्श्वोदर हृन्नाभेस्तृष्णोद्गार विसूचिकाः । कासः कण्ठास्यशोषश्च श्वासश्चामाशयस्थिते ॥ पक्वाशयस्थोऽन्त्रकूजं शूला-

every thing appears of a yellowish colour, the sputa is of the same colour, and the eyes appear red. The patient has great thirst, and every thing feels hot, and as if enveloped in flames.

When *phlegm* is deranged the symptoms are whiteness of the countenance and body, the saliva and foam are of the same colour, the body is cold, and the patient shivers. The person sees every thing white, and as it appears to approach near him, he faints. These fits cease very slowly.

When *air*, *bile*, and *phlegm* are deranged together, all the symptoms of the separate forms are present. This disease is incurable if not recent, as the person becomes weak and emaciated, and the fits are frequent, and accompanied with severe convulsive movements of the body. The eye-brows contract frequently with the eyelids, and the eyes move rapidly. In such cases the patient will die. The fits come after ten days, a fortnight, or monthly. In other cases they occur very often. As some seeds thrown in the ground during the rains do not germinate for a long time after, so in this disease the deranged air, bile, and phlegm produce the disease after long intervals.

टोपौ करोति च। कृच्छ्रमूत्र-पुरीषत्व मानाहं त्रिकवेदनाम्। श्रोत्रादिष्विन्द्रियवधं कुर्य्याद्दुष्टसमीरणः॥

त्वग्रुक्षा स्फुटिता सुप्ता कृशा कृष्णा च तुद्यते। आतन्यते सरागा च पर्व्वरुक् त्वग्गतेऽनिले॥ रुजास्तीव्राः ससन्तापा वैवर्ण्यं कृशतारुचिः॥ गात्रे चारूंसि भुक्तस्य स्तम्भश्चासृग्गतेऽनिले॥ गुर्व्वङ्गं तुद्यतेऽत्यर्थं दण्डमुष्टिहतं यथा॥ सरुक् श्रमितमत्यर्थं मांसमेदोगतेऽनिले। भेदोऽस्थिपर्व्वणां सन्धि शूलं मांसबलक्षयः। अस्वप्नः सन्तता रुक् च मज्जास्थिकुपितेऽनिले॥ क्षिप्रं मुञ्चति बध्नाति शुक्रं गर्भमथापि वा॥ विकृतिं जनयेच्चापि शुक्रस्थः कुपितोऽनिलः। कुर्य्यात्सिरागतः शूलं शिराकुञ्चनपूरणम्॥ स वाह्या-

Nervous Diseases, (*Báta Byadhi.*)

These diseases are produced by the continued use of dry, cold, or light articles of food, taken in unusually small quantities; excessive venery, and watching; improper and violent exercise; fasting; and copious discharges of blood, or other evacuations. They are also produced by much jumping, swimming, or fighting, wearing wet clothes, or wanting to do impossibilities, as raising weights, &c. Any cause producing the absorption of parts by which the individual is weakened, and swoons; too much thinking, sorrow, grief, fear, and other diseases producing emaciations; sleeping uncomfortably during the day, or in an unusual position; anger, or not attending to the calls of nature; the accumulation of indigestable food, or certain injuries of vital parts, produce these diseases. They are also caused by the person falling from a height, by riding very fast on an elephant, horse, or camel, or whatever goes very fast. These causes derange air, filling the empty vessels in one part, or over all the body, and thus produce the symptoms of the disease.

अन्तरायामं खल्लीं कौब्ज्यमथापि वा ॥ सर्व्वाङ्गैकाङ्गरोगांश्च कुर्य्यात् स्नायुगतोऽनिलः। हन्ति सन्धिगतः सन्धीन् शूलटोपौ करोति च ॥

प्राणे पित्तावृते च्छर्द्दिर्दाहश्चैवोपजायते। दौर्ब्बल्यं सदनं तन्द्रा वैरस्यञ्च कफावृते। उदाने पित्तयुक्ते तु दाहो मूर्च्छा भ्रमः क्लमः ॥ अस्वेदहर्षौ मन्दोऽग्निः शीतता च कफावृते ॥ स्वेद-दाहौष्ण्यमूर्च्छाः स्युः समाने पित्तसंवृते ॥ कफेन सङ्गे विण्मूत्रे गात्रहर्षश्च जायते। अपाने पित्तयुक्ते तु दाहौष्ण्यं रक्तमूत्रता। अधःकाये गुरुत्वञ्च शीतता च कफावृते। व्याने पित्तावृते दाहो गात्रविक्षेपणं क्लमः। स्तम्भनो दण्डकश्चापि शूलशोथौ कफावृते।

When air is so deranged it produces the following symptoms: the muscles of the small joints are contracted with rigidity, and cannot be moved. These symptoms are accompanied with so much pain, that they seem as if broken by force. The skin becomes rough, the person speaks nonsense, and complains of pain in the joints of the hand, back, and head; he cannot sleep, nor walk with vigour, and is deformed, and the members become thin. When women are so affected, they have miscarriages, and it diminishes the semen, and stops menstruation. The parts affected shake, there is no feeling in the part, the person has severe pain in the head, and no smell; the eyes become dry and dull, and a painful weight is felt in the pit of the stomach, and stiffness of the nape of the neck. These symptoms are accompanied with spasm of different parts, with loss of sense and great fatigue.

These different causes, and the different parts of the body affected, produce various forms of the disease. When the air is deranged in the abdomen, the dejections and urine are constipated, pain is felt in the abdomen and its sides, and diseases of the heart, hysteria (*gulma*), and piles (*arsha*), are produced.

यदा तु धमनी सर्व्वाः कुपितोऽभ्येति मारुतः । तदाक्षिपत्याशु
मुहुर्म्मुहुर्देहं मुहुश्चरः ॥ मुहुर्म्मुहुश्चाक्षेपणादाक्षेपक इति स्मृतः ।

क्रुद्धः स्वैः कोपनैर्वायुः स्थानादूर्द्ध्वं प्रपद्यते । पीड़यन् हृदयं
गत्वा शिरःशङ्खौ च पीड़यन् ॥ धनुर्व्वन्नमयेद्गात्राण्याक्षिपेन्मोहये-
त्तदा । स कृच्छ्रादुच्छ्वसेच्चापि स्तब्धाक्षोऽथ निमीलकः । कपोत
इव कूजेच्च निःसंज्ञः सोऽपतन्त्रकः ॥ दृष्टिं संस्तभ्य संज्ञाञ्च हत्वा
कण्ठेन कूजति ॥ हृदि मुक्ते नरः स्वास्थ्यं याति मोहं वृते
पुनः ॥ वायुना दारुणं प्राहुरेके तदपतानकम् ॥ कफान्वितो
भृशं वायुस्तास्वेव यदि तिष्ठति ॥ दण्डवत् स्तम्भयेद्देहं स तु
दण्डापतानकः । धनुस्तुल्यं नमेद् यस्तु स धनुस्तम्भसंज्ञकः ।

When air is deranged generally there is much pain over the body, which shakes with pain in the joints. They feel as if broken. When situated in the pelvis it stops the usual evacuations, with great pain and flatulency, and produces gravel, and the stone. In women it produces deformities in the fœtus, and the plurality of children. When air is deranged in the anus, the legs, thighs, *os coccygus*, hands, and breast are painful, and the body is thin. When deranged air is situated in the *stomach*, the sides, back, scrobiculus cordis, and navel are painful, with thirst, belching, and cholera; the person complains of cough, and the throat and mouth are dry, with asthma. When air is deranged in the small intestines (*paukáshay*), they make a noise, with scanty dejections, and little urine. Such a person has uneasy choliky pains in the abdomen, with pain in the lower part of the back.

When air is deranged in the *organs* of *sense* it destroys their functions. When deranged in the skin it becomes dry, rough, and has no feeling; has a black colour, and is painful. In some cases it is stretched over the body without wrinkles, and is of a red colour, accompanied with pains in the joints, and slight chops in the skin over the body.

When air is deranged in the *blood*, great pain is felt in the body which is hot, and the colour of the skin is unnatural.

अङ्गुलीगुल्फजठरहृद्वक्षोगलसंश्रितः। स्नायुः प्रतानमनिलो यदाक्षिपति वेगवान्। विष्टब्धाक्षः स्तब्धहनुर्भग्नपार्श्वः कफं वमन्। अभ्यन्तरं धनुरिव यदा नमति मानवम्॥ तदास्याभ्यन्तरायामं कुरुते मारुतो बली। बाह्यस्नायु प्रतानस्थो बाह्यायामं करोति च। तमसाध्यं बुधाः प्राहुः र्वक्षःकट्यूरुभञ्जनम्। कफपित्तान्विते वायु र्वायुरेव च केवलः॥ कुर्युरादाक्षेपकं त्वन्यं चतुर्थमभिघातजम्। गर्भपातनिमित्तश्च शोणितातिस्रवाच्च यः। अभिघातनिमित्तश्च न सिद्ध्यत्यपतानकः॥

The body is thin, the person has no appetite, and the skin has red eruptions over it, and after eating the body is unwieldy, and the person cannot work. When air is deranged in the *flesh* or *fat* the body is heavy, with pain, as if beaten with a stick, and the person is much fatigued.

When air is deranged in the *bones* and *marrow* the long bones and joints are very painful ; his strength and flesh become diminished ; the person has no sleep, and pain is very severe and continued.

When air is deranged in the *semen* it is quickly discharged, or is constipated, and in women it retains the fœtus long in the uterus, or abortions are produced. The semen in such cases has an unusual colour, and produces twins.

When air is deranged in the *vessels* it produces painful contraction, or fulness of the vessel.

When air is deranged in the *nerves* (tendons ?) the whole body may be diseased, or it may be confined to one situation. It produces episthotonos, with lameness, spasm, and cramps of the leg, with hemiplegia.

गृहीतार्द्धं तनो र्वायुः शिराःस्नायु विशोष्य च। पत्तमन्यतरं हन्ति सन्धिबन्धान् विमोचयन्॥ कृत्स्नार्द्धकाय स्तस्य स्याद-कर्म्मण्यो विचेतनः॥ एकाङ्गरोगं तं केचि दन्ये पत्तवधं विदुः। सर्व्वाङ्गरोग स्तद्वच्च सर्व्वकायाश्रित ऽनिले॥ दाहसन्तापमूर्च्छाः स्यु र्वायौ पित्तसमन्विते। शैत्यशोथगुरुत्वानि तस्मिन्नेव कफान्विते। शुद्धवातहतं पत्तं कृच्छ्रसाध्यतमं विदुः। साध्यमन्येऽन संयुक्त मसाध्यं क्षयहेतुकम्॥

उच्चैर्व्याहरतोऽत्यर्थं खादतः कठिनानि वा। हसतो जृम्भतो वापि भाराद्विषमशायिनः॥ अर्द्दयत्यनिलो वक्त्र मर्द्दितं जनयत्यतः॥ वक्रीभवति वक्त्रार्द्धं ग्रीवा चाप्यपवर्त्तते॥ शिरश्चलति

When in the *joints* it produces swellings, and pain in the joints.

When the vital air (*prán báyu*), which is situated in the thorax, is deranged with bile, it produces vomiting with a burning sensation of the parts. When this air is mixed with phlegm it produces weakness, debility, languor, and drowsiness; and the taste for food is deranged.

Vital air in the throat (*udán báyu*), when mixed with *bile* produces great heat in the body, swooning, fainting, and languor. When mixed with *phlegm* there is no perspiration, horripilation is felt over the body; the person becomes melancholy, has little internal heat in the stomach, and the body feels cold.

Vital air in the umbilical region (*samána báyu*), when mixed with bile, produces much perspiration, a burning sensation of the body, fainting, and swooning. When mixed with phlegm constipation of the dejections and urine, and a state of goose-skin over the surface may be remarked.

Vital air in the anus (*apána báyu*). When mixed with bile the body is very hot, or is only slightly warm, and the

---

वाक्सङ्गो नेत्रादीनाञ्च वैकृतम् ॥ ग्रीवाचिबुकदन्तानां यस्मिन् पार्श्वे च वेदना ॥ तमर्दितमिति प्राहुर्व्याधिं व्याधिविचक्षणाः । क्षीणस्यानिमिषाक्षस्य प्रसक्ताव्यक्तभाषिणः । न सिद्ध्यत्यर्दितं नाढं त्रिवर्षं वेपनस्य च ॥ गते वेगे भवेत् स्वास्थ्यं सर्व्वेष्वाक्षेपकादिषु ॥

जिह्वानिर्लेखनाच्छुष्कभक्षणादभिघाततः । कुपितो हनुमूलस्थः स्रंसयित्वानिलो हनुः ॥ करोति विवृतास्यत्वमथवा संवृतास्यताम् । हनुग्रहः स तेन स्यात् कृच्छ्राच्चर्व्वणभाषणम् ॥ दिवा स्वप्नासमस्थान विवृतोर्द्ध्वनिरीक्षणैः । मन्यास्तम्भं प्रकुरुते स एव श्लेष्मणावृतः ॥ वाग्वाहिनीशिरासंस्थो जिह्वां स्तम्भयतेऽनिलः ।

urine is bloody. When mixed with phlegm the person has a sense of heaviness in the lower part of the trunk, and the body feels cold.

Vital air over the body (*byán báyu*), when mixed with bile the body is very hot, and there are convulsions of the extremities, with great fatigue. When mixed with phlegm the person remains stupid, and rigid, and he feels pain, and swelling of the body.

Different varieties of nervous diseases are thus supposed to be produced by the derangements of the air (*báyu*). In *Bhábaprakásha* eighty varieties are described. The following may be considered the most important :—

1. When air is much deranged, and passes into the different vessels of the body it produces contractions of the body. This form is called *akhyepaka*, or spasmodic convulsions.

2. When air is deranged, and rises from its situation, it produces pain in the chest, head, and temples. The body and members are bent like a bow; and it produces convulsions. The person has difficulty in breathing, the eyes are fixed and shut. The person moans, and has little sense. This form is called *apatántraka* or rigid spasms. In this disease the body is drawn up either backwards or forwards, or to either side.

जिह्वास्तम्भः स तेनान्नपानवाकेष्वनीशता । रक्तमाश्रित्य पवनः कुर्य्यान्मूर्द्धधराः शिराः । रुक्षाः सवेदनाः कृष्णाः सोऽसाध्यः स्यात् शिरोग्रहः । स्फिक्पूर्व्वा कटिपृष्ठोरु जानुजंघापदं क्रमात् । गृध्रसी स्तम्भरुक् तोदैर्गृह्णाति स्पन्दते मुहुः । वाताद्वातकफात्तन्द्रा गौरवारोचकान्विता । तलं प्रत्यङ्गुलीनां याः कण्डरा बाहुपृष्ठतः । बाह्वोः कर्म्मक्षयकरी विश्वची चेति सोच्यते ॥

वातशोणितजः शोथो जानुमध्ये महारुजः । ज्ञेयः क्रोष्टुकशीर्षस्तु स्थूलः क्रोष्टुकशीर्षवत् । वायुः कट्याश्रितः सक्थ्नः कण्डरामाक्षिपेद् यदा । खञ्जस्तदा भवेज्जन्तुः पङ्गुः सक्थ्नोर्द्वयो

3. When the eye remains fixed, with loss of sense, the person makes a peculiar noise, the air is dislodged from the chest with relief, and is followed by weakness of the senses ; it is called *dáruna* or *apantánaka.*

4. When air is mixed with phlegm, and is situated in the vessels, the person is rigid like a stick, hence its name is *dandápatánaka.*

5. When the body is bent like a bow it is called *dhanustambha.*

6. When the air is deranged in the fingers, ankles, belly, chest, or neck, the air contracts the nerves of these parts, and forces the body forward, accompanied with Tetanus, and vomiting of phlegm ; the eyes are fixed, and severe pain is felt in the sides ; this form is called *ámbotreama.*

7. When the air affects the veins of the back it produces *apostrotonas* (*bájhyá-áma*) ; this form is incurable, as the breast and back joints are broken by the violence of the symptoms. This variety of the disease is produced by external injuries, in miscarriages, and great hemorrhages.

र्वधात् ॥ प्रक्रामन् वेपते यस्तु खञ्जन्निव च गच्छति ॥ कलायखञ्जं तं विद्यात् मुक्तसन्धिप्रबन्धनम् ॥ रुक् पादे विषमन्यस्ते श्रमाद्वा जायते यदा । वातेन गुल्फमाश्रित्य तमाहुर्वातकण्टकम् । पादयोः कुरुते दाहं पित्तासृक्सहितोऽनिलः । विशेषतश्चंक्रमतः पाददाहं तमादिशेत् ।

हृष्येते चरणौ यस्य भवतश्चापि सुप्तकौ । पादहर्षः स विज्ञेय कफवातप्रकोपतः ॥ अंसदेश-स्थितो वायुः शोषयेदंसबन्धनम् । शिराश्चाकुञ्च्य तत्रस्थो जनयेदवबाहुकम् । आवृत्य वायुः सकफो धमनीः शब्दवाहिनीः ॥ नरान् करोत्यक्रियकान् मूकमिन्मिणगद्गदान् ।

8. *Pakshyághátá* (paralysis, *hemiplegia*). There are two varieties of this disease, one affecting one side of the body, and another affecting one half of the body taken transversely. When air affects the vessels and nerves of one side, it produces this disease; when the person loses the power of that part, which is without feeling, and with looseness of the joints. When deranged air alone produces *hemiplegia,* the disease will be cured with difficulty. When air and bile, or air and phlegm produce this disease it may be cured ; but when there is great weakness of the essential parts of the body, as after hemorrhagia in parturition or injuries, the disease is incurable.

9. When all the body is palsied it is called *sarbánga-rog.* When air and bile are both deranged, it produces great heat of the body, and fainting. When air is deranged with phlegm, the body is cold, is swelled, and heavy.

10. *Arddata,* or *hanustambha,* (Tetanus and Trismus ?) When the air is deranged by a person speaking very loud, or by eating large mouthfuls of meat, or hard things, or laughing much, or gaping or sleeping uncomfortably, or bearing heavy weights, it affects the lower jaw or half the face and

---

अधो या वेदना याति वर्च्चोमूत्राशयोत्थिता। भिन्दन्तीव गुदोपस्थं सा तूनी नाम नामतः॥ गुदोपस्थोत्थिता या तु प्रतिलोमं प्रधाविता। वेगैः पक्वाशयं याति प्रतीतूनीति सोच्यते। साटोपमत्युग्ररुज माध्मातमुदरं भृशम्। आध्मानमिति तं विद्याद्घोरं वातनिरोधजम्। विमुक्तपार्श्वहृदयं तदेवामाशयोत्थितम्। प्रत्याध्मानं विजानीयात् कफव्याकुलितानिलम्॥ नाभेरधस्तात् संजातः सञ्चारी यदि वा चलः॥ अष्ठीलावद्घनग्रन्थिरूर्द्धमायतः उन्नतः। वाताष्ठीलां विजानीयाद् बहिर्मार्गाविरोधिनीं एतामेव रुजोपेतां वातविन्मूत्ररोधिनीम्॥ प्रत्यष्ठीलामिति वदेज्जठरे तिर्य्यगुत्थिताम्। मारुतेऽविगुणे वस्तौ मूत्रं सम्यक् प्रव-

neck, which it draws laterally, and the head shakes. The person cannot speak, there is a deformity of the eye, nose, mouth, and neck, with pain in these parts, as also in the chin and teeth, and the senses are in an unhealthy state. The dangerous symptoms of this disease are when the person is weak, the pain severe, and he cannot move his eyelids, nor speak distinctly; when the mouth is turned to one side, and with the shaking of the part of the body, as the head, has continued for three or more years. In all these spasmodic diseases the symptoms for a time disappear, and again recur.

11. Sometimes while cleaning the tongue with the tongue scraper, when eating dry and hard food, or by external injury, the air is deranged in the joints of the jaw, and are sometimes dislocated, when the mouth remains open. In other cases the jaw is locked, when the patient is unable to speak or eat.

12. When sleeping in the day time, especially in an unnatural attitude, or when regarding intensely an object above the person, *air* may be so deranged, and mixed with phlegm as to produce the stiffness of the neck, which remains straight and rigid. This is called *manyástambha.*

र्त्तते। विकारा विविधा स्यात्र प्रतिलोमे भवन्ति च॥ सार्व्वाङ्गकम्पः शिरसो वायुर्व्वेपथुसंज्ञकः। खल्लौ तु पादजंघोरुकरमूलावमोटनौ।

स्थाननामानुरूपैश्च लिङ्गैः शेषान् विनिर्द्दिशेत्। सर्व्वेष्वेतेषु संसर्गं पित्तादेरुपलक्षयेत्। हनुस्तम्भार्द्दिताक्षेपपक्षाघातापतानकाः। कालेन महता वातानां यत्नात् सिध्यन्ति वा न वा। नवान् बलवतस्त्वेतान् साधयेन्निरुपद्रवान्। विसर्पदाहरुक्सङ्गमूर्च्छारुच्यग्निमार्द्दवैः। क्षीणमांसबलं वाता घ्नन्ति पक्षवधादयः॥ शूनं सुप्तत्वचं भग्नं कम्पाध्माननिपीड़ितम्॥ रुजार्त्तिमन्तञ्च नरं वातव्याधिर्विनाशयेत्॥ अव्याहतगतिर्यस्य स्थानस्थः प्रकृतिस्थितः। वायुः स्यात् सोऽधिकं जीवेद्वीतरोगः समाः शतम्॥

13. When the air affects the nerve of the tongue, it becomes rigid and immoveable, and the person cannot speak, eat, or drink. This disease is named *jihwástambha.*

14. When air enters the blood-vessels of the head, the vessels becomes dry, black, and painful, producing headache or the disease called *shirograha.*

15. When air attacks the buttocks, back, loins, hip, thigh, knees, legs, and feet, it produces pain in these parts; passes from one to the other, often without the pain being properly defined. In other cases the affected parts shake; sometimes when air is mixed with phlegm it produces heaviness of the part, dyspepsia and drowsiness. This variety is called *gridhrasi.*

16. *Bishwáchi.* When air affects the tendons of the back of the hand and arm, it produces this disease, in which there is no motion in the hand or arm.

17. When air and blood are changed in a part, it swells with severe pain. In this manner the knee-joint may be affected, and become large, like a jackal's head. This disease is called *kustakashirsha.*

अथ वातरक्तनिदानम् ।

लवणाम्लकटुक्षारस्निग्धोष्णाजीर्णभोजनैः । क्लिन्नशुष्काम्बूजानूपमांसपिण्याकमूलकैः ॥ कुलत्थमाषनिष्पावशाकादिपललेक्षुभिः ॥ दध्यारनालसौ वीर शुक्ततक्रसुरासवैः । विरुद्धाध्यशनक्रोध दिवास्वप्नप्रजागरैः । प्रायशः सुकुमाराणां मिथ्याहारविहारिणाम् ॥ स्थूलानां सुखिनाञ्चापि कुप्यते वातशोणितम् ॥ हस्त्यश्वोष्ट्रैर्गच्छतश्चाश्नतश्च विदाह्यन्नं सविदाहोऽशनस्य । कृत्स्नं रक्तं विदहत्त्वाशु तच्च दुष्टं स्रुतं पादयोश्चीयते तु । तत्संपृक्तं वायुना दूषितेन तत्प्राबल्यादुच्यते वातरक्तम् ॥

स्वेदोत्यर्थं न वा कार्ष्ण्यं स्पर्शाज्ञत्वं क्षतेऽतिरुक् । सन्धिशैथिल्यमालस्यं सदनं पिड़कोद्गमः ॥ जानुजङ्घोरुकट्यंस हस्त-

18. When air is deranged in the sides of the thighs, it draws the tendons of these parts, which contract, and the person walks feebly. This disease is called *khanja.*

19. If both sides are affected the person cannot walk, this disease is called *pangu.*

20. When in walking the person limps, his body shakes, or as if the person was walking over *kálai,* a kind of pea, and is feeble, it is called *kaláskhanja* (chorea sanctir viti).* In this disease the parts seem as if loosened from their natural binding. The disease is characterized by the person feeling in the commencement a trembling or shivering sensation through his body, accompanied with a dimness of sight, and a pain in the neck, jaw, or teeth, or of the part affected. These symptoms are followed by involuntary twitching of the head, neck, and jaw, often of one side, especially of one leg. The patient speaks indistinctly, and then the involuntary motions extend to the whole voluntary muscles of progression, producing a

---

पादाङ्ग-सन्धिषु। निस्तोदः स्फुरणं भेदो गुरुत्वं सुप्तिरेव च। कण्डूः सन्धिषु रुग् भूत्वा भूत्वा नश्यति चासकृत्। वैवर्ण्यं मण्डलोत्पत्ति र्वातासृक् पूर्व्वलक्षणम्॥

वातेऽधिकेऽधिकं तत्र शूलस्फुरणभञ्जनम्। शोथस्य रौक्ष्यं कृष्णत्वं श्यावता॥ वृद्धिहानयः॥ धमन्यङ्गुलिसन्धीनां सङ्कोचोऽङ्गग्रहोऽतिरुक्॥ शीतद्वेषानुपशयौ स्तम्भवेपथुसुप्तयः॥ रक्ते शोथोऽतिरुक् तोद स्ताम्रश्चिमिचिमायते। स्निग्धरुक्षैः शमं नैति कण्डूक्लेदसमन्वितः॥ पित्ते विदाहः सम्मोहः स्वेदो मूर्च्छा मदस्तृषा। स्पर्शासहत्वं रुग्रागः शोथः पाको भृशोष्मता। कफे स्तैमित्यगुरुता सुप्तिस्निग्धत्वशीतता। कण्डू मन्दा च रुग्द्वन्द्वं सर्व्वलिङ्गञ्च सङ्करात्॥

---

* In some works the term *Ardita* is given to this disease, and others apply the term *Ardita* to Tetanus and Trismus.

dancing motion. When the disease extends over the body, and has continued long, it is considered incurable. Its existing cause is considered to be irregularity in the bowels from eating indigestable food, too much walking or laughing, carrying great loads &c.

21. When the ankle joint is strained in walking it produces pain in the ankle with stiffness, it is called *bátakantaka.* The pain resembling that of a thorn piercing the flesh.

22. Air, bile, and blood accumulated in the feet produce a burning sensation of the part, particularly when the person is walking, it is called *pádadáha.* This is one of the most distressing and intractable diseases peculiar to this country. It is called "Fever in the feet."

23. When *phlegm* and *air* are deranged in the two feet they become cold, with insensibility, as when sitting very long in a particular position, when the leg feels dead with a disagreeable numb feeling. It is called *pádaharsha* (foot numb-

---

पादयोर्मूलमास्थाय कदाचिद्धस्तयोरपि। आखोर्विषमिव क्रुद्धं तद्देहमुपसर्पति॥ आजानु स्फुटितं यच्च प्रभिन्नं प्रस्रुतञ्च यत्। उपद्रवैश्च यज्जुष्टं प्राणमांसक्षयादिभिः॥ वातरक्तमसाध्यं स्यात्-याप्यं संवत्सरोत्थितम्। अस्वप्नारोचकश्वास मांसकोथशिरोग्रहाः। मूर्च्छातिमदरुक्तृष्णा ज्वरमोहप्रवेपकाः॥ हिक्कापांगुल्य वीसर्पपाकतोदभ्रमक्लमाः॥ अङ्गुलीवक्रतास्फोटदाहमर्म्मग्रहार्बुदाः। एतैरुपद्रवैर्व्वर्ज्जं मोहेनैकेन वापि यत्। अकृत्स्नोपद्रवं याप्यं साध्यं स्यान्निरुपद्रवम्। एकदोषानुगं साध्यं नवं याप्यं द्विदोषजम्। त्रिदोषजमसाध्यं स्यात् यस्य च स्युरुपद्रवाः॥

अथोरुस्तम्भनिदानम्।

शीतोष्णद्रवसंशुष्कगुरुस्निग्धैर्निषेवितैः। जीर्णाजीर्णे तथायास संक्षोभस्वप्नजागरैः॥ सश्लेष्ममेदःपवनः साममत्यर्थसञ्चितम्॥

ness) ; and is a frequent complaint among us, from our sitting on the ground, in often constrained positions.

24. When air is deranged in the shoulder-joint, it dries the ligaments and tendons of the part. They are contracted, and the arm becomes fixed. It is called *apabáhuka*, or stiff arm.

25. When the air is mixed with phlegm, and enters into the air-vessels (*dhamani*) the person cannot speak, or speaks slowly, and indistinctly. This disease is called *múka* (dumbness), and *minmina* and *gadgada* (indistinct speech).

26. When pain commences from the bowels and bladder, and passes to the anus and urinary passages, producing great pain in these parts, which feel as if torn asunder, the disease is called *tunie.*

27. When it commences from the anus and urinary passages, and passes up to the intestines with great violence, it is called *pratunie.*

28. Swelling and pain, with a rumbling noise of the abdomen, produced by the air being confined in the abdomen, is called *ádhyána*, or drumb-belly.

अभिभूयेतरं दोषमूरू चेत् प्रतिपद्यते। सक्थ्यस्थिनी प्रपूर्य्यान्तः श्लेष्मणा स्तिमितेन च। तदा स्तभ्नाति तेनोरू स्तब्धौ शीतावचेतनौ॥ परकीयाविव गुरू स्यातामतिभृशव्यथौ। ध्यानाङ्गमर्द्द स्तैमित्य तन्द्रा छर्द्द्यरुचि ज्वरैः॥ संयुक्तौ पादसदनकृच्छ्रोद्धरणसुप्तिभिः। तमुरुस्तम्भमित्याहुराढ्यवातमथापरे॥

प्राग् रूपं तस्य निद्रातिध्यानं स्तिमितता ज्वरः। लोमहर्षोऽरुचिश्छर्द्दिर्जङ्घोरू: सदनं तथा॥ वातशङ्किभिरज्ञानात्तस्य स्यात् स्नेहनात् पुनः। पादयोः सदनं सुप्तिः कृच्छ्रादुद्धरणं तथा॥ जङ्घोरुग्लानिरत्यर्थं शश्वच्चादाहवेदने। पादञ्च व्यथते न्यस्तं शीतस्पर्शं न वेत्ति च॥ संस्थाने पीड़ने गत्यां चालने चाप्यनीश्वरः। अन्यनेयौ हि संभग्नावरू पादौ च मन्यते॥ यदा दाहार्त्ति-

29. When the swelling is confined to the stomach with pain and noise, it is called *pratyádhyána* ; and is produced by the air being mixed with phlegm.

30. When a hard oblong swelling is felt under the navel, which passes from one part to another, or rests stationary, and becomes prominent, and air, urine, and dejections are constipated, it is called *ashthilá* or *bátashthilá.*

31. When the hard swelling is longitudinal, and is accompanied with much pain, and the urine and dejections are constipated, it is called *pratashthilá.* These derangements of air produce diseases in various situations ; when deranged in the bladder, it causes the stoppage of urine, &c.

32. When air is deranged in the head, it is always shaking. The disease is called *bapati.*

33. When air is affected in the feet, legs, thighs, and wrist, it produces spasm and is called *kuli.* The other diseases of air are named according to the part particularly affected. In all these nervous diseases it is of importance that the Physician observe whether the symptoms of bile and phlegm, &c.

तोदर्त्तो वेपनः स्फुरणो भवेत्। उरुस्तम्भ स्तदा ह्यनयात् साधयेदनया नवम्॥

अथामवातनिदानम्।

विरुद्धाहारचेष्टस्य मन्दाग्नेर्निश्चलस्य च। स्निग्धं भुक्तवतोऽह्यन्न व्यायामं कुर्व्वतस्तथा॥ वायुना प्रेरितो ह्यामः श्लेष्मस्थानं प्रधावति। तेनत्यर्थं विदग्धोऽसौ धमनीः प्रतिपद्यते॥ वातपित्तकफैर्भूयो दूषितः सोऽन्नजो रसः। स्रोतांस्यभिष्यन्दयति नानावर्णोऽतिपिच्छिलः॥ जनयत्याशु दौर्ब्बलं गौरवं हृदयस्य च। व्याधीनामाश्रयो ह्येष आमसंज्ञेति दारुणः॥ युगपत् कुपितावन्तस्त्रिकसन्धिप्रवेशकौ। स्तब्धं वा कुरुते गात्र मामवातः स उच्यते।

are present, as they will affect his prognosis, and treatment. In *hanugraha* (lock-jaw), *ardito* (or paralysis of the face), *akhepoká* (spasmodic diseases), *pakhyághóta* (hemiplegia), *apatánaka* (epilepsy), our prognosis may be rather favourable, when the person is strong, the disease is recent, and is not accompanied with any bad symptoms. This is particularly the case when the patient is rich, as the treatment will generally be tedious.

The unfavourable symptoms are when the disease is accompanied with erysipelas (*bisarpa*), or with severe burning sensations, with great heat and pain, as if the body was torn, and with constipation, fainting, and loss of appetite, or when the digestion is very weak. In such cases the patient will die. This disease is also dangerous when the person is swollen, when the parts are without feeling, and are accompanied with flatulency and shaking of the body, with great pain and weakness.

Should the air not be deranged, and be confined to its usual situation, the person will live for a hundred years free from disease.

अङ्गमर्द्दोऽरुचिस्तृष्णा चालस्यं गौरवं ज्वरः। अपाकः शूनताङ्गानामामवातस्य लक्षणम्। स कष्टः सर्व्वरोगाणां यदा प्रकुपितो भवेत्॥

हस्तपादशिरोगुल्फ-त्रिकजानूरुसन्धिषु। करोति सरुजं शोथं यत्र दोषः प्रपद्यते॥ स देशो रुज्यतेऽत्यर्थं व्याविद्ध इव वृश्चिकैः। जनयेत् सोऽग्निदौर्व्बल्यं प्रसेकारुचिगौरवम्॥ उत्साहहानिं वैरस्यं दाहञ्च बहुमूत्रताम्। कुक्षौ कठिनतां शूलं तथा निद्राविपर्य्ययम्॥ तृट्छर्द्दिभ्रममूर्च्छाश्च हृद्ग्रहं विड्विबन्धताम्। जाड्यान्त्रकूजमानाहं कष्टांश्चान्यानुपद्रवान्॥ पित्तात् सदाहरागञ्च सशूलं पवनानुगम्। स्तिमितं गुरुकण्डूञ्च कफदुष्टं तमादिशेत्॥

A kind of Leprosy,* (*Bátc-rakta.*)

This disease is produced by the blood being diseased with *air* (*báyu*). Its exciting causes are using sour food, and alkaline salts. In like manner spices, or other hot articles, indigestable articles of food, putrified, or dry meats, as the flesh of crocodiles, of the buffalo, of the rhinoceros, or the like. Til oil-cake, and other indigestable articles of food, curdled or butter-milk, bad wines, and excess in eating and drinking, the passions, unhealthy and improper mixtures of food, eating too often, or sleeping during the day produce this disease. Delicate constitutions, and fat people, who lead a sedentary life are predisposed to this disease. Long continued riding on horses, elephants, or camels, and whatever produces great heat of the body ; by these causes the blood is diseased, and is conveyed by the air to the feet, where it accumulates, and produces this disease, first in the feet, and then in other parts of the body. *Báta-rakta* is ushered in sometimes by free, at other times by a cessation of perspirations ; the body becomes of a dark hue,

---

एकदोषानुगः साध्यो द्विदोषो याप्य उच्यते। सर्व्वदेहचरः शोथः सकृच्छ्रः सान्निपातिकः ॥

अथ शूलपरिनामशूलान्नद्रवशूलनिदानम्।

दोषैः पृथक् समस्तामद्वन्द्वैः शूलोऽष्टधा भवेत्। सर्व्वेष्वेतेषु शूलेषु प्रायेण पवनः प्रभुः ॥ व्यायामयानादतिमैथुनाच्च प्रजागरात् शीतजलातिपानात्। कलाय मुद्गाढ़किकोरदूषादत्यर्थरुक्षाध्यशनाभिघातात् ॥ कषाय-तिक्तातिविरूढ़जान्न विरुद्धवल्लुरशुष्कशाकात्। विट्शुक्रमूत्रानिलवेगरोधात् शोकोपवासादतिहास्यभाष्यात् ॥ वायुः प्रवृद्धो जनयेद्धि शूलं हृत्पार्श्वपृष्ठ-

---

* Under this head several diseases are described ; such as certain forms of rheumatism, abscesses ; and such cachectic states as may terminate in true leprosy.

and parts have no feeling. If there are sores they are very painful; the joints are loose, the person feels languid, and cannot work; and small pimples appear over the body, with pain of a gnawing or lancinating kind, as if ants were eating the flesh, or needles thrust into the skin. The knees, legs, thighs, loins, shoulders, hands, and arms, are so affected. The pain intermits, and these parts become heavy, without feeling, and the skin has patches of an unusual colour.

When *air* is much deranged there is severe pain of the body, as if ants were eating the flesh, and the vessels, nails, fingers, and joints are contracted. The patient has no appetite, and if not treated the symptoms increase. The person cannot work, and the body shakes, with rigidity of the joints.

When *blood* is much deranged swellings appears over the body, with much pain. The skin is of a copperish colour with slight stinging pain (*chin chin*).

When *bile* is deranged the body feels hot, with a burning sensation, and dulness of intellect. He perspires much, has fainting fits, with an appearance of drunkenness and

---

त्रिकवस्तिदेशे। जीर्णे प्रदोषे च घनागमे च शीते च कोपं समुपैति गाढ़म्॥ मुहुर्मुहुश्चोपशम-प्रकोपौ विड्वातसंस्तम्भन-तोदभेदैः। संस्वेदनाभ्यञ्जनमर्द्दनाद्यैः स्निग्धोष्णभोजैश्च शमं प्रयाति॥

क्षारातितीक्ष्णोष्णविदाहि-तैल-निष्पावपिण्याककुलत्थयूषैः। कट्वम्लसौवीर-सुराविकारैः क्रोधानलायासरविप्रतापैः॥ ग्राम्यातियोगादशनैर्विदग्धैः पित्तं प्रकुप्याशु करोति शूलम्। तृष्णोहदाहार्त्तिकरं हि नाभ्यां संस्वेदमूर्च्छाभ्रम-चोषयुक्तम्॥ मध्यन्दिने कुप्यति चार्द्धरात्रे विदाहकाले जलदात्यये च। शीते च शीतैः समुपैति शान्तिं सुस्वादुशीतैरपि भोजनैश्च॥

thirst; pressure of the part produces great pain, with redness, heat, swelling, and sometimes abscesses are formed.

When *phlegm* is deranged the body is very cold, as if a cold wet cloth was applied over the body, which feels heavy, and without feeling. The skin is smooth, shining and itchy, and feels cold, with slight pain.

When two or three of the above humours are affected the symptoms resemble the two or three forms, as above enumerated.

In some cases the ankles and wrists are first affected, and then it extends over the body like the poison of certain animals.

The disease is incurable, when accompanied with a sore from the ankle to the knee, or when it is opened and pus escapes in large quantities. When the person is very weak and reduced the disease will be fatal; but if the person lives for a year, or it is chronic, he will live. When the disease is severe the person cannot obtain sleep, has no appetite, has a difficulty in breathing, parts of the body slough, he complains of head-ache, fainting, delirium, pain in the body, thirst, fever, has no sense, with shaking, hiccough, contraction of the fingers and toes, so that he cannot walk nor work,

---

आनुपवारिजकिलाट-पयोविकारै मांसेक्षुपिष्टकृशरातिलशष्कुलीभिः। अन्यैर्बलासजनकैरपि हेतुभिश्च श्लेष्मा प्रकोपमुपगमय्य करोति शूलम्॥ हृल्लासकास-सदनारुचि-सम्प्रसेकै रामाशये स्तिमितकोष्ठ-शिरोगुरुत्वैः। भुक्ते सदैव हि रुजं कुरुतेऽतिमात्रं सूर्य्योदयेऽथ शिशिरे कुसुमागमे च॥ सर्व्वेषु दोषेषु च सर्व्वलिङ्गं विद्याद्भिषक् सर्व्वभवं हि शूलम्। सुकष्टमेनं विषवज्रकल्पं विवर्ज्जनीयं प्रवदन्ति तज्ज्ञाः॥

आटोपहृल्लास-वमीगुरुत्व-स्तैमित्य-मानाह-कफप्रसेकैः। कफस्य लिङ्गेन समानलिङ्गं मामोद्भवं शूलमुदाहरन्ति॥ वस्तौ हृत्पार्श्व-

and erysipelas appears with vascular eruptions. Severe pain is felt in the vital parts, tumours appear over the body, want of memory, fatigue, and delirium follow, and precede death. When all the symptoms of this severe form of the disease are not present, the disease may not be fatal. If none of the severe symptoms are present, the disease may be cured. When only one of the humours is deranged; as air, bile, &c., and the disease is recent, it may be cured; but, if two of the humours are deranged, the disease will remain, when three are affected the disease is incurable, and when all the severe symptoms are present the disease will be fatal.

Diseases of the Extremities.

The diseases of the upper extremities are few, and of little importance, compared to those of the lower extremities; to which the following remarks are principally confined. These diseases are *Urustambha* and *Slipada*, or swellings of the extre-

---

पृष्ठेषु सशूलः कफवातिकः कुक्षौहृन्नाभिमध्येषु सशूलः कफपैत्तिकः। दाहज्वरकरो घोरो विज्ञेयो वातपैत्तिकः॥

एकदोषोत्थितः साध्यः कृच्छ्रसाध्यो द्विदोषजः। सर्व्वदोषोत्थितो घोरस्त्वसाध्यो भूर्य्युपद्रवः॥ स्वैर्निदानैः प्रकुपितो वायुः सन्निहितस्तदा। कफपित्ते समावृत्य शूलकारी भवेद्बली॥ भुक्ते जीर्य्यति यच्छूलं तदेव परिणामजम्। तस्य लक्षणमप्येतत् समासेनाभिधीयते॥ आध्मानाटोपविण्मूत्र-विबन्धारतिवेपनैः। स्निग्धोष्णोपशमप्रायं वातिकं तद्वदेद्भिषक्॥ तृष्णादाहारतिस्वेदं कट्वम्ललवणोद्भवम्। शूलं शीतशमप्रायं पैत्तिकं लक्षयेद्बुधः॥ छर्द्दिहृल्लासमम्मोहं स्वल्परुग्दीर्घसन्तति। कटुतिक्तोपशान्तौ चं तच्च

mities, diseases of the nails, of the soles of the feet, and ulcers of the axilla, and groin. The other diseases of the extremities have been already considered under those of *Bátabyadhi.*

Urustambha (large abscess). These are produced under the fascia of the thigh by cold, hot, or very liquid or dry food, heavy oleaginous or indigestable food, or other articles of the like kind, fatigue, grief, agitation, sleeping during the day, and watching at night. By these means the air, phlegm, and fat are deranged and mixed with bile, which accumulates in the thighs, and in the external parts of the thigh-bone. The thigh then becomes senseless like a dead part, and is very painful.

This disease produces lowness of spirits, pain over the body, drowsiness, and chilliness, cold, vomiting, loss of appetite and fever. The thigh cannot be moved, and it is raised with difficulty, and as if asleep. Other practitioners call the disease *Adabáta.*

Befere the accumulation of humours in the thigh, the person feels sleepy, is in low spirits, the body cold, with fever, loss of

---

ज्ञेयं कफात्मकम् ॥ संसृष्टलक्षणं बुद्धा द्विदोषं परिकल्पयेत् । त्रिदोषज मसाध्यन्तु क्षीणमांसबलानलम् ॥

जीर्णे जीर्यत्यजीर्णे वा यच्छूल मुपजायते । पथ्यापथ्यप्रयोगेण भोजनाभोजनेन च ॥ न शमं याति नियमात् सोऽन्नद्रव उदाहृतः । अन्नद्रवाख्यशूलेषु न तावत् स्वास्थ्यमश्नुते ॥ वान्तमात्रे जरत् पित्तं शूलमाशु व्यपोहति ॥

अथोदावर्त्तनाहनिदानम् ।

वातविन्मूत्रजृम्भाश्रुक्षवोद्गारवमीन्द्रियः । क्षुत्तृष्णोच्छ्वासनिद्राणां धृत्योदावर्त्तसम्भवः ॥ वातमूत्रपुरीषाणां सङ्गाध्मानं क्लमो रुजा । जठरे वातजाश्चान्ये रोगाः स्युर्व्वातनिग्रहात् ॥ आटोपशूलौपरिकर्त्तिकां च सङ्गः पूरीषस्य तथोर्द्धवातः । पुरीषमास्यादथवा

appetite and vomiting. Both legs and thighs are heavy and weak. When the pain is supposed to be rheumatic, and the part is rubbed with oleaginous medicines, the disease increases, affects the feet and prevents the person walking; and is accompanied with much pain, swelling, and inflammation, followed by insensibility, and the leg feels as if it was broken. When there is much lancinating pain, inflammation, and shivering, the patient will die. When these symptoms are absent, or the disease is recent, the patient may be cured by the practitioner, as the disease under this circumstance is not always fatal.

Acute Rheumatism (*Ambát.*)

This disease is produced in dyspeptic patients who lead a sedentary life, taking improper food, or are intemperate. All indigestable food has this effect; such as oleaginous articles, particularly when the person, at the same time, takes much

---

निरेति पुरीषवेगेऽभिहते नरस्य ॥ वस्तिमेहनयोः शूलं मूत्रकृच्छ्र शिरोरुजा । विनामो वङ्क्षणानाहः स्याल्लिङ्गं मूत्रनिग्रहे ॥ मनग्रा-गलस्तम्भशिरोविकारा जृम्भोपघातात् पवनात्मकाः स्युः । तथा-क्षिणाघ्रावदनामयाश्च भवन्ति तीव्राः सह कर्णरोगैः ॥

आनन्दजं वाप्यथ शोकजं वा नेत्रोदकं प्राप्तममुञ्चतो हि । शिरो गुरुत्वं नयनामयाश्च भवन्ति तीव्राः सह पीनसेन ॥ मन्या-स्तम्भः शिरःशूलमर्द्दितार्द्धावभेदकौ । इन्द्रियाणाञ्च दौर्ब्बल्यञ्च क्षवथोः स्याद्धिनिग्रहात् ॥ कण्ठास्यपूर्णत्वमतीव तोदः कूजश्च वायोरथवा प्रवृत्तिः । उद्गारवेगेऽभिहते भवन्ति घोरा विकाराः पवनप्रसूताः ॥ कण्डुकोठारुचिव्यङ्गशोथपाण्ड्वामयज्वराः । कुष्ठ-वीसर्पहृल्लासा च्छर्द्दिनिग्रहजा गदाः ॥ मूत्राशये वै गुदमुष्कयोश्च

exercise. By such causes the chyle is not properly prepared, and indigested food (*Am*) is formed in the stomach. This *Am* is carried into the great abdominal vessels. The deranged chyle produced in this manner, by the morbid condition of air, bile, or phlegm is like mucilage, and deranges all the abdomen. This (*Amras*) morbid chyle is the cause of all the varieties of this disease. The deranged phlegm and air are accumulated in the loins producing pain and rigidity of the body, and hence it is called *Ambát*, (air mixed with morbid chyle.) From the loins it extends over all the body.

The general symptoms are pain over the body, loss of appetite, thirst, want of appetite, languor, heaviness, fever, and there is a deadened sensation of the parts. When this disease is in such an aggravated form, it is most difficult to cure.

When the deranged phlegm and air with the morbid chyle passes to the wrist, ankle, neck, hip, knee, loins, it produces a burning sensation, much pain, like the bite of the centipede, with swelling. The person feels great lassitude with a copious flow of urine; he cannot sleep, and complains of pain in the abdomen, and is distressed with thirst, vomiting, giddiness, fainting, pain in the chest, costiveness, &c.

शोथो रुजामूत्रविनिग्रहश्च। शुक्राश्मरी तत् स्रवणं भवेच्च ते ते विकारा विहते च शुक्रे॥ तन्द्राङ्गमर्द्दावरुचिः श्रमश्च क्षुधाभिघातात् कृशता च दृष्टेः। कण्ठास्यशोषः श्रवणावरोध-तृष्णाविघातात् हृदयव्यथा च॥ श्रान्तस्य निश्वासविनिग्रहेण हृद्रोगमोहावथ-वापि गुल्मः। जृम्भाङ्गमर्द्दोऽक्षिशिरोतिजाड्यं निद्राभिघातादथ-वापि तन्द्रा॥ वायुः कोष्ठानुगो रुक्षैः कषायकटुतिक्तकैः। भोजनैः कुपितः सद्य उदावर्त्तं करोति च॥ वातमूत्रपुरीषासृक् कफमेदो वहानि वै। स्रोतांस्युदावर्त्तयति पुरिषं चातिवर्त्तयेत्॥ ततो हृद्बस्तिशूलार्त्तो हृल्लासारतिपीड़ितः। वातमूत्रपुरीषाणि

When bile is much deranged in this disease there is a burning sensation and redness of the part; and when air is principally deranged, the pain is very severe. When phlegm is much deranged, the itching and rigidity of the part is considerable, and it feels as if it was covered with a wet cloth. When one humour is alone affected, it is curable, when two it is difficult to cure, and when three, and the whole body is affected the cure is very difficult, tedious, and the disease is even fatal in some cases.

Sul, Colic, (*Gastroperiodynia.*)

This disease is called *Sul,* from the pain resembling that produced by piercing the abdomen with the deadly *Trisula* or three-pointed instrument in the hands of *Shiva*, the destroying power of the Triad, and it is said to be sometimes so incurable

---

कृच्छ्रेण लभते नरः ॥ श्वासकास-प्रतिश्याय-दाहमोहतृषा ज्वरान्। वमि-हिक्काशिरोरोग मनः श्रवणविभ्रमान्॥ बहू-नन्यांश्च लभते विकारान् वातकोपजान्।

आमं शकृद्वा निचितं क्रमेण भूयो विबद्धं विगुणानिलेन। प्रवर्त्तमानं न यथास्वमेनं विकारमानाहमुदाहरन्ति॥ तस्मिन् भवन्त्यामसमुद्भवे तु तृष्णा प्रतिश्यायशिरोविदाहाः। आमाशये शूलमथो गुरुत्वं हृत्स्तम्भ-उद्गारविघातनञ्च॥ स्तम्भः कटी पृष्ठ-पुरीषमूत्रे शूलोऽथ मूर्च्छा शकृतश्च छर्द्दिः। शोथश्च पक्वाशयजे भवन्ति तथालसोक्तानि च लक्षणानि॥

अथ गुल्मनिदानम्।

दुष्टा वातादयोऽत्यर्थं मिथ्याहारविहारतः। कुर्वन्ति पञ्चधा गुल्मं कोष्ठान्तर्ग्रन्थिरूपिणम्॥ तस्य पञ्चविधं स्थानं पार्श्व-

that even *Shiva* himself cannot remove it. It frequently happens that the individual, in despair of being cured, commits suicide, as the only means left of relieving himself, and of propitiating the anger of the deity. Such fancies have a pernicious effect upon the progress of medical knowledge, for instead of endeavouring to discover the cause and nature of the disease, and the means of alleviating the sufferings of the afflicted, the practitioner finds a ready excuse for his indifference and ignorance in what he declares to be the will of God.

There are eight varieties of *Sul*, produced by derangement of air, bile, and phlegm; by two being deranged together; by the three being deranged together, and the last form is by indigestion. In all these forms, however, air is more or less deranged.

1. The causes of Air Colic (*Báyu-Sul*) are violent exercise, as fighting, riding, frequent intercourse with women, watching at night, drinking too much cold water, eating peas (especially *Kalái, Mudga, Araki)*, dry food, as dry flesh, vegetables, and fish, overeating, or eating too often; injuries, and bitter or

---

हृन्नाभिवस्तयः। हृन्नाभ्योरन्तरे ग्रन्थिः सञ्चारी यदि वाचलः॥ वृत्तश्चयापचयवान स गुल्म इति कीर्त्तितः। स व्यस्तैर्जायते दोषैः समस्तैरपि चोच्छ्रितैः॥ पुरुषाणां तथा स्त्रीणां ज्ञेयो रक्तेन चापरः। उद्गारबाहुल्यपुरीषवन्ध तृप्त्यक्षमत्वान्त्र-विकुजनानि॥ आटोपमाध्मानमपक्तिशक्ति रासन्नगुल्मस्य वदन्ति चिह्नम्। अरुचिः कृच्छ्रविण्मुत्र-वातताऽन्त्रविकुजनम्॥ आनाहश्चोर्द्ध्ववातत्वं सर्व्वगुल्मेषु लक्षयेत्।

रुक्षान्नपानं विषमातिमात्रं विचेष्टनं वेगविनिग्रहश्च। शोकोऽभिघातोऽतिमलक्षयश्च निरान्नता चानिलगुल्महेतुः॥ यः स्थानसंस्थानरुजा विकल्पं विड्वातसङ्गं गलवक्त्रशोषम्। श्यावारुणत्वं शिशिरज्वरश्च हृत्कुक्षि-पार्श्वांस-शिरोरुजश्च॥ करोति जीर्णे

astringent food. When rice is eaten, and other grain that have vegetated, or an improper mixture of food is taken, as milk and flesh, &c., or when the calls of nature are not attended to, and the semen, urine, air, fæces are constipated; or by grief, fasting, much and loud laughing or speaking, they produce *Sul* by deranging the air. When air is so deranged the accession of pain occurs at intervals when the person drinks cold water on an empty stomach, when the food has been digested, towards the evening in the rainy season, when the sky is overcast, and during the winter months.

The pain is in the chest, sides of the abdomen, back, in the joining of the lumbar vertebræ with the os coccygis, and in the pelvic region. It is accompanied with difficulty in breathing, rigidity of the body, and scanty evacuations.

2. When deranged bile produces this disease, it is caused by eating nitre or heating salts of the same kind, hot food like white mustard-seed, pepper, or the like; different kinds of wines, roasted articles or oils, or shoots of the young bamboo, or oil cake, sour or bitter articles; great anger, remaining

---

त्वधिकं प्रकोपं भुक्ते मृदुत्वं समुपैति यश्च। वातात् स गुल्मो न च तत्र रूक्षं कषायतिक्तं कटु चोपशेते॥ कट्वम्लतीक्ष्णोष्णविदाहिरूक्ष क्रोधातिमद्यार्क-हुताशसेवा। आमाभिघातो रुधिरञ्च दुष्टं पैत्तस्य गुल्मस्य निमित्तमुक्तम्॥ ज्वरः पिपासा वदनाङ्गरागः शूलं महज्जीर्यति भोजने च। स्वेदो विदाहो व्रणवच्च गुल्मः स्पर्शासहः पैत्तिकगुल्मरूपम्। शीतं गुरु स्निग्ध मचेष्टनञ्च संपूरणं प्रस्वपनं दिवा च॥ गुल्मस्य हेतुः कफसम्भवस्य सर्व्वस्तु दुष्टो निचयात्मकस्य। स्तैमित्य-शीतज्वरगात्रसाद-हृल्लासकासारुचिगौरवाणि। शैत्यं रुगल्पा कठिनोन्नतत्वं गुल्मस्य रूपाणि कफात्मकस्य॥ निमित्तरूपाण्युपलभ्य गुल्मे द्विदोषजे दोषबलाबलञ्च॥

near the fire, exposure to the sun, great fatigue, excess in venery, or any thing that is very heating is to be carefully avoided. These different causes derange bile, and produce that form of *Sul* when is felt in the umbiliacus. In this case it produces thirst, his senses are dull, body hot, with great grief, and severe pain in the umbiliacus. He perspires much, and he is giddy and sometimes faints, with dryness of the mouth, is eager to remain in a cold situation, and to take cold articles of food. Accessions of pain occur at noon and midnight, during great heat of the weather, and at the beginning of the rains. The pain is diminished during the cold hours of the day, when the body is cool; and when cold or bitter things are taken, especially when they feel grateful they mitigate the symptoms.

3. When deranged phlegm produces *Sul*, it is caused by eating the flesh of the rhinoceros or buffalo, fish or any kind of food obtained from water, whey, milk, or butter-milk; or sugarcandy, rice cakes, or sesamum-seed, oil, rice, and other

---

व्यामिश्रलिङ्गानपरांश्च गुल्मांस्त्रीनादिशेदौषधकल्पनार्थम्। महारुजं दाहपरीतमश्मवद्घनोन्नतं शीघ्रविदाहि दारुणम्॥ मनःशरीराग्निवलापहारिणं त्रिदोषजम् गुल्ममसाध्यमादिशेत्॥

नवप्रसूताहितभोजना या या चामगर्भं विसृजेदृतौ च। वायुर्हि तस्याः परिगृह्य रक्तं करोति गुल्मं सरुजं सदाहम्॥ पैत्तस्य लिङ्गेन समानलिङ्गं विशेषणञ्चापरपरं निवोध। यः स्पन्दते पिण्डित एव नाङ्गैश्चिरात् सशूलः समगर्भलिङ्गः। स रौधिरस्त्रीभव एव गुल्मो मासे व्यतीते दशमे चिकित्स्यः॥

सञ्चितं क्रमशो गुल्मो महावास्तुपरिग्रहः। कृतमूलः शिरानद्धो यदा कूर्म्म इवोत्थितः। दौर्व्वल्यारुचिहृल्लासकासच्छर्द्यरति ज्वरैः। तृष्णा तन्द्रा प्रतिश्यायै र्युज्यते स न सिद्ध्यति॥ गृहीत्वा सजरं- श्वास छर्द्यतीसारपीड़ितम्॥ हृन्नाभि हस्तपादेषु

articles of food which are of a cooling or heavy nature, as *Más-kalái*. All these articles increase phlegm, and thus may produce *Sul*. In these cases the patient complains of nausea, cough, languor, and want of appetite, phlegm proceeds from his nose and mouth, the pit of the stomach is cold, and his body is very heavy with head-ache. In such cases after eating great pain occurs, especially at sun-rise, and during the spring or dew months. (*Sishira.*)

4. When air, bile and phlegm are deranged together the symptoms of the three above forms are combined in one person. When so deranged in one spot a physician will know it by examining the part. This form gives much distress, like poison or thunder, and such a person should be avoided by the physician as incurable.

5. When *Sul* is produced by indigestion the symptoms are the same as produced by deranged phlegm. There is a rumbling noise heard in the abdomen, nausea and vomiting, the body feels heavy and cold, as if covered with a wet cloth, and the breathing is difficult. The person can get neither

---

शोथः कर्षति गुल्मिनम् ॥ श्वासः शूलं पिपासान्नविद्वेषो ग्रन्थिमूढ़ता । जायते दुर्व्वलत्वञ्च गुल्मिनो मरणाय वै ॥

अथ हृद्रोगनिदानम् ।

अत्युष्णगुर्व्वन्नकषायतिक्त-श्रमाभिघाताध्यशनप्रसङ्गैः । संचिन्तनैर्वेगविधारणैश्च हृदामयः पञ्चविधः प्रदिष्टः ॥ दूषयित्वा रसं दोषा विगुणा हृदयं गताः । हृदि वाधां प्रकुर्व्वन्ति हृद्रोगं तं प्रचक्षते ।

आयम्यते मारुतजे हृदयं तुद्यते यथा । निर्म्मथ्यते दीर्य्यते च स्फोट्यते पाट्यतेऽपि च ॥ तृष्णोषादाहचोषाः स्युः पैत्तिके हृदयक्लमः ॥ धुमायनञ्च मूर्च्छा च स्वेदः शोषो मुखस्य च । गौरवं कफसंस्रावोऽरुचिस्तम्भोऽग्निमार्द्दवम् ॥ माधुर्य्यमपि चास्यस्य बला-

appetite nor sleep, he is costive with severe pain in the abdomen, and there is a discharge of phlegm, from the nose, mouth, &c.

In order to distinguish the different forms of *Sul* the practitioner should know that air is chiefly affected when the pain is principally confined to the pelvic region. When bile is much deranged, the pain is principally felt in the umbiliacal region; and when phlegm is deranged it produces pain in the breast, sides of the abdomen, and in the scrobiculus cordis. When air, bile, and phlegm are deranged the pain is felt in all the above situations. When phlegm and air are deranged there is severe pain in the pelvic region, sides of the abdomen, and back. When bile and phlegm are deranged the pain is in the scrobiculus cordis, and between the chest and the umbiliacus. When air and bile are deranged there is great heat of the body, and inflammatory fever. *Sul* may be cured when it is produced by either air, bile, or phlegm, being deranged singly. When two are diseased, with difficulty; but when all the three are deranged at the same time it is incurable. In *Sul* some other forms of disease may accompany and complicate it; such as severe pain, thirst,

---

सावतते ह्वदि। विद्याविद्दोषन्त्वपि सर्व्वलिङ्गं तीव्रार्त्तितोदं क्रिमिजं सकण्डुम्। उत्क्लेदः ष्ठीवनं तोदः शूलं ह्वल्लासकस्तमः। अरुचिः श्यावनेवत्वं शोथश्च क्रिमिजे भवेत्। क्लमः सादो भ्रमः शोषो ज्ञेयास्तेषामुपद्रवाः। क्रिमिजे क्रिमिजातीनां श्लैष्मिकानाञ्च ये मताः।

अथ मूत्रकृच्छ्रनिदानम्।

व्यायाम-तीक्ष्णौषध-रुक्षमद्य प्रसङ्गनित्य-द्रुतपृष्ठयानात्। आपूपमांसाध्यशनादजीर्णात् स्युर्मूत्रकृच्छ्राणि नृणां तथाष्टौ। पृथक् मलाः स्वैः कुपिता निदानैः सर्व्वेऽथवा कोपमुपेतग्र वस्तौ। मूत्रस्य मार्गं परिपीडयन्ति यदा तदा मूत्रयतीह कृच्छ्रात्॥

fainting fits, spasm of the intestines with costiveness, the body is heavy and there is no appetite, with cough, asthma, and hiccough. Other *shástras* enumerate the following symptoms, severe pain in the abdomen, vomiting, fever, thirst, and the body seems to swim round. When the person becomes thin, and has no strength, he will not recover.

6. *Parinám Sul* * is the variety produced during the digestion of food. When air is deranged by the usual causes it affects also bile and phlegm, and *Sul* is the consequence. After eating, when degestion has taken place, severe fever occurs. The symptoms of this variety are, when air is deranged, the abdomen swells, a gurgling noise is heard in the abdomen, the dejections and urine are constipated, with lassitude and shivering. Bile, when much deranged in this form of *Sul*, produces thirst, heat, restlessness, and copious perspirations; and when sour, pungent, or salt things are eaten the pain is increased, and when cold food is eaten they give relief.

तीव्रार्त्तिरुग्वङ्क्षणवस्तिमेढ्रे स्वल्पं मुहुर्मूत्रयतीह वातात् पीतं सरक्तं सरुजं सदाहं कृच्छ्रं मुहुर्मूत्रयतीह पित्तात्। वस्तेः सलिङ्गस्य गुरुत्वशोथौ मूत्रं सपिच्छं कफमूत्रकृच्छ्रे॥ सर्व्वाणि रूपाणि तु सन्निपातात् भवन्ति तत् कृच्छ्रतमं हि कृच्छ्रम्। मूत्रावाहिषु शल्येन चतेष्वभिहतेषु वा॥ मूत्रकृच्छ्रं तदाघाताज्जायते भृशदारुणम्। वातकृच्छ्रेण तुल्यानि तस्य लिङ्गानि निर्द्दिशेत्॥

---

* *Parinám Sul.* This variety had not been described before 1836, (see the *Indian Journal* for March, page 114,) by European Physicians, which induced me to add the following particulars of this curious disease.

Gastroperiodynia, or periodical pain in the stomach, often commences with symptoms of indigestion and heart-burn, succeeded by a feeling of uneasiness in the scrobiculus cordis, slight at first, and occurring at irregular intervals, and these lessening gradually while the pain increases in violence In severer cases, the paroxysm of acute pain generally occurs rather suddenly, when the stomach is empty; sometimes early in the morning, or three or four hours after dinner; increasing slowly when the digestive process is finished, and the activity of the abdominal organs has ceased.

When phlegm is much deranged there is vomiting, nausea and dulness of the intellect, with pain, not severe, but remains many hours. When two of these are deranged the respective symptoms are combined, and when three are deranged the person will die. When such a person's flesh, strength and internal fire are much diminished the disease will be fatal.

Retention of Discharges. (*Adábarta*).

If a man wish long life he should attend to the calls of nature, while he avoids indulgence of the passions, particularly anger, pride, lust, revenge, and covetousness.

There are thirteen kinds of diseases produced by checking the efforts of nature to relieve herself. As by stopping the evacuation of air, fæces, urine, by yawning, tears, sneezing, belching, vomiting, semen, appetite, thirst and abstaining from liquids, the stopping of breath, watching, and another variety of

---

शकृतन्तु प्रतीघाताद्वायुर्विगुणतां गतः। आध्मानं वातशूलञ्च मूत्रसङ्गं करोति च॥ अश्मरीहेतु तत्पूर्व्वं मूत्रकृच्छ्रमुदाहरेत्। शुक्रे दोषैरुपहते मूत्रमार्गे विधाविते॥ सशुक्रं मूत्रयेत् कृच्छ्रात् वस्तिमेहन शूलवान्। अश्मरी शर्करा चैव तुल्य सम्भवलक्षणे॥ विशेषं शर्करायाश्च शृणु कीर्त्तयतो मम। पच्यमानाश्मरी पित्तात् शोष्यमाना च वायुना। विमुक्तकफसन्धाना क्षरन्ती शर्करा मता। हृत्पीड़ा वेपथुः शूलं कुक्षावग्निश्च

The excruciating pain is confined to the pit of the stomach, particularly towards the right hypocondrium, although the neighbouring parts often participate, as the muscles of the loins, &c. The pain is of a cutting or gnawing nature; and during the paroxysm is intense, from which the patient generally obtains temporary relief from pressure. For this purpose he often turns upon his breast and places a hard ball in the pit of the stomach, on which he rests his body, and keeps rolling from side to side. A few days since I ordered an unfortunate person, in this position, to turn round for me to examine him; but such was the agony, that he could not remain without the soothing influence of pressure. As a substitute, he drew from under his clothes a piece of prepared bamboo, an inch in diameter, and a cubit in length, round at one end.

indisposition is produced by taking bad food. When these are not indulged in, it produces the constipation which forms this class of diseases.

1. When air *(Apanna báyu)* is stopped in its passage through the anus it produces a swelling in the abdomen, severe pain, difficulty of breathing, head-ache, hiccough, cough, discharge of mucus, difficulty of diglutition and a vomiting of bile, phlegm, or fæces with constipation, and severe pain in the anus followed by a discharge of air.

2. *Dejections.* When the fæces are confined a gurgling noise is heard in the abdomen, with pain in the anus, as if the part was cut; the dejections are confined, as air ascends, and sometimes stercoraceous vomiting occurs.

3. *Urine.* When confined, there is severe pain in the pelvis, urethra, anus, scrotum, groins, navel, and sometimes in the head, when the urine is discharged in small quantities with pain. The bladder swells, and the body remains bent forward.

दुर्व्वलः। तया भवति मूर्च्छा च मूत्रकृच्छ्रञ्च दारुणम्। मूत्रवेगनिरस्ताभिः प्रथमं याति वेदना। यावदस्याः पुनर्नैति गुड़िका स्रोतसो मुखम्॥

अथ मूत्राघातनिदानम्।

जायन्ते कुपिते दोषे मूत्राघातास्त्रयोदश। प्रायो मूत्रविघातादैर्व्वातकुण्डलिकादयः। रौक्षाद्वेगविघाताद्वा वायुर्व्वस्तौ सवेदनः। मूत्रमाविश्य चरति विगुणः कुण्डलीकृतः॥ मूत्रमल्पाल्पमथवा सरुजं संप्रवर्त्तते। वातकुण्डलिकां तान्तु व्याधिं विद्यात्

This extremity he placed to the pit of the stomach while he rested the other on the floor; and by bending the body over it, produced such a degree of violent pressure, that at first I feared he would injure himself, and even penetrate the abdomen. He continued in this position while I gained the necessary information of his state, and then returned to his former position, commenced rolling from side to side upon the hard ball, placed in the pit of the stomach, and his low wailing proved how intense were his sufferings. This was an acute form of the disease, and until checked by remedies, it occurred daily about 4 o'clock, and he continued in dreadful agony the whole night.

15

4. When *gaping* is checked the diseases of the neck, throat, and of the head are produced; with other diseases of air, such as diseases of the eyes, nose, ears, and mouth.

5. When *tears* are confined they flow when the person is very happy, or very sorrowful; and when confined the head becomes heavy, and various severe eye diseases are produced. In such patients the phlegm discharged from the nose and mouth is without smell or taste.

6. When *sneezing* is confined, diseases of the head, eyes, nose, and ears are produced.

7. When *belching* is confined, the throat and mouth feel as if distended, and very painful; the person's speech is not intelligible, are is confined by the mouth, anus, &c., and the disease produces the diseases of air.

8. Should *vomiting* be impeded it produces leprosy, loss of appetite, jaundice, fever, great sensibility of the skin and nausea.

9. When *semen* is confined, the bladder, rectum, and testicles swell, and become painful. The urine is confined and is

---

सुदारुणम् ॥ आध्मापयन् वस्तिं गुदं रुद्ध्वा वायुश्चलोन्नताम् ॥ कुर्य्यात्तीव्रार्त्तिमष्ठीलां मूत्रविण्मार्गरोधिनीम् ॥ वेगं विधारयेत् यस्तु मूत्रस्याकुशलो नरः। निरुणद्धि मुखं तस्य वस्ते र्वस्तिगतोऽनिलः। मूत्रसङ्गो भवेत्तेन वस्तिकुक्षिनिपीड़ितः। वातवस्ति स विज्ञेयो व्याधिः कृच्छ्रप्रसाधनः ॥

चिरं धारयतो मूत्रं त्वरया न प्रवर्त्तते। मेहमानस्य मन्दं

These paroxysms usually occur at intervals of a day or two, and remain from two hours to as many days, with occasional intervals of ease. During these accessions the state of the pulse, although full, continues slow and natural, and there is not usually more heat of body than is occasioned by a continual movement.

In the intermissions the patient feels well, and all the functions are performed as when in perfect health. The tongue is clean, but sometimes parched, appetite good, and alvine secretions healthy and regular.

I have not been able to obtain any certain evidences of the causes which produce this disease. It appears to be the effect of a combination, individually discharged in small quantities with pain, or the urine has a white deposit, and the semen is discharged involuntary. The other diseases may occur that deranged semen produces.

10. When the *appetite* is not gratified, it is followed by drowsiness, pain as if the part was crushed, loss of appetite, fatigue, and the eye is dim.

11. When the *thirst* is not gratified, the mouth and throat are dry, the hearing becomes dull, and pain is felt in the breast.

12. When the *breathing* is difficult from being confined from the fatigue produced by severe exercise, the food appears to stick in the throat, the understanding is impaired which produces (*Gulma*), and there is a feeling of hard lumps in the abdomen.

13. When *sleep* is not gratified, it is followed by yawning, and pain of the body, as if it was crushed. The eyes and head feel heavy, and coma supervenes.

वा मूत्रातीतः स उच्यते। मूत्रस्य वेगेऽभिहते तदुदावर्त्तहेतुकः। अपानः कुपितो वायुरुदरं पूरयेद्भृशम्॥ नाभेरधस्तादाध्मानं जनयेत्तीव्रवेदनम्। तन्मूत्रजठरं विद्यादधोवस्तिनिरोधनम्॥ वस्तौ वाप्यथवा नाले मणौ वा यस्य देहिनः॥ मूत्रं प्रवृत्तं सज्येत सरक्तं वा प्रवाहतः। स्रवेच्छनैरल्पमल्पं सरुजं वाथ नीरुजम्। विगुणानिलजो व्याधिः स मूत्रोत्सङ्गसञ्ज्ञितः।

रुक्षस्य क्लान्तदेहस्य वस्तिस्थौ पित्तमारुतौ। मूत्रक्षयं सरुग्दाहं जनयेत्तां तदाह्वयम्॥ अन्तर्वस्ति मुखे वृत्तः स्थिरोऽल्पः

---

slight; but when occurring in a peculiar constitution, produces this distressing complaint. I have generally known it to occur in the young and robust male; to be aggravated by exposure to the weather, and by eating indigestable food, sleeping on the damp ground, &c. The accession seems oftener to occur when the organs are in a state of inactivity, than from causes increasing the nervous susceptibility. I have not seen it in females, although there is no reason why they should not be also effected; and I am informed that they are sometimes attacked but in a less violent degree. Persons of a nervous temperament are in general not so liable to this disease as might be supposed.

The air of the stomach when dry, astringent, sour, or bitter food is eaten, produces quickly *Udábarta*, and deranges the canals of air, urine, fæces, blood, phlegm, fat, and the vessels which feed them. Air closes these canals and produces pain in the breast and pelvis, with heaviness of the body, and no appetite, with scanty evacuations.

The retention of the above discharges produces pain of the chest and abdomen, nausea, laziness, and the air, urine, and dejections are evacuated with pain. If produced by phlegm there is difficult and noisy breathing, and the phlegm is discharged from the mouth and nose. *(Coryza)*. In this case there is neither taste nor smell ; and the body feels hot, with dejection of mind. The person is insensible, and complains of thirst, fever, vomiting, hiccough, and head-ache. The person is deaf, the body swims round, followed by the other symptoms produced by

---

सहसा भवेत् ॥ अश्मरी तुल्यरुग्ग्रन्थिर्मूत्रग्रन्थिः स उच्यते ॥ मूत्रितस्य स्त्रियं यातो वायुना शुक्र मुद्धतम्। स्थानाच्च्युतं मूत्रयतः प्राक् पश्चाद्वा प्रवर्त्तते ॥ भस्मोदकप्रतीकाशं मूत्रशुक्रं तदुच्यते ॥ व्यायामाध्वातपैः पित्तं वस्तिं प्राप्यानिलान्वितम्। वस्तिं मेढ्रं गुदञ्चैव प्रदहेत् स्रावयेदधः ॥ मूत्रं हारिद्र मथवा सरक्तं रक्तमेव वा। कृच्छ्रात् पुनः पुनर्जन्तोरुष्णावातं ब्रुवन्ति तम् ॥ पित्तं कफो द्वावपि वा संहन्येतेऽनिलेन चेत् ॥ कृच्छ्रान्मूत्रं तदा पीतं श्वेतं रक्तं घनं सृजेत् ॥ सदाहं रोचना शङ्खचूर्णवर्णं भवेत्तु तत्। शुष्कं समस्तवर्णं वा मूत्रसादं वा वदन्ति तम्। रूक्षदुर्व्वलयो वातेनोदावर्त्तं शकृद् यदा ॥ मूत्रस्रोतोऽनुपद्येत विट्संसृष्टं तदा नरः। विड्गन्धं मूत्रयेत् कृच्छ्रात् विड्विघातं विनिर्द्दिशेत् ॥

deranged air. The life of such a person should be considered hopeless, when there is much thirst, great weakness, and languor, severe pain in the abdomen, and stercoraceous vomiting.

Gulma, (*Swellings in the Abdomen.*)

When air, bile, and phlegm are deranged by eating bad food, at irregular times, or by unsuitable exercise, this disease is produced, which resembles a ball in the abdomen. There are five kinds and situations of this disease. One in either side of the abdomen, one in the umbiliacus, another in the pelvis, and one between the chest and the abdomen, (scrobiculus cordis,) sometimes the swelling is fixed, and at other times it is moveable* there are four kinds of this disease in the male, three by the derangement of air, bile, and phlegm, another by the morbid mixture of the three, and the fifth kind is peculiar to females from the retention of the menses.

द्रुताध्वलङ्घनायासैरभिघातात् प्रपीड़नात्। स्वस्थानाद्वस्तिरुद्वृत्तः स्थूलस्तिष्ठति गर्भवत्॥ शूलस्पन्दनदाहार्त्तो विन्दुं विन्दुं स्रवत्यपि। पीड़ितस्तु सृजेद्धारां संस्तम्भोद्वेष्टनार्त्तिमान्॥ वस्तिकुण्डलमाहुस्तं घोरं शस्त्रविषोपमम्॥ पवनप्रबलं प्रायो दुर्निवारमबुद्धिभिः। तस्मिन् पित्तान्विते दाहः शूलं मूत्रविवर्णता॥ श्लेष्मणा गौरवं शोथः स्निग्धं मूत्रं घनं सितम्। श्लेष्मरुद्धविलो वस्तिः पित्तोदीर्णो न सिध्यति। अविभ्रान्तविलः साध्यो न तु यः कुण्डलीकृतः। स्याद्वस्तौ कुण्डलीभूते तृण्मोहः श्वास एव च।

अथाश्मरीनिदानम्।

वातपित्तकफैस्तिस्रश्चतुर्थी शुक्रजा परा। प्रायःश्लेष्माश्रयाः सर्वा अश्मर्य्यः सुर्य्यमोपमा। विशोषयेद्वस्तिगतं सशुक्रं मूत्रं सपित्तं पवनं

* Under the term *Gulma* are arranged very different diseases : as tumours of the pylorus, partial enlargements of the liver, and diseases of the large intestines.

Gulma is ushered in by much belching, costiveness, loss of appetite, difficulty of making water, fulness of the body, with flatulence, and indigestion. These symptoms are followed by others produced by the use of food and drink of a dry nature, by a kind of wine which produces roughness of the surface of the body, by improper food, or by eating it at irregular times, or eating too much, by taking unsuitable exercise, and by neglecting the calls of nature, such as sneezing, and dejections, grief, accidents, bruises, or by too great evacuations or fasting. The symptoms of *Gulma*, produced by air, are its being situated in the abdomen, in the umbiliacus, or sides, and its moving about. It is sometimes small, and at other times large; sometimes round, at other times long; sometimes the pain is slight, at other times severe, with constipation, dryness of the throat and mouth; the skin of the body having a dark yellow colour, and fever commencing with chilliness. The pain in the breast and sides of the abdomen, shoulders, or head are considerable, particularly after the food is digested, but the person feels better immediately after eating. Astringent, dry, bitter, or pungent things increase the complaint.

कफं वा। यदा तदाश्मर्युपजायते तु क्रमेण पित्तेष्विव रोचना गोः॥ नैकदोषाश्रयाः सर्व्वाः अथासां पूर्व्वलक्षणम्। वस्त्याध्मानं तदासन्नदेशेषु परितोऽतिरुक्॥ मूत्रे वस्तसगन्धित्वं मूत्रकृच्छ्रं ज्वरोऽरुचिः। सामान्यलिङ्गं रुङ्नाभिसेवनी वस्तिमूर्द्धसु॥ विशीर्ण-धारमूत्रः स्यात् तया मार्गनिरोधने। तद्व्यपायात् सुखं मेहेदच्छं गोमेदकोपमम्॥ तत्संक्षोभात् क्षते सास्रमायासाच्चातिरुग् भवेत्।

तत्रवाताद्भृशं चार्त्तो दन्तान् खादति वेपते। मृद्नाति मेहनं नाभिं पीड़यत्यनिशं क्वणन्। सानिलं मुञ्चति शकृत् मुहुर्मेहति विन्दुशः। श्यावारुणाश्मरी चास्य स्याच्चिताकण्टकैरपि॥ पित्तेन दह्यते वस्तिः पच्यमान इवोष्मवान्॥ भल्लातकास्थिसंस्थान रक्ता-

Bile. When the disease is produced by eating sour, bitter, hot, or other things of the same kind; by living on dry food; by anger; by drinking much wine, remaining much in the sun, or near the fire; by collections of indigested food, or diseased blood in the abdomen, the bile is deranged producing the *Pitta Gulma*, with the following symptoms. The disease commences with fever, thirst, and a red colour of the mouth and skin. When digestion is going on, there is much pain, and perspiration, with a severe burning sensation in the pit of the stomach, which is tender on being touched, or it is followed by a swelling in the stomach, which is painful like a boil.

Phlegm is deranged by cold, or by eating indigestable or oleaginous articles of food; particularly when the person does not take exercise, eats too much, and sleeps too long during the day. When *phlegm* is thus deranged it produces coldness and languor of the body, with low fever, nausea, cough, no appetite, and heaviness of the body, without much pain. The ball gradually becomes harder, and larger.

पीतासिताश्मरी। वस्तिर्निस्तुद्यत इव श्लेष्मणा शीतलो गुरुः॥ अश्मरी महती श्लक्ष्णा मधुवर्णा खरा सिता॥

एता भवन्ति बालानां तेषामपि च भुयसा। आश्रयोपचयाल्पत्वात् ग्रहणाहरणे सुखा॥ शुक्राश्मरी तु महतां जायते शुक्रधारणात्। स्थानाच्च्युतममुक्तं हि मुष्कयोरन्तरेऽनिलः॥ शोषयत्युपसंगृह्य शुक्रं तच्छुक्रमश्मरी। वस्तिरुग्वकृच्छ्रत्वं मुष्कश्वयथुकारिणी। तस्यामुत्पन्नमात्रायां शुक्रमेति विलीयते॥ पीड़िते त्ववकाशेऽस्मिन्नश्मर्य्येव च शर्करा। अणुशो वायुना भिन्ना सा तस्मिन्ननुलोमगे। निरेति सह मूत्रेण प्रतिलोमे निरुध्यते। मूत्रस्रोतः प्रवृत्ता सा सिक्ता कुर्य्यादुपद्रवान्॥ दौर्ब्बल्यं सदनं कार्श्यं कुक्षिशूल मथारुचिम्। पाण्डुत्वमुष्णवातञ्च तृष्णां हृत्पीड़नं

When air, bile, and phlegm are deranged, and are produced by the causes given above, there will be severe pain, great heat of body, and the *Gulma* or swelling feels hard like a stone, and is large, and quickly produces the heat of the body; so severe is this form of the complaint that the person is in great distress. His body becomes thin, with a bad colour, and he has no appetite, nor strength. Such a disease is incurable.

There is a kind of *Gulma*, so like pregnancy that it may deceive physicians, unless they observe the precaution of not giving medicine until after the tenth month, (the supposed time of utero-gestation.) *

The unfavourable symptoms of *Gulna* are its enlarging so as to fill the abdomen; and the increase being rapid, and the swelling being surrounded by vessels, with much pain in the breast, as well as in the part. When the swelling is of the figure of a turtle, when there is much debility, loss of appetite, nausea, cough, vomiting, restlessness, fever, thirst, coma, and the discharge of mucus from the mouth and nose, without either taste or smell, such a person will not recover.

वमिम् ॥ प्रसूननाभिद्वषसं वद्धमूत्रं रुजातुरम् ॥ अश्मरीच्चपथ्यात्याशु सिकता शर्कराान्विता ॥

अथ प्रमेह-मधुमेह-पीड़का-निदानम् ।

आस्यासुखं स्वप्नसुखं दधीनि ग्राम्यौदकानुपरसाः पयांसि। नवान्नपानं गुड़वैकृतञ्च प्रमेहहेतुः कफकृच्च सर्व्वम् ॥ मेदश्च मांसञ्च शरीरजञ्च क्लेदं कफो वस्तिगतं प्रदुष्य। करोति मेहान् समुदीर्ण मुष्णैस्तानेव पित्तं परिदुष्य चापि ॥ क्षीणेषु दोषेष्ववकृष्य धातून् संदुष्य मेहान् कुरुतेऽनिलश्च ॥

* There is an instructive case in point. A young woman became pregnant, and for the uncomfortable sensations attending that state consulted a physician, who after trying various remedies, without effect, one of which was thrusting a red hot iron into the tumour, which is frequently done for spleen, and sometimes with good effect by raising its activity; but in the present case

When a person with *Gulma* has fever, asthma, vomiting, diarrhœa, and swelling of the breast, umbiliacus, with swelling of the hand or feet, the disease will be fatal.

When after asthma, cough, thirst, with no appetite, much pain, and the swelling has suddenly disappeared with much weakness, the person will soon die.

Diseases of the Heart.

Painful affections of the heart *Ridraga* (Angina pectoris?) are produced by want of attention to the calls of nature, the use of hot and dry food; the improper mixture of food; an intemperance in eating, or unusual food; which causes indigestion, and deranges the humours. The impure chyle is received into the heart, and produces this painful disease; of which there are five varieties. When produced by deranged *air* the patient feels various acute kinds of pains, sometimes it is lancinating, at other times as if the heart was cut or torn. When produced by deranged *bile* there is much pain in the heart, with thirst, heart-burning and dryness. This is succeeded by

---

साध्याः कफोत्था दश पित्तजाः षट् याप्या न साध्यः पवनाच्च-
तुष्कः । समक्रियत्वाद्विषमक्रियत्वान्महात्ययत्वाच्च यथाक्रमं ते ॥
कफः सपित्तः पवनश्च दोषा मेदोऽस्र शुक्राम्बु-वसालसीकाः ।
मज्जारसौजः पिशितञ्च दूष्याः प्रमेहिणां विंशतिरेव मेहाः ॥
दन्तादीनां मलाढ्यत्वं प्राग्रूपं पाणिपादयोः । दाहश्चिक्क-
णता देहे तृट् स्वाद्वास्यञ्च जायते ॥ सामान्यं लक्षणं तेषां

the woman escaped. The physician finding that the disease did not yield to his treatment declared the case to be one of *Gulma*, for which nothing could be done, and that it would increase, and she would die with much pain, and violent shrinking. As this frightened very much the other females the patient was removed to a distant room, and in that state of anxiety passed some months, until parturition commenced. That was considered as the approach of death, and not to defile the house she was put out into the compound upon a mat, and her female friends deserted her. In this state she was delivered of a female child to the astonishment of all, and to the disgrace of the medical man.

fainting, much sweating, dryness of the mouth, and smoke appears to come out of the mouth. When produced by *phlegm* the patient feels a heaviness of the heart, a discharge of mucus from the mouth and nose, loss of appetite, and a sweet taste in the mouth.

When produced by *worms* there is a lancinating, or piercing pain in the region of the heart; nausea, vomiting, belching and loss of appetite. The eyes become dark greenish, with emaciation of the body. All these diseases of the heart terminate in emaciation, languor, loss of appetite and strength, with giddiness.

Strangury, (*Mutrakriehchhra.*) *

This disease is produced by wrestling, or other violent kinds of exercise, hot spices, dry food, wines, excessive venery, riding on horseback very quickly; eating the flesh of the buffaloes, of the rhinoceros, &c., or other indigestable food; another cause is eating too frequently, or it may be produced by bad digestion.

प्रभूताविलमूत्रता। दोषदुष्या विशेषेऽपि तत्संयोगविशेषतः। मूत्रवर्णादिभेदेन भेदो मेहेषु कल्पते॥

अच्छं बहुसितं शीतं निर्गन्धमुदकोपमम्। मेहत्युदकमेहेन किञ्चिदाविल-पिच्छिलम्॥ इक्षोरस मिवात्यर्थं मधुरंश्चेक्षु मेहतः॥ सान्द्री भवेत् पर्युषितं सान्द्रमेहेन मेहति॥ सुरामेहि सुरातुल्य मुपर्यच्छमधोघनम्। संहृष्टरोमा पिष्ठेन पिष्टवत् बहुलं सितम्॥ शुक्राभं शुक्रमिश्रं वा शुक्रमेही प्रमेहति। मुर्त्तानुन् सिकतामेही सिकतारूपिणो मलान्॥ शीतमेही सुबहुशो मधुरं भृशशीतलम्। शनैः शनैः शनैर्मेही मन्दं मन्दं प्रमेहति। लालातन्तुयुतं मूत्रं लालामेहेन पिच्छिलम्॥

* From *Muta*, urine, and *Krichchhra*, slow and painful.

There are eight forms of this disease. The derangements of air, bile and phlegm separately or combined, when they occur in the bladder, produce this and diseases in the urinary passages, when the urine is discharged with pain. This disease is also produced by injuries of the parts, by constipation of the bowels, and by calculi.

1. When the deranged air produces the disease it causes severe pain in the pelvis, in the testicles, and in the penis. The patient has a frequent desire for making water, and the urine passes in drops accompanied with pain.

2. When the bile of the part is deranged the urine is of a yellow or red colour. There is much scalding or burning pain in the passages, the urine is discharged in small quantities frequently, accompanied with heat and uneasiness.

3. When the phlegm is deranged the pelvis, bladder, urinary passages, and testicles feel heavy; they are swelled, and the urine is cold, shining like oil, and soon dries up.

4. When the air, bile, and phlegm are deranged the separate symptoms of each variety appear in the same person, and is cured with difficulty.

5. *Salajah.* When the parts are injured by external violence, the disease is accompanied with much pain, followed by other symptoms of deranged air.

गन्धवर्णरसस्पर्शैः क्षारेण क्षारतोयवत्। नीलमेहेन नीलाभं कालमेही मसीनिभम्॥ हारिद्रमेही कटुकं हरिद्रासन्निभं दहत्। विस्रं माञ्जिष्ठमेहेन मञ्जिष्ठासलिलोपमम्॥ विस्रमुष्णं सलवणं रक्ताभं रक्तमेहतः॥

वसामेही वसामिश्रं वसाभं मूत्रयेन्मुहुः। मज्जाभं मज्जमिश्रं वा मज्जमेही मुहुर्मुहुः॥ कषायं मधुरं रूक्षं क्षौद्रमेहं वदेद्बुधः। हस्ती मत्त इवाजस्रं मूत्रं वेगविवर्जितम्॥ सलसीकं विबद्धञ्च हस्तिमेही प्रमेहति॥

6. *Sakripratikatajah*, when the bowels are very costive, from air being deranged, it is accompanied with much swelling and pain in the abdomen, with difficulty in mictirition.

7. *Asarijah* is produced by calculi, with a difficulty and pain in mictirition.

When a person runs quickly or jumps, is much fatigued, is fasting, or the part is injured, the bladder rises out of the pelvis of a round form, and large like the gravel uterus. It is accompanied with much pain and moves from side to side, and the urine is very hot, and passes in drops. If the swelling is pressed, above the pubis, the urine passes easily, and in a continued stream. When the person cannot move, it is called *Bastikundala*, and is a severe and dangerous disease.

When bile produces the disease it is incurable; when phlegm it may be cured, especially if it continues to be discharged, except in the case of "*Kundali báta*." When the bladder is round above pelvis, with thirst and insensibility and noisy breathing, it is incurable.

अविपाकोऽरुचिश्छर्द्दिर्निद्रा कासः सपीनसः। उपद्रवाः प्रजायन्ते मेहानां कफजन्मनाम्॥ वस्तिमेहनयोस्तोदो मुष्कावदरणं ज्वरः। दाहस्तृष्णाम्लिका मूर्च्छा विड्भेदः पित्तजन्मनाम्॥ वातजानामुदावर्त्तः कम्पहृद्ग्रहलोलताः। शूलमुन्निद्रता शोषः कासः श्वासश्च जायते॥

यथोक्तोपद्रवारिष्टमतिप्रस्नुतमेव च। पिड़कापीड़ितं गाढ़ं प्रमेहो हन्ति मानवम्॥ जातः प्रमेही मधुमेहिना वा न साध्य उक्तः स हि वीजदोषात्। ये चापि केचित् कुलजा विकारा भवन्ति तांश्च प्रपदन्त्यसाध्यान्॥ सर्व्वे एव प्रमेहास्तु कालेनाप्रतिकारिणः॥ मधुमेहत्वमायान्ति तदासाध्या भवन्ति हि॥

8. *Sarajah,* when the semen is affected by deranged humours, and carried into the passage of the urine, it is discharged with much difficulty and pain.

9. *Asari* and *Sakará* produced by stone or gravel. They are produced by the same causes, and the symptoms of both are the same. When the stone is broken and dried up with bile and air, it is discharged through the urethra. When stone is retained in the bladder, it forms the peculiarity of the two diseases.

In *Sakará* there is shivering with severe pain in the chest and sides, loss of appetite, and fainting. This is followed by a fit of strangury, which is a severe disease, the pain being only mitigated when the urine is not discharged, and the suffering is very acute, as the gravel is passing through the urethra.

Suppression of Urine, (*Mutraghata.*)

The derangements of air, bile, and phlegm in the bladder produce the thirteen forms of this disease.

मधुमेहे मधुसमं जायते स किल द्विधा। क्रुद्धे धातुक्षया-द्वायौ दोषावृतपथेऽथवा॥ आवृतो दोषलिङ्गानि सोऽनिमित्तं प्रदर्शयन्। क्षणात् क्षीणः क्षणात् पूर्णो भजते कृच्छ्रसाध्यताम्। मधुरं यच्च मेहेषु प्रायो मध्विव मेहति। सर्व्वेऽपि मधुमेहाख्या माधुर्य्याच्च तनोरतः॥

शराविका कच्छपिका ज्वालिनी विनतालजी। मसूरिका सर्षपिका पुत्रिणी सविदारिका॥ विद्रधिश्चेति पिड़काः प्रमेहोपेक्षया दश। सन्धिमर्म्मसु जायन्ते मांसलेषु च धामसु॥ अन्तोन्नता तु तद्रूपा निम्नमध्या शराविका। गौरसर्षपसंस्थाना तत्प्रमाना च सर्षपी। सदाहा कूर्म्मसंस्थाना ज्ञेया कच्छपिका बुधैः। ज्वालिनी तीव्रदाहा तु मांसजालसमावृता। अवगाढ़रुजा, क्लेदा

Bátakundaliká. This disease is produced by eating dry articles of food, by retention of the natural discharges; by which the air is deranged in the bladder, which mixes with the urine producing pain, and they turn round in a circle, and the urine is retained, or it is discharged in drops. The person is very fearful in this disease.

Astila. When the air is deranged between the rectum and bladder it forms a large ball like a stone (prostate gland?) and produces suppression of the urine, fæces, and air; and is accompanied with swelling in the bladder and much pain. This disease is also called *Bátastila.*

Batabasti. When an ignorant person stops the evacuation of the urine or dejections, which deranges the air stops up the neck of the bladder, and produces retention. This disease produces pain in the pelvis, and in the sides; which form is cured with much difficulty.

When a person allows the urine to flow for some time, and then stops, it produces the disease called *Mutrátita,* or retention, when the urine is only discharged in small quantities.

पृष्ठे वापुरदरेऽपि वा। महती सरुजा नीला विनता नाम सा स्मृता। महतगल्पचिता ज्ञेया पिड़का चापि पुत्रिणी॥ मसूराकृतिसंख्याना विज्ञेया तु मसूरिका॥

प्रमेहनिदानम्।

रक्तासिता स्फोटचिता विज्ञेया ललजी भवेत्। विदारीकन्दवद्वृत्ता कठिना च विदारिका॥ विद्रधे र्लक्षणैर्युक्ता ज्ञेया विद्रधिका तु सा। ये यन्मयाः स्मृता मेहा तेषामेतास्तु तन्मयाः॥ विना प्रमेहमप्येता जायन्ते दुष्टमेदसः। तावच्चैता न लक्ष्यन्ते यावद्वास्तुपरिग्रहाः॥ गुदे हृदि शिरस्यंसे पृष्ठे मर्म्मसु चोत्थिताः। सोपद्रवा दुर्व्वलाग्नेः पिड़काः परिवर्ज्जयेत्॥

When urine is retained by such causes as produced the same effect as the retention of air, which is situated near the rectum, it produces swelling of the abdomen, with much pain under the umbiliacus. This disease is called *Mutrajathara*.

When the urine stops by impediments in the urethra, near the glans penis or elsewhere; or when expelled with great force mixed with blood, sometimes with much pain, in other cases with no pain. This variety is called *Mutrasanga*.

When the body is dried up by the free use of stimulants, and dry food, and great fatigue, the air and bile are deranged in the bladder, and the urine, which becomes scanty is of a black colour, and produces severe pain and heat. This disease is called *Mutrakia*.

When there is a small hard round ball at the neck of the bladder, accompanied with much pain, it may prevent the passage of the urine, and produce the symptoms of stone. It is called *Mutragrinti*.

When at the proper time urine is not discharged, and the patient has connection with woman, the semen is discharged

---

अथ मेदोनिदानम् ।

अव्यायाम-दिवास्वप्न-श्लेष्मलाहारसेविनः । मधुरोऽन्नरसः प्राय स्नेहान्मेदः प्रवर्द्धयेत् ॥ मेदसावृतमार्गत्वात् पुष्यन्त्यन्ये न धातवः । मेदस्तु चीयते तस्मादशक्तः सर्व्वकर्म्मसु । क्षुद्रश्वास तृषा मोह स्वप्न क्रथनसादनैः ॥ युक्तः क्षुत्स्वेददुर्गन्धै रल्पप्राणोऽल्पमैथुनः । मेदस्तु सर्व्वभूताना मुदरेऽन्वस्थिसंस्थितम् ॥ अतएवोदरे वृद्धिः प्रायो मेदस्विनो भवेत् ॥

मेदसावृतमार्गत्वाद्वायुकोष्ठे विशेषतः । चरन् सन्धुक्षयत्यग्नि माहारं शोषयत्यपि ॥ तस्मात् सशीघ्रं जरयत्याहार मभिकाङ्क्षति विकारांश्चाप्नुते घोरान् कांश्चित् कालव्यतिक्रमात् । एतानुपद्रव-

with the urine, sometimes before, and in other cases after the urine. This urine is of a white colour, as if mixed with chalk, and the disease is called *Mutrasukra.*

When violent exercise is taken, as in fighting, travelling, or great heat, the bile is deranged in the bladder with air, which passes mixed with urine, and produces a burning pain in the bladder, penis, and anus. The urine becomes yellow as if mixed with tamarinds, or blood; it is discharged with difficulty, and is called *Usnabáta.*

When deranged air produces this disease it is accompanied with great pain and heat, on its being discharged.

When the urine is yellow from bile, it causes in its passage a burning pain in the part, and there is much sediment.

When phlegm produces the disease the urine is white, like the powder of shells, and is of different consistence. This variety is called *Mutrakasáda.*

When the body is very dry and weak, and the fæces is collected for some time, it may be evacuated with the urine, have the smell of fæces, and pass with difficulty and much pain. This is most probably the recto-vaginal fistula, which is only described in modern books; and is called *Bierbigáta.*

करौ विशेषादग्निमारुतौ ॥ एतौ तु दहतः स्थूलं वनदावो वनं यथा। मेदस्यतीव संवृद्धे सहसैवानिलादयः। विकारान् दारुणान् कृत्वा नाशयन्त्याशु जीवितम् ॥ मेदोमांसातिवृद्धत्वाच्चलस्फिगुदरस्तनः। अयथोपचयोत्साहो नरोऽतिस्थूल उच्यते ॥

अथोदरनिदानम्।

रोगाः सर्व्वेऽपि मन्देऽग्नौ सुतरामुदराणि च। अजीर्णान्मलिनैश्चान्नै र्जायन्ते मलसञ्चयात् ॥ रुद्ध्वा स्वेदाम्बुवाहीनि दोषाः स्रोतांसि सञ्चिताः। प्राणाग्न्यपानान् संदूष्य जनयन्त्युदरं नृणाम् ॥ आध्मानं गमने शक्ति र्दौर्व्वल्यं दुर्व्वलाग्निता। शोथः सदनमङ्गानां

Urinary Calculi, (*Ashmari.*)

When air, bile, and phlegm are deranged it produces different forms of calculi ; and another kind is produced from semen. Phlegm is the chief cause of the disease in all its different forms.

This disease is produced in those who live on hard indigestable food, and do not use evacuating remedies, by which the phlegm is deranged, and mixing with urine passes into the bladder and forms the stone.

Others suppose that the calculi are produced by collections of the impurities of the urine which sink down and form, by being dried with the internal fire, calculi in the bladder. Others suppose they are formed as hailstones are formed in the sky.

This disease is ushered in by pain in the bladder, especially in its neck, scrotum, and penis. In some cases languor and fever are present, and the urine has the smell of goat's urine. When formed the pain is in the umbiliacus, bladder, perineum, penis, particularly during mictirition. The urine does not pass in a stream, but in drops: it also stops suddenly. It is

---

सङ्गो वातपुरीषयोः ॥ दाहस्तन्द्रा च सर्व्वेषु जठरेषु भवन्ति हि । पृथग्दोषैः समस्तैश्च प्लीहबद्धक्षतोदकैः । सम्भवन्त्युदराण्यष्टौ तेषां लिङ्गं पृथक् शृणु ॥

तत्र वातोदरे शोथः पाणिपान्नाभिकुक्षिषु । कुक्षिपार्श्वोदरकटीपृष्ठरुक्पर्व्वभेदनम् । शुष्ककासोऽङ्गमर्द्दोऽधो गुरुता मलसंग्रहः । श्यावारुणत्वगादित्वमकस्माद्वृद्धिह्रासवत् ॥ सतोदभेदमुदरं तनुकृष्णशिराततम् आध्मातदृतिवच्छब्द माहतं प्रकरोति च । वायुश्चात्र सरुक्शब्दो विचरेत् सर्व्वतो गतिः ॥

पित्तोदरे ज्वरो मूर्च्छा दाहस्तृट् कटुकास्यता । भ्रमोऽतीसारः पीतत्वं त्वगादावुदरं हरित् ॥ पीतताम्रशिरानद्धं सस्वेदं

sometimes mixed with blood, in other cases it is clear or mixed with gravel. The pain is increased by walking, jumping, and riding.

Four different forms of this disease are observed. The following are the peculiarities of each form.

When produced by *air* it is always accompanie l with deranged phlegm, and this forms the stone. This stops near the neck of the bladder, and suddenly impedes the flow of urine; and is accompanied with much pain. To assist the evacuation of the urine the patient presses the parts particularly the umbiliacus, penis, and anus. The colour of the calculi are black, rough, and unequal; and are surrounded with elevations like the *kadam*.

Bile. In this case the bile being mixed with deranged phlegm, become a thick mass, increases in size, passes to the neck of the bladder, and prevents the passage of the urine. In the bladder there is a burning pain, as if produced by the application of heat. The air from the anus is hot, and the stone is yellow and sometimes red, black, or greyish, and resembles the stone of the "marking-nut."

शोष दह्यते। धूमायते मृदुस्पर्शं क्षिप्रपाकं प्रदूयते॥

श्लेष्मोदरेऽङ्गसदनं स्वाप-श्वयथु-गौरवम्। निद्रोत्क्लेशोऽरुचिः श्वासः कासः शुक्लत्वगादिता॥ उदरं स्तिमितं स्निग्धं शुक्लराजीततं महत्। चिराभिवृद्धं कठिनं शीतस्पर्शं गुरु स्थिरम्॥

स्त्रियोऽन्नपानं नखलोममूत्र-विड़ार्त्तवैर्युक्त मसाधुवृत्ताः। यस्मै प्रयच्छन्त्यरयो गरांश्च दुष्टाम्बुदूषी विषसेवनाद्वा॥ तेनाशु रक्तं कुपिताश्च दोषाः कुर्युरः सुघोरं जठरं त्रिलिङ्गम्। तच्छीतवाते भृशदुर्द्दिने च विशेषतः कुप्यति दह्यते च॥ स चातुरो मुह्यति हि प्रसक्तं पाण्डुः कृशः शुष्यति तृष्णाया च॥

Phlegm. A person who eats much of those articles of diet which produce diseases of phlegm is liable to have this form of stone. In such cases the phlegm becomes thick, and a stone is formed in the bladder. It produces a sudden stop of the flow of the urine, with severe pain in the bladder, and the person feels as if beaten. The bladder feels heavy and cool; and the stone is white, shining, large, like the appearance of a hen's egg.

The fourth kind of stone is produced by excesses in venery, or by the stoppage of semen which collects between the scrotum and penis. There it dries, and stops the passage of urine. This produces pain in bladder and scrotum, and a difficulty in mictirition. In such cases the scrotum sometimes swells.

The three first forms frequently attack children, and old people; by sleeping during the day, and using improper food and sweetmeats. The stone is easily extracted in the young, as the parts are small. In old people the disease is produced by derangements of air, bile and phlegm.

Stone is a dangerous disease, being like poison, or thunder. When recent it may be cured by medicines; but when of long standing an operation is required.

दूष्योदरं कीर्त्तितमेतदेव प्लीहोदरं कीर्त्तयतो निबोध। विदाह्यभिष्यन्दिरतस्य जन्तोः प्रदुष्टमत्यर्थं मसृक् कफश्च॥ प्लीहाभिवृद्धिं कुरुतः प्रवृद्धौ प्लीहोत्थमेतज्जठरं वदन्ति। तद्वामपार्श्वे परिवृद्धिमेति विशेषतः सीदति चातुरोऽत्र। मन्दज्वराग्निः कफपित्तलिङ्गैरुपद्रुतः क्षीणबलोऽतिपाण्डुः॥ सव्यान्यपार्श्वे यकृति प्रवृद्धे ज्ञेयं यकृद्दाल्युदरं तदेव॥ उदावर्त्तरुजानाहैर्मोहतृड्दहनज्वरैः। गौरवारुचिकाठिन्यैर्विद्यात्तत्र मलान् क्रमात्॥

यस्यान्त्रमन्नैरुपलेपिभिर्वा बालाश्मभिर्वा पिहितं यथावत्। सञ्चीयते तस्य मलः सदोषः शनैः शनैः शङ्करवच्च नाड्याम्॥ निरु-

Diseases of the Urinary Organs.

Under this head will be considered the diseases of the Urine, Bladder and Uretha.

Morbid Secretion of Urine, (*Prameha.*)

This disease is produced by a sedentary life, as sitting, lying down, or sleeping in the day time, using too much curdled milk, various kinds of fish, amphibious animals, or the flesh of buffaloes, new rice, or new water, such as rain or fresh river water, or food with different preparations of jagry, or whatever produces phlegm. It is also produced by the deranged phlegm of the bladder which affects the fat, flesh, or serum of the body; but particularly the region of the bladder. The bile is deranged by its peculiar causes, and in like manner the air may produce the disease, when the other humours are deranged, and convey them to the bladder.

There are twenty varieties of diseased urine; of which phlegm forms ten varieties which are curable, bile forms six varieties which are cured with great difficulty, but do not destroy life;

ध्यते तस्य गुदे पुरीषं निरेति कृच्छ्रादपि चाल्पमल्पम्। हृन्नाभिमध्ये परिवृद्धिमेति तस्योदरं बद्धगुदं वदन्ति॥

शल्यं तथान्नोपहितं यदन्त्रं भुक्तं भिनत्त्यागत मन्यथा वा। तस्मात् स्रुतोऽन्त्रात् सलिलप्रकाशः स्रावः स्रवेद्वै गुदतस्तु भूयः॥ नाभे रधश्चोदर मेति वृद्धिं निस्तुद्यते दाल्यति चातिमात्रम्। एतत् परिस्राव्युदरं प्रदिष्टं दकोदरं कीर्त्तयतो निबोध॥

यः स्नेहपीतोऽप्यनुवासितो वा वान्तो विरिक्तोऽप्यथवा निरूढः। पिबेज्जलं शीतलमाशु तस्य स्रोतांसि दूष्यन्ति हि तद्वहानि॥ स्नेहोपलिप्तेष्वथवापि तेषु दकोदरं पूर्ब्बवदभ्युपैति॥ स्निग्धं महत्तत् परिवृत्तनाभि समाततं पूर्णमिवाम्बुना च। यथा दृतिः क्षुभ्यति कम्पते च शब्दायते चापि दकोदरं तत्॥

and air forms four varieties, which are incurable. The causes of the different degrees of facility of removing these different varieties are that all the forms are accompanied with deranged phlegm, and when combined with deranged bile the cure of the disease is difficult, as those remedies which diminish bile will increase the phlegm. In like manner those remedies which decrease the air increase the phlegm therefore the cure is difficult; and on this account the disease produced by air is dangerous even from the beginning. These twenty kinds of disease are produced by derangements of air, bile and phlegm, fat, blood, semen, serum *(Amba)*, lymph *(Basá)*, the essential parts of all the humours *(Ozzo)*, the flesh and the chyle.

This order of diseases is ushered in by the appearance of morbid secretions about the teeth, ears, nose, and eyes. The hands and feet are very hot and burning, and the surface of the skin is shining as if oil had been applied to it. This is accompanied with thirst, and a sweet taste in the mouth. The different varieties of this disease are distinguished from each other by the symptoms of deranged humours, and by the colour of the urine.

जन्मनैवोदरं सर्व्वं प्रायः कृच्छ्रतमं मतम्। वलिन स्तद्-जाताम्बु यत्नसाध्यं नवोत्थितम् ॥ पच्चाद्बद्धगुदं तूर्द्ध्वं सर्व्वं जातोदकं तथा ॥ प्रायो भवत्यभावाय छिद्रान्त्रं चोदरं नृणाम्। शूनाक्षं कुटिलोपस्थ मुपक्लिन्नतनुत्वचम् ॥ वलशोणितमांसाग्नि परि-क्षीणञ्च वर्ज्जयेत्। पार्श्वभङ्गान्नविद्वेषः शोथातिसारपीड़ितम् ॥ विरिक्तञ्चाप्युदरिणं पूर्य्यमानं विवर्ज्जयेत् ॥

अथ शोथनिदानम्।

रक्त-पित्त-कफान् वायु र्दुष्टादुष्टान् वहिः शिराः। नीत्वा रुद्धगति स्तैर्हि कुर्य्यात्त्वं मांससंश्रयम्। उत्सेधं संहतं शोथं तमाहु र्निचयादतः ॥ सर्व्वं हेतुविशेषैस्तु रूपभेदान्नवात्मकम्।

In the disease produced by phlegm, insects approach the urine; the person is languid, his body becomes fat, and there is a discharge of mucus from the nose and mouth, with dispeptic symptoms, and looseness of the skin. He is always sleepy, with cough and difficult breathing.

When the disease is produced by bile, there is a cutting pain in the scrotum, bladder, and penis, with fever, dispepsia, vomiting, heat of the body, thirst, want of sleep, and yellowness of the excretions. In some cases it is accompanied with jaundice.

When produced by diseased *air* there is pain in the chest, the patient has a desire to eat every thing, there is watching, shivering, pain and costiveness. The following are the names and characteristic symptoms of the twenty varieties of diseased urine :—

1. *Udakameha.* In this disease the urine is nearly of the natural colour, without any sediment. It is white, cold, has no smell, and is like water.

2. *Ekhyumeha.* The urine is like the juice of sugar-cane in colour and taste.

दोषैः पृथगद्वयैः सर्व्वै रभिघाताद्विषादपि ॥ तत्पूर्व्वरूपं द्वयथुः शिरायामङ्गगौरवम् ॥

शुद्ध्रामयाभुक्त-कृषाबलानां चाराम्लतीक्ष्णोष्ण गुरूपसेवा। दध्याम मृच्छाकविरोधि दुष्ट गरोपसृष्टान्ननिषेवणाच्च। अर्शांस्यचेष्टा न च देहशुद्धि र्मर्म्मोपघातो विषमा प्रसूतिः। मिथ्योपचारः प्रतिकर्म्मणाञ्च निजस्य हेतुः श्वयथोः प्रदिष्टः ॥

सगौरवं स्यादनवस्थितत्वं सोत्सेधमुष्माथ शिरातनुत्वम्। सलोमहर्षश्च विवर्णता च सामान्यलिङ्गं श्वयथोः प्रदिष्टम् ॥ चलस्तनुत्वक् परुषोऽरुणोऽसितः सुसुप्तिहर्षार्त्तियुतोनिमित्ततः। प्रशाम्यति प्रोन्नमति प्रपीड़ितो दिवाबली च श्वयथुः समीरणात्।

3. In *Sáṇdrameha* the urine becomes thick after standing sometime.

4. When the urine is of a white colour, is thin and pure above, and thick below, it is named *Surámeha.*

5. *Pishtameha.* At the time of micturition the hair over the body is erect, and the urine has a copious white powder; as if flower had been mixed with it.

6. *Sukrameha.* In this variety the urine is the colour of semen, which sometimes appears mixed with it.

7. When the urine lets fall a hard and small deposit like sand it is called *Sikatameha.*

8. In *Swetameha* there is a copious secretion of urine which is sweet and cold.

9. When there are frequent calls to make urine, which is discharged in small quantities, the disease is called *Shanairmeha.*

10. *Lálameha,* When the urine is like mucilage, and has long adhesive fibrous matter mixed with it, the disease is named *Lálameha.*

11. In *Khármeha* the urine has the colour, taste, and smell of potassa, and is like it to the touch.

मृदुः सुगन्धोऽसितपीतरागवान् भ्रमज्वर-स्वेद-तृषा मदान्वितः। य उष्यते स्पृष्टरुगर्च्चिरागकृत् सपित्तशोथो भृशदाहपाकवान्॥ गुरुः स्थिरः पाण्डुररोचकान्वितः प्रसेक निद्रा वमिवह्निमान्द्यकृत्। सकृच्छ्रजन्मप्रशमो निपीड़ितो नचोन्नमेद्रात्रिबली कफात्मकः॥ निदानाकृतिसंसर्गात् श्वयथुः स्याद्विदोषजः। सर्व्वाकृतिः सन्निपाताच्छोथो व्यामिश्रलक्षणः॥

अभिघातेन शस्त्रादि छेदभेदक्षतादिभिः। हिमानिलोदध्यनिलैर्भल्लात-कपिकच्छुजैः॥ रसैः शूकैश्च संस्पर्शाच्छ्वयथुः स्याद्विसर्पवान्। भृशोष्म लोहिताभासः प्रायशः पित्तलक्षणः॥ विषजः सविषप्राणि परिसर्पणमूत्रणात्। दंष्ट्रा दन्तनखाघातादविषप्राणि-

12. In *Nilamcha* the urine is of a blue colour.

13. In *Kálameha* the urine is of a black colour, like ink.

14. In *Haridrameha* the urine is bitter and of a yellow colour like tamarind water, and there is great heat in passing the urine.

15. In *Manjistameha* the urine has the smell of indigested food, and is of the colour of the water of madder.

16. *Raktamcha.* The smell is like that of indigested food, is hot, is saltish to the taste, and is of a red colour.

17. *Basámeha.* The urine in this variety is of a light colour like fat, and seems as if mixed with it. It is discharged frequently.

18. *Majjámeha.* The urine in this form is like the colour of marrow, and appears as if mixed with it. It is discharged frequently.

19. *Kandrameha.* The urine is astringent and sweet to the taste. It has a troubled appearance.

20. *Hastimeha.* In this disease there is an incontinence of urine, which is discharged involuntary. It appears mixed with fat.

नामपि ॥ विन्मूत्र-शुक्रोपहतमलवद्दस्त्वशङ्करात् ॥ विषवृक्षानिल-स्पर्शात् गरयोगावचूर्णनात् ॥ मृदुश्चलोऽवलम्बी च शीघ्रो दाह-रुजाकरः ॥

दोषा श्वयथु मुद्धं हि कुर्व्वन्त्यामाशयस्थिताः । पक्काशयस्था मध्ये तु वर्च्चःस्थानगतास्त्वधः ॥ कृत्स्नदेहमनुप्राप्ता कूर्युः सर्व्व-सरं तथा ।

यो मध्यदेशे श्वयथुः स कष्टः सर्व्वगश्च यः । अर्द्धाङ्गे रिष्ट-भुतः स्याद यश्चोर्द्धं परिसर्पति ॥ श्वासः पिपासा छर्द्दिश्च दौर्व्वल्यं ज्वर एवच । यस्य चान्ने रुचिर्नास्ति श्वयथुतं विवर्ज्जयेत् ॥ अनग्रोपद्रवकृतः शोथः पादसमुत्थितः ॥ पुरुषं हन्ति नारीञ्च

The unfavourable symptoms of the above varieties of disease are when they are congenital; when the seven forms of diseased air, bile, and phlegm are present; when accompanied with a great discharge of the humours; when accompanied with large deep-seated abscesses; and when accompanied with *Madhumeha*, or sweet urine. These forms destroy the patient. All hereditary diseases being incurable, the congenital forms are such. All these different forms of *Prameha* if not properly treated, terminate in *Madhumeha*; or sweet urine, and they are then incurable.

The following forms of *Prameha* may be cured; when the urine is of the natural colour, is neither shining on the surface, nor white, and is of the usual taste, or is bitter and pungent. The following eruptions and abscesses may occur in the course of this disease in joints, and in vital or sensible parts; as the temples, or where there is much muscle.

1. *Sarābika*; with a central hollow, with high edges.
2. *Kachchhapika* are hot, and are in the form of a turtle, in appearance.
3. *Jwalini* is hot, and part appears irregular in its surface.

मुखजो गुदजो द्वयम् । नवोऽनुपद्रवः शोथः साध्योऽसाध्यः पुरोरितः । विवर्ज्जयेत् कुक्षुदराश्रितञ्च तथा गले मर्म्मणि संस्थितञ्च स्थूलः खरश्चापि भवेद्विवर्ज्ज्यो यश्चापि बालस्थविराबलानाम् ॥

अथ वृद्धिनिदानम् ।

क्रुद्धोऽनुर्द्धोगतिर्वायुः शोथशूलकरश्चरन् । मुष्कौ वङ्क्षणतः प्राप्य फलकोषाभिवाहिनीः ॥ प्रपीड्य धमनीर्वृद्धिं करोति फलकोषयोः । दोषास्रमेदोमूत्रान्त्रैः स वृद्धिः सप्तधा गदः । मूत्रान्त्रजावप्यनिलाद्धेतुभेदस्तु केवलम् ॥

वातपूर्णदृतिस्पर्शो रूक्षो वातादहेतु रुक् । पक्कोडुम्बरसंकाशः पित्ताद्दाहोष्मपाकवान् ॥ कफाच्छीतो गुरुः स्निग्धः कण्डूमान्

4. *Binatá* eruption is of a blue colour, and is accompanied with severe pain. It appears in the back or abdomen, and is accompanied with a copious secretion of urine.

5. *Alagi* is of a red and dark colour, in spots.

6. *Masuriká* is of a small figure with a central depression of a yellow colour.

7. *Sarsapika* is of a light yellow colour, and has the figure of mustard seed.

8. *Patirni* is elevated, and is surrounded with small eruptions.

9. *Bidáriká* like a bulbous root, hard, and hot.

10. *Bridadi* is a kind of abscess.

These various forms of eruptions may be produced by the derangements of fat without the presence of *Prameha*; and they are not observable until they have arrived at their full size, as it does not affect the pulse, etc. When they appear about the anus, breast, head, shoulders, back, and other sensible or vital parts, and if accompanied with bad symptoms they are dangerous.

कठिनोऽल्परुक् । कृष्णास्फोटावृतः पित्तैः वृद्धिलिङ्गश्च रक्तजः । कफवन्मेदसा वृद्धि र्मृदुस्तालफलोपमः ॥ मूत्रधारणशीलस्य मूत्रजः स तु गच्छतः । अम्भोभिः पूर्णदृतिवत् क्षोभं याति सरुङ् मृदुः । मूत्रकृच्छ्रमधः स्याच्च चलयन् फलकोषयोः ॥

वातकोपिभि राहारैः शीततोयावगाहनैः । धारने रणभाराध्व-विषमाङ्गप्रवर्त्तनैः ॥ क्षोभनैः क्षुभितोऽन्यैश्च क्षुद्रान्त्रावयवं यदा पवनो विगुणीकृत्य स्वनिवेशादधो नयेत् ॥ कुर्याद्वङ्क्षणसन्धिस्थो ग्रन्थ्याभं श्वयथुं तथा । उपेक्ष्यमाणस्य च मुष्कवृद्धिमाध्मानरुक् स्तम्भवतीं सवायुः । प्रपीड़ितोऽन्तः स्वनवान् प्रयाति प्रध्मापयन्नेति पुनश्च मुक्तम् । अन्त्रवृद्धिरसाध्योऽयं वातवृद्धिसमाकृतिः ।

When boils, are severe, and the internal heat is diminished, the physician is to give the case over as desperate. At the termination of the eruption, when there is thirst, cough, sloughing of the flesh, fainting, hiccough, delirium, slight fever, erysipelas in the temples, and the other sensible parts are very painful, so that the patient cannot be moved, the case will be fatal. Females are not liable to these diseases, as by the monthly discharge the body and humours are purified.

Samarogá or Bahumutra, is a disease only mentioned in modern books, most probably by its being classified as a variety of *Prameha*. Some manuscripts state that it is a disease peculiar to woman and is probably mistaken for Lucoreah, although generally considered to be Diabetes*

It is produced by excessive venery, grief, much exertion, and poison. In this disease all the humours are deranged, and pass through the vessels of the urinary passages; and are discharged copiously, without pain, and pure like water. The woman becomes weak suddenly, and the discharge of urine becomes involuntary. The patient becomes uneasy with

---

अथ गलगण्डगण्डमालापचीग्रन्थ्यर्व्वुदनिदानम्।

निबद्धः श्वयथुर्यस्य मुष्कवल्लम्बते गले। महान् वा यदि वा ह्रस्वो गलगण्डं तमादिशेत्॥ वातः कफश्चापि गले प्रदुष्टो मन्ये च संश्रित्य तथैव मेदः। कुर्व्वन्ति गण्डं क्रमशः स्वलिङ्गैः समन्वितं तं गलगण्डमाहुः॥ तोदान्वितः कृष्णशिरावनद्धः श्यावोऽरुणो वा पवनात्मकस्तु। पारुष्ययुक्तश्चिरवृद्धपाको यदृच्छया पाकमियात् कदाचित्॥ वैरस्यमास्यस्य च तस्य जन्तोर्भवेत्तथा तालुगलप्रशोषः। स्थिरः सवर्णो गुरुरुग्रकण्डुः शीतो महांश्चापि कफात्मकस्तु॥ चिराभिवृद्धिं भजते चिराद्वा प्रपच्यते मन्दरुजः

*See *Chikitsa Ratnasangraha*, or the jewels of treatment

giddiness, and the mouth and palate become dry, followed by fainting and delirium. The skin is dry and rough, with great thirst.

Great Fatness, (*Medah.*)

Cause. When persons remain without exercise, sleep during the day, take too much ghee, milk, and preparations of sweetmeats, rice, and different kinds of indigestable cakes, the chyle becomes oily, and sweeter than natural, and as it circulates it produces fatness. It is accompanied by the following symptoms :—The person feels a difficulty of breathing, thirst, is not sensitive, is always sleepy and uneasy, and cannot excite the body or work; such a person has always a good appetite, his perspiration has a disagreeable smell, he has less inclination for women. He speaks indistinctly; and the other essential parts of the body are not nourished. The fat is alone inflamed, and such a person usually dies of diabetis, carbuncle, fever, fistula-in-ano, or large internal abscesses. He is also subject to disease of the air (báyu), and the diseases he may contract are always severe.

कदाचित्। माधुर्य्यमास्यस्य च तस्य जन्तो र्भवेत्तथा तालुगल-प्रलेपः॥ स्निग्धोः गुरु पाण्डुरनिष्टगन्धो मेदोभवः कण्डुयुतोऽल्परुक् च। प्रलम्बतेऽलावुवदल्पमूलो देहानुरूपक्षयवृद्धियुक्तः॥ स्निग्धास्यता तस्य भवेच्च जन्तो र्गलेनु शब्दं कुरुते च नित्यम्। कृच्छ्राच्छ्वसन्तं मृदु सर्व्वगात्रं संवत्सरातीत मरोचकार्त्तम्॥ क्षीणञ्च वैद्यो गलगण्डयुक्तं भिन्नस्वरञ्चापि विवर्ज्जयेच्च।

कर्कन्धुकोलामलकैः प्रमाणैः कक्षांस-मन्या-गलवङ्क्षणेषु। मेदःकफाभ्यां चिरमन्दपाकैः स्याद्गण्डमाला बहुभिश्च गण्डैः॥ ते ग्रन्थयः केचिदवाप्तपाकाः स्रवन्ति नश्यन्ति भवन्ति चान्ये।

Enlargement of the Abdomen, (*Udara.*)

This disease is divided into eight varieties, three of these are produced by derangements of the air, bile, and phlegm, and one by the combination of the three. The fifth is accompanied by enlargement of the spleen; the sixth is called *Baddaguda*, concretions; they seventh *Parisrábyudara*, or *Agantuka*, or accidental; and the eighth *Dakodara*, or Asitis.

This disease (*Udara*) is produced by eating bad food without an appetite; eating dry putrid food, and the improper administration of purgatives, emetics, and other active medicines by which the air, bile, and phlegm are deranged in the abdomen. The first symptoms of this disease resemble *Gulma*; followed by swelling of the abdomen. It is produced by the taking up of the fluid part of the chyle, which is conveyed by air into the surface, and produces swelling under the skin, and enlargement of the abdomen.

The disease is ushered in by weakness, unhealthy colour of the skin, languor, and want of appetite. There are no wrinkles on the abdomen, which swells, while the rest of the body is thin,

---

कालानुबद्धं चिरमादधाति सैवापचीति प्रवदन्ति तज्ज्ञाः ॥ साध्याः स्मृताः पीनस-पार्श्वशूल-कास-ज्वरच्छर्दियुता स्त्वसाध्याः ।

वातादयो मांस-मसृक्-प्रदुष्टाः संदुष्य मेदश्च तथा शिराश्च । वृत्तोन्नतं विग्रथितञ्च शोथं कुर्वन्त्यतो ग्रन्थिरिति प्रदिष्टः ॥ आयम्यते दूयति तुद्यते च प्रत्यस्यते मथ्यति भिद्यते च । कृष्णो मृदुर्वस्तिरिवाततश्च भिन्नः स्रजेच्चानिलजास्र मच्छम् ॥ दंदह्यते धुपयपि दूयते च पापच्यते प्रज्वलतीव चापि ॥ रक्तः स पीतोऽप्यथवापि पित्तात् भिन्नं स्रवेदुष्ण मतीव चास्रम् । शीतो विवर्णोऽल्परुजोऽतिकण्डुः पाषाणवत् संहननोपपन्नः ॥ चिराभिवृद्धिश्च कफप्रकोपाद्भिन्नस्रवेच्छुक्लघनञ्च पूयम् । शरीरवृद्धि क्षयवृद्धि

and prominent veins appear over the surface of the abdomen. He has pain in the pelvis; fulness in the abdomen, with burning; the feet swell, and the person is weak and cannot walk. By degrees the body swells, the air and dejections are stopped, the body is hot, and the person complains of faintness. The forms of this disease, called *Busrabi,* and *baddaguda* are incurable; the other forms are cured with much difficulty. In the latter stages of this disease manual assistance or operations are sometimes required for the cure of the disease.

1. When diseased *air* produces this disease, the hands, feet, and abdomen are swelled, with pain in the sides of the abdomen, pit of the stomach, loins, and back, with pain in the joints as if they were broken. He complains of cough without expectoration, stretching and heaviness about the loins, the dejections and urine are constipated, the skin and eyes are of a dark yellow colour. The swelling is not always the same; sometimes it increases, and at other times decreases, with severe pain in, and over the abdomen. Dark coloured vessels are prominent over the abdomen, which is swelled like a leather bottle, and makes a noise like it when it is struck.

हानिः स्निग्धो महान् कण्डुयुतो रुजश्च ॥ मेदःकृतो गच्छति चात्र भिन्ने पिण्याक सर्पिः-प्रतिमं तु मेदः । व्यायामजातै रबलस्य तैस्तैराचिप्य वायुस्तु शिराप्रतानम् ॥ संकुच्य संपीड्य विशोष्य चापि ग्रन्थिं करोत्युन्नतमाशु वृत्तम् । ग्रन्थिः शिराजः स तु कृच्छ्रसाध्यो भवेद् यदि स्यात् सरुजश्चलश्च । सचारुजश्चाप्यचलो महांश्च मर्म्मोत्थितश्चापि विवर्ज्जनीयः ॥

गात्रप्रदेशे क्वचिदेव दोषाः संमूर्च्छिता मांस मसृक् प्रदूष्य । वृत्तं स्थिरं मन्दरुजं महान्त मनल्पमूलं चिरवृद्ध्यपाकम् ॥ कुर्व्वन्ति मांसोच्छ्रयमत्यगाधं तदर्ब्बुदं शास्त्रविदो वदन्ति वातेन पित्तेन कफेनञ्चापि रक्तेन मांसेन च मेदसा वा तज्जायते तस्य च लक्ष-

2. *Bile.* The symptoms of this variety are fever, faintness, burning, thirst, and an acid taste in the mouth; the head swings round, looseness is produced, the eyes and skin are of a yellow colour, the abdomen is of a green colour, and small yellow vessels appear upon the surface, with much perspiration; the body burns, there is a feeling as if smoke was rising in his throat, and the symptoms of bilious diseases; as well as the peculiar symptoms of this disease are quickly developed.

3. *Phlegm (Shleshmodara)* when much deranged the person cannot work, is always sleepy, the abdomen swells, and there is no feeling in the abdomen, heaviness, sickness, no appetite, difficulty of breathing, cough, the eyes and skin are pale, abdomen cold, and the bowels are constipated; and white vessels appear upon its surface. After many days the swelling is completely formed, and is very difficult to remove. The body feels cold and hard, and the abdomen heavy.

When there is much pain, constipation and swelling of the abdomen, it proves that air is deranged; when faintness, thirst, heat, and fever are present, the bile is deranged; and when there is a sense of weight with no appetite, and hard abdomen, the phlegm is deranged.

यानि ग्रन्थेः समानानि तदा भवन्ति। दोषः प्रदुष्टो रुधिरं शिराश्च संकूच्य संपीड्य ततस्तपाकम्॥ सास्रावमुन्नह्यति मांसपिण्डं मांसाङ्कुरै राचित माशु वृद्धिम्॥ करोत्यजस्र रुधिरप्रवृत्ति समाध्य मेतद्रुधिरात्मकन्तु। रक्तक्षयोपद्रव-पीड़ितत्वात् पाण्डुर्भवेदर्व्वुद पीड़ितस्तु॥ मुष्टिप्रहारादिभिरर्द्दितेऽङ्गे मांसं प्रदुष्टं जनयेद्धि शोयम्। अवेदनं स्निग्धमनन्यवर्णं मपाकमश्मोप मप्रचाल्यम्॥ प्रदुष्टमांसस्य नरस्य गाढ़ मेतद्भवेन्मांसपरायणस्य। मांसार्व्वुदं ते तदसाध्यमुक्तं साध्येश्वपीमानि तु वर्ज्जयेच्च॥ संप्रस्रुतं मर्म्मणि यच्च यातं स्रोतःसु वा यच्च भवेदचाल्यम्। यज्जाययेऽन्यत् खलु

4. The derangements of the *air*, *bile*, and *phlegm* are said by the moderns to be often caused by enchantment, or by the use of Philters, as of a woman to her husband, or lover. For this purpose the parings of nails, the cuttings of hair, fæces, urine, menstrual blood, etc, are used, on the absurd supposition of increasing their love towards them. Certain poisons administered by an enemy are said also to produce this disease. These causes not only derange the three humours, but also the blood. This form of disease is increased by cloudy weather, when the abdomen is swelled; and when the air is cold, it is also increased in violence, and the person becomes faint, the body yellow, the person very thin and dry, and he complains of thirst. This form of disease is called *Dakodara*.

5. *Plihodara* (*spleen*). This is a swelling of the abdomen with an enlargement of the spleen. It is produced by eating indigestable food, or of a heavy nature, as also articles which produce cold; as curdled milk, and articles which increase phlegm. These substances when frequently eaten derange blood and cough, and swell the spleen. In this disease there is

---

[illegible] ज्ञेयं तदध्यर्ब्बुदमर्ब्बुदज्ञैः ॥ यद्द्वन्द्वजातं युगपत् क्रमाद्वा द्विरर्ब्बुदं तच्च भवेदसाध्यम्। न पाकमायान्ति कफाधिकत्वात् मेदो बहुत्वाच्च विशेषतस्तु॥ दोषस्थिरत्वात् ग्रहणाच्च तेषां सर्व्वार्ब्बुदान्तेव निसर्गतस्तु।

अथ श्लीपदनिदानम्।

यः सज्वरो वङ्क्षणजो भृशार्त्तः शोथो नृणां पादगतः क्रमेण। तत्श्लीपदं स्यात् करकर्णनेत्र शिश्नौष्ठनासास्वपि केचिदाहुः॥ वातजं कृष्णरूक्षञ्च स्फुटितं तीव्रवेदनम्। अनिमित्तरुजं तस्य बहुशो ज्वर एवच॥ पित्तजं पीतसङ्काशं दाहज्वरयुतं मृदु। श्लैष्मिकं स्निग्धवर्णञ्च श्वेतं पाण्डु गुरु स्थिरम्। वल्मीकमिव संजातं कण्टकै रुपचीयते॥ अब्दात्मकं महत्तच्च वर्ज्जनीयं विशे-

languor, loss of appetite, and symptoms of deranged phlegm, etc. The person becomes very weak, and the body of a yellow colour. When the liver is swelled it is called *Jukrit Udara.* In this form the air, bile, and phlegm are deranged, and the disease is severe.

6. *Baddaguda.* This form is produced by the accumulation of indigestable matter with the food, such as hair, gravel, etc. These form balls which produce constipation, and swelling occurs between the chest and umbiliacus. The person has stercoral vomiting, as a drain is stopped by an accumulation of filth. The air, bile, and phlegm are deranged at the obstructed part, and the fæces is confined. The stools are in small quantities, and are evacuated with great pain, the umbiliacus, and breast are much swelled.

7. *Parisrábyudara* is produced by sharp substances, such as fish bones, portions of wood, etc. being taken with the food, and wounding the canal. A watery discharge is evacuated by the anus, proceeding from the wounded surface. The abdomen increases in size under the umbiliacus with much pain and burning. It is to be treated as the last; but both are generally incurable. The other forms are cured with difficulty.

षतः। त्रीण्यपेतानि जानीयात् श्लीपदानि कफोच्छ्रयात्॥ गुरुत्वञ्च महत्वञ्च यस्मान्नास्ति कफं विना। पुरानोदकभूयिष्ठाः सर्व्वर्त्तुषु च शीतलाः॥ ये देशास्तेषु जायन्ते श्लीपदानि विशेषतः। शास्त्रावमतुग्नन्तसर्व्वलिङ्गं सकण्डुरं श्लेष्मयुतं विवर्ज्जयम्॥

अथ विद्रधिनिदानम्।

त्वग्रक्तमांसमेदांसि संदूष्यास्थि-समाश्रिताः। दोषाः शोथं शनैर्घोरं जनयन्तुग्रच्छ्रिता भृशम्॥ महामूलं रुजावन्तं वृत्तं वाप्यथवायतम्। स विद्रधिरिति ख्यातो विज्ञेयः षड्विधश्च सः॥ पृथग्दोषैः समस्तैश्च क्षतेनाप्यसृजा तथा। षण्णामपि हि तेषान्तु

8. *Asitis*, (*Jalodara, or Dakodara.*) When a person has taken a large quantity of prepared ghee, or has had frequent enemas, or after emetics or purgatives he drinks large quantities of cold water, they stop the absorbent vessels, and produce this disease. In this case the abdomen becomes large, the umbiliacus prominent, and appears shining as if anointed and full of water, and like it moves about, and gives a sound like a leather bag.

In all these forms of diseases there is swelling, weakness, loss of appetite, languor, and swelling of different parts of the body, constipation, burning, and great thirst. When with these symptoms water collects, the disease is incurable.

Swellings, (*Shotha.*)

Under this head is considered swellings of different kinds. When air is deranged, and mixes with the diseased blood, bile, and phlegm, it conveys them to the external parts of the body, stops the air-vessels, and their contents, which accumulate, and produce swellings.

लक्षणं संप्रचक्ष्यते ॥ कृष्णोऽरुणो वा विषमो भृशमत्यर्थवेदनः । चित्रोत्थान-प्रपाकश्च विद्रधि र्वातसम्भवः ॥ पक्वोडुम्वरसङ्काशः श्यावो वा ज्वरदाहवान् । क्षिप्रोत्थान-प्रपाकश्च विद्रधिः पित्तसम्भवः ॥ शरावसदृशः पाण्डुः शीतः स्निग्धोऽल्प-वेदनः । चिरोत्थानप्रपाकश्च विद्रधिः कफसम्भवः ॥ तनुपीतासिताश्चैषा मास्रावाः क्रमशः स्मृताः । नानावर्णो रुजास्रावो घाटालो विषमो महान् ॥ विषमं पच्यते चापि विद्रधिः सान्निपातिकः ।

तै स्तै र्भावै रभिहते क्षते वा पथ्यकारिणः । क्षतोष्मावायु-विसृतः सरक्तं पित्तमीरयेत् ॥ ज्वर स्तृष्णा च दाहश्च जायते तस्य देहिनः । आगन्तुविद्रधि र्ह्येष पित्तविद्रधिलक्षणः ॥

This disease is caused by great fatigue in walking, with fasting; by eating much indigestable cakes, sour articles of food, vegetables, or clay; by salt, which debilitates the humours, and by other indigestable, or unhealthy articles of food and mixtures. In other cases it is produced by leading a sedentary life, personal neglect of medicines, uncleanness, injuries to vital parts, untimely parturition, the improper use of emetics and purgatives, and piles. These cause a swelling of the body, which is accompanied with pain and heaviness, restlessness, heat, and discolouration of the body.

According to *Charaka* there are nine varieties of *Shotha*, three being produced by air, bile, and phlegm, when affected separately; three when two humours are deranged; one when three are deranged at the same time; one when caused by an injury, and one by poison. *Sushruta* does not allow that three varieties are produced by the combination of two diseased humours; and consequently considers this disease as having only five varieties produced by general, and one by a local, or accidental cause.

कृष्णास्फोटावृतः श्याव स्तीव्रदाह रुजाकरः पित्तविद्रधिलिङ्गस्तु रक्तविद्रधिरुच्यते ।

पृथक् सम्भूय वा दोषाः कुपिता गुल्मरूपिणम् । वल्मीकवत् समुन्नद्ध मन्तः कुर्व्वन्ति विद्रधिम् गुदे वस्तिमुखे नाभ्यां कुक्षौ वङ्क्षणयोस्तथा । वृक्कयोः प्लीह्नि यकृति हृदि वा क्लोम्नि वाप्यथ ॥ तेषामुक्तानि लिङ्गानि वाह्यविद्रधिलक्षणैः अधिष्ठानविशेषेण लिङ्गं शृणु विशेषतः ॥ गुदे वातनिरोधश्च वस्तौ कृच्छ्राल्पमूत्रता । नाभ्यां हिक्का तथाटोपः कुक्षौ मारुतकोपनम् ॥ कटीपृष्ठग्रहस्तीव्रो वङ्क्षणोत्थे तु विद्रधौ । वृक्कयोः पार्श्वसंकोचः प्लीह्न्युच्छ्वासावरोधनम् ॥ सर्व्वाङ्ग-प्रग्रहस्तीव्रो हृदि कासश्च जायते । श्वासो यकृति हिक्का च क्लोम्नि पेपीयते पयः ।

1. When *air* is deranged the swelling passes from one part to another, the skin is thin, the surface dry and soft, of a red or black colour, with dullness of feeling. The parts when pressed pit, but they recover the level on the pressure being removed. The symptoms increase in the day time.

2. When the swelling is produced by deranged *bile* the swelling is moist, and has a bad smell, is of a yellow, red, and black colour, produces various kinds of pain, and ripens soon. In such cases the body is soon fatigued, the patient is feverish, perspires much, complains of thirst, and dullness, the pulse is very frequent, his eyes of a red colour, and the pain is severe.

3. *Phlegm. Dropsy* is characterized by always remaining in one place, is of a yellowish pale, and shining colour, is cold and hard, and painfully itchy. The patient has no appetite, and cough is discharged from the mouth and nose, the person is always sleepy, the swelling and the internal heat are diminished, and when the disease occurs it causes much uneasiness to the person, and is cured slowly. Pressure does not diminish this variety, the symptoms of which increase at night.

नाभेरुपरिजाः पक्वा यान्तूर्द्ध मितरे त्वधः। अधःस्रुतेषु जीवेत्तु स्रुतेवर्द्धं न जीवति॥ हृन्नाभिवस्तिवर्ज्ज्या ये तेषु भिन्नेषु वाह्यतः। जीवेत् कदाचित् पुरुषो नेतरेषु कदाचन॥ साध्या विद्रधयः पञ्च विवर्ज्ज्यः सान्निपातिकः। आमपक्व विदग्धत्वं तेषां शोथवदादिशेत्॥ आध्मातं वद्धनिष्यन्दं छर्द्दिहिक्कातृषान्वितम्। रुजाश्वाससमायुक्तं विद्रधिर्नाशयेन्नरम्॥

अथ व्रणशोथनिदानम्।

एकदेशोत्थितः शोथो व्रणानां पूर्व्वलक्षणम्। षड्विधः स्यात् पृथक् सर्व्वं रक्तजागन्तुजस्तथा॥ शोथाः षडेते विज्ञेयाः प्रागुक्तैः शोथलक्षणैः। विशेषः कथ्यते चैषां पक्वापक्वादिनिश्चये॥ विषमं

4, 5, 6, 7. When two of the above humours are deranged, the symptoms of both forms of the two humours, stated above, are present; and when three are deranged, all the symptoms are present in the separate varieties.

8. *Accidental Swellings* (*Abhighátaja shotha*), when the body is wounded by a cutting instrument, by injuries; or when bruised by an accident, bréathing cold air, and the air of the ocean is of much use. The vapour or juice of the marking-nut (*bhallátaka*) applied to the body, or rubbing the part with cowach (*kapikachchhú*) will be of use. These produce swelling, heat, and redness, accompanied with the other symptoms of diseased bile. Bad water, either drank, or with which the body is washed, produces such swellings of parts.

9. *Bishaja-shotha.* When the poison of any animal is taken by the mouth, is introduced into the system by a wound, or by contact; when urine is applied to a wound, or the person wears a cloth that is dirty, is covered with excrement, or he breathes air coming from a poisonous tree it produces this form of swelling. The application of the powder of different poisonous

---

पच्यते वातात् पित्तोत्थश्चाचिराच्चिरम्। कफजः पित्तवच्छोथो रक्तागन्तुसमुद्भवः॥

मन्दोष्मताल्पशोथत्वं काठिन्यं त्वक् सवर्णता। मन्दवेदनता चैतत् शोथानामामलक्षणम्॥ दह्यते दहनेनेव क्षारेणेव च पच्यते। पिपीलिकागणेनेव दश्यते छिद्यते तथा॥ भिद्यते चैव शस्त्रेण दण्डेनेव च ताड्यते। पीड्यते पाणिनेवान्तः सूचीभिरिव तुद्यते॥ सोषाचोषो विवर्णः स्यात् अङ्गुल्येवावघट्यते। आसने शयने स्थाने शान्तिं वृश्चिकविद्धवत्॥ न गच्छेदाततः शोथो भवेदाध्मातवस्तिवत्। ज्वरस्तृष्णारुचिश्चैवं पच्यमानस्य लक्षणम्॥ वेदनोपशमः शोथो लोहिताल्पो न चोन्नतः। प्रादुर्भावो वलीनाञ्च तोदः कण्डू र्मुहुर्मुहुः॥ उपद्रवाणां प्रशमो निम्नता पुठनं त्वचाम्। वस्ताविवाम्ब-

articles, or of certain animals walking over the body, produce the same effect. Thus if frogs, etc. discharge their urine upon a part, it swells. The poison is either discharged from the trunk, teeth, or nails of the animal into the wound. By such causes the part swells, becomes pendulous, and is accompanied with pain. These swellings are soft, rise quickly, and are not fixed in one place, but move about. Sometimes they are quickly produced, and increase downwards (*distid*) ; and are very hot, and painful. When air, bile, and phlegm are deranged in the stomach (*ámásiya*), the swelling occurs in the head and upper extremities, when deranged in the small intestines (*paukashaya*), the swelling will occur in the trunk, and when in the rectum (*andaka*), the swelling will occur in the lower extremities. When air, bile, and phlegm are deranged over the body, it will swell the whole body, and pass from one part to another.

When the swelling occurs in the trunk of the body it will be cured with difficulty, and also when the swelling is over the body. When the upper or lower half of the body is affected the disease is dangerous, or when the swelling proceeds proximated from the part first affected.

सञ्चारः स्याच्छोथेऽङ्गुलिपीड़िते ॥ पूयस्य पीड़यतेऽक मन्तमन्ते च पीड़िते। भक्ताकाङ्क्षा भवेच्चैतच्छोथानां पक्कलक्षणम् ॥ नर्त्तेऽनिलाद्रुङ्न विना च पित्तं, पाकः कफञ्चापि विना न पूयः। तस्माद्धि सर्व्वं परिपाककाले पचन्ति शोथा स्त्रिभिरेव दोषैः ॥

कक्षं समाश्रितऽ यथैव वह्निः वायूरितः संदहति प्रसह्य। तथैव पुयो ह्यविनिःसृतो हि मांसं शिराः स्नायु च खादतीह ॥ यश्छिनत्त्यामममज्ञानात् यो वा पक्क मुपेक्षते। श्वपचाविव मन्तव्यौ तावनिश्चितकारिणौ ॥ आमं विदह्यमानञ्च सम्यक् पक्कञ्च यो भिषक्। जानीयात् स भवेद्वैद्यः शेषा स्तस्करवृत्तयः ॥

The swelling will not be cured when the person breathes with noise and difficulty, when accompanied with thirst, vomiting, weakness, hiccough and fever, and when he has no appetite, and is affected with diarrhœa and severe pain (*sul*). Such a diseased person will die. When the swelling commences in the feet of the male, or in the face of the female, both are very dangerous. It is also very dangerous in both sexes, when the swelling is about the anus.

When the swelling is recent, with no bad symptoms, it will be cured. When the throat and vital parts are swelled with much pain ; or when it attack infants, or old persons, or very weak persons, the disease will be fatal.

Shlipada, (*Elephantiasis.*)

In the *Mádhab Nidán* it is stated that the patient's groin first swells, and become very painful, with fever. The swelling then slowly descends to the foot, producing this disease. In other books, it is stated that the same disease may occur in the hands,

---

अथ शारीरव्रणनिदानम् ।

द्विधा व्रणः स विज्ञेयः शारीरागन्तुभेदतः । दोषै राद्य स्तयोरन्त्यः शस्त्रादिक्षतसम्भवः ॥ स्तब्धः कठिनसंस्पर्शो मन्दस्रावो महारुजः । तुद्यते स्फुरति श्यावो व्रणो मारुतसम्भवः ॥ तृष्णा मोहज्वरक्लेद-दाह-दुष्ट्यवदारणैः । व्रणं पित्तकृतं विद्यात् गन्धैः स्रावैश्च पूतिकैः बहुपिच्छो गुरुः स्निग्धः स्तिमितो मन्दवेदनः ॥ पाण्डुवर्णोऽल्पसंक्लेद श्चिरपाकी कफव्रणः । रक्तो रक्तस्रुतीरक्ताद्द्वित्रिजः स्यात्तदन्वयैः ॥

त्वङ्मांसजः सुखे देशे तरुणस्यानुपद्रवः । धीमतोऽभिनवः काले सुखैः साध्यः सुखं व्रणः ॥ गुणैरन्यतमैर्हीनस्ततः कृच्छ्रो व्रणः स्मृतः । सर्व्वैर्विहीनो विज्ञेय स्त्वसाध्यो भूर्य्युपद्रवः ॥

ears, eye-lids, nose, lips, and penis. When it occurs in the groin, and descends to the leg and foot, or when situated in the hand it is produced by bad flesh and fat ; and the parts affected become hard and rough.

When air produces this disease the swelling is of a black colour, rough, dry, with cracks and small sores. This form is very painful, and occurs suddenly, with much fever.

When produced by diseased bile it is of a yellowish colour, hot, soft, and accompanied with fever.

When produced by diseased phlegm, the skin is shining, of a white or grey colour, the part is very heavy, hard, fixed to one place, and has the appearance of a large white-ant's hill, of an irregular sharp-pointed appearance. This form is difficult to cure after it has been present a year, when very large, when it discharges continually, is itchy, and when all the above symptoms are present, as this indicates that air, bile, and phlegm are diseased.

Elephantiasis is most frequent in those countries where there is much stagnant water, and in cold damp situations, such as Rungpore, Farridpore, etc.

पूतिः पूयातिदुष्टासृक् स्राव्युत्सङ्गी चिरस्थितिः। दुष्टो व्रणोऽतिदुर्गन्धः शुद्धलिङ्गो विपर्य्ययः॥ जिह्वातलाभो मृदु श्लक्ष्णः स्निग्धो विगतवेदनः। सुव्यवस्थो निरास्रावः शुद्धो व्रण इति स्मृतः॥ कपोतवर्णप्रतिमा यस्यान्ताः क्लेदवर्जिताः। स्थिराश्च पिड़कावन्तो रोहतीति तमादिशेत्॥ रूढ़वर्त्मानमग्रन्थिमशूलमरुजं व्रनम्। त्वक्सवर्णं समतलं सम्यग्रूढ़ं विनिर्दिशेत्॥

कुष्ठिनां विषजुष्टानां शोषिणां मधुमेहिनाम्। व्रणाः कृच्छ्रेण सिध्यन्ति येषाञ्चापि व्रणे व्रणाः॥ वसां मेदोऽथ मज्जानं मस्तुलुङ्गञ्च यः स्रवेत्। आगन्तुजो व्रणः सिद्ध्येत् न सिद्ध्येद्दोषसम्भवः॥ मद्यागुर्व्वाज्यसुमनःपद्मचन्दनचम्पकैः। सगन्धा दिव्यगन्धाश्च

In the above description the marked accessions and remissions are not mentioned, but it is stated that the damp and cold situations produce this disease, that it attacks different parts of the body, and that it is incurable, after it has remained upwards of a year, or is very large. It is also observed that it is incurable, when the skin is much affected, as indicated by the continual discharge, the itchy or painful nature of the swelling, and its discolouration.

Diseases of the Male Organs of Generation.

Diseases of the Scrotum (*Briddhi*).—There are seven varieties of swelling of the scrotum produced by air, bile, phlegm, blood, fat, urine, and by the descent of the intestine. Any of those deranged humours may produce the swelling of the scrotum, or the testicle. The bowel only causes the swelling of the scrotum. The preceding symptoms are pains in the loins, pelvic region, and penis, followed by the swelling of the scrotum.

Symptoms. When the swelling is produced by deranged *air* the scrotum is extended as a bag of air, the surface is rough, and the peculiar pain produced by air is felt in the scrotum.

मुमूर्षूणां व्रणाः स्मृताः ॥ ये च मर्म्मसु सम्भूता भवन्त्यत्यर्थ-वेदनाः । दह्यते चान्तरत्यर्थं वहिः शीताश्च ये व्रणाः । दह्यते वहिरत्यर्थं भवन्त्यन्तश्च शीतलाः ॥ प्राणमांसक्षयश्वासकासारोचक-पीड़िताः । प्रवृद्धपूयरुधिरा व्रणा येषाञ्च मर्म्मसु ॥ क्रियाभिः सम्यगारब्धा न सिध्यन्ति च ये व्रणाः । वर्ज्जयेदपि तान् वैद्यः संरक्षन्नात्मनो यशः ॥

अथ सद्योव्रण-निदानम् ।

नानाधारामुखैः शस्त्रै र्नानास्थान-निपातितैः । भवन्ति नाना-कृतयो व्रणास्तां स्तान्निबोध मे ॥ छिन्नं भिन्नं तथा विद्धं क्षतं पिच्छिलमेव वा । घृष्टमाहु स्तथा षष्ठं तेषां वक्ष्यामि लक्षणम् ॥

When produced by *bile* the swelling is red like the red fig, has a burning sensation and is accompanied with fever. In this form suppuration soon takes place.

When caused by diseased *phlegm*, the swelling is hard, is not painful, the surface is cool, it is itchy, and is not accompanied with fever.

Produced by *blood* the swelling is surrounded with black tubercles, and is accompanied with the symptoms of bile.

Fat produces the disease which is characterized by softness, shining, itchiness, and little pain. It becomes like the fruit of the palm tree ; that is rough and tuberculated.

The form produced by *urine* (yellow serum), collected between the testicle and its external covering, moves like a bag of water.

The last form is hernia which is produced by carrying heavy weights, by fighting with strong persons, falling or jumping, and the like. By such causes air is deranged, which propels the intestine downwards, it remains in the groin, and if not treated for some days it descends still lower, and pro-

---

तिर्य्यक् छिन्नमृजुर्वापि यो व्रणस्त्वायतो भवेत्। गात्रस्य पातनं तद्धि छिन्नमित्यभिधीयते॥ शक्तिदन्तेषु खड्गाग्रविषाणै राशयो हतः। यत् किञ्चित् प्रस्रवेत्तद्धि भिन्नलक्षणमुच्यते॥ स्थानान्यामाग्निपक्वानां मूत्रस्य रुधिरस्य च। हृदुण्डुकफुप्फुसश्च कोष्ठ इत्यभिधीयते॥ तस्मिन् भिन्ने रक्तपूर्णे ज्वरो दाहश्च जायते।

मूत्रमार्गगुदास्येभ्यो रक्तं घ्राणाच्च गच्छति। मूर्च्छा श्वास तृषाध्मात मभक्तच्छन्द एव च॥ विण्मूत्रवातसङ्गश्च स्वेदास्रावोऽक्षिरक्तता। लोहगन्धित्वमास्यस्य गात्रदौर्गन्ध्यमेव च॥ हृच्छूलं पार्श्वयोश्चापि विशेषञ्चात्र मे शृणु। आमाशयस्थे रुधिरे रुधिरं छर्द्दयत्यपि॥ आध्मानमपिमात्रञ्च शूलञ्च भृशदारुणम्। पक्वाशयगते चापि रुजा गौरवमेव च॥ अधःकाये विशेषेण

duces a swelling of the scrotum. The tumor is oblong, and when pressed it passes upwards with a peculiar noise, and again descends when the pressure is removed.

Antrabriddhi (Hernia) is incurable, unless when it is recent and situated in the groin.

Brishanakachchhú, (itchiness of the scrotum *pruzigo.*) This is a common and troublesome disease. Medical authors say that it is produced by not attending to cleanliness, by which the perspiration is accumulated, which irritates and produces an eruption on the part. This sometimes degenerate into sores.

Scrofulous swellings (*Gandamálá*).

When many small tumors like plums appear in the axilla, neck, back, and groins, they are produced by diseased fat, and phlegm. They suppurate slowly, and continue to appear and suppurate for a long period, when it is called *Apachi.* When not attended by any bad constitutional disease it is curable, but when accompanied with *Coriza,* with pain in the sides, cough, fever, and vomiting, it is incurable.

शीतता च भवेदिह। मूत्त्रास्य मलग्राभितं यद्दङ्गस्त्वाशयं विना॥ उत्खण्डितं निर्गतं वा तद्विद्ध मितिनिर्द्दिशेत्। नातिच्छिन्नं नातिभिन्नं उभयो र्लक्षणान्वितम्॥ विषमं व्रणमङ्गे यत् तत्क्षत्वभिधीयते। प्रहारपिड़नाभ्यान्तु यदङ्गं पृथुतां गतम्॥ सास्थि तत् पिच्छितं विद्यात् मज्जरक्त-परिप्लुतम्।

घर्षणादभिघाताद्वा यदङ्गं विगतत्वचम्। उषास्रावान्वितं तच्च घृष्टमित्यभिधीयते॥ श्यावं सशोथं पिड़काचितञ्च मूहुर्मुहुः शोणितवाहिनञ्च। मृदुन्नतं बुद्बुदतुल्यमांसं व्रणं सशल्यं सरुजं वदन्ति॥ त्वचोऽतित्य शिरादीनि भित्वा वा परिच्छिद्य वा।

Goitre (*Galaganda.*)

The swelling of the throat, whether it be small or large, is called by this name. It is of an oblong form like the scrotum. It is produced when air and phlegm are diseased in the throat, and diseased fat slowly produces it.

When *air* is diseased there is pain in the throat, and black veins spread over it. The swelling is of a green or red colour, dull and irregular. This form increases slowly and rarely suppurates; but, when it does it is without any apparent cause. The person has a bad taste in his mouth, with dryness of the palate and throat.

Phlegm. In this variety the swelling is hard, fixed, cold, and the colour is not altered. It increases slowly, is heavy, itchy, and large, and sometimes suppurates. The taste of the mouth is sweetish, and the palate and throat is as if covered with some matter.

When produced by diseased *fat* it is slow in its increase, and suppurates with little pain, and is of the shape of a pumpkin (*kadu*), with a small root. The swelling increases, and

---

कोष्ठे प्रतिष्ठितं शल्यं कुर्य्यादुक्तानुपद्रवान् ॥ तत्रान्तर्लोहितं पाण्डु शीतपादकराननं शीतोच्छ्वासं रक्तनेत्रमानद्धञ्च विवर्ज्जयेत् ।

भ्रमः प्रलापः पतनं प्रमोहो विचेष्टनं ग्लानिरथोष्णता च । स्रस्ताङ्गता मूर्च्छनमूर्द्ध्ववात स्तीव्रा रुजो वातकृताश्च तास्ताः ॥ मांसोदकाभं रुधिरञ्च गच्छेत् सर्व्वेन्द्रियार्थोपरमस्तथैव । दशार्द्धसंख्येष्वथ विक्षतेषु सामान्यतो मर्म्मसु लिङ्गमुक्तम् ॥ सुरेन्द्रगोपप्रतिमं प्रभुतं रक्तं स्रवेत्तत्क्षतजश्च वायुः । करोति रोगान् विविधान् यथोक्तान् शिरासु छिन्नास्वथ वाक्षतासु ॥ कौब्जं शरीरावयवावसादः क्रियास्वशक्तिस्तुमुला रुजश्च । चिराद्व्रणो रोहति यस्य चापि तं स्नायुविद्धं पुरुषं व्यवस्येत् ॥

diminishes with changes in the size of the body. The face is shining as if anointed. The swelling is heavy, of a yellowish colour, and of a bad smell. It is itchy and painful, accompanied with a peculiar change in the voice. The unfavourable symptoms are difficulty in breathing, softness of the part, and after it has continued for one year, it is accompanied with dyspepsia, and hoarseness. When the person is thin and weak he will die.

Bhagandara (*Fistula-in-Ano.*)

This disease is called *Bhagandara*, because the anus, vagina, bladder, and its surrounding parts, are affected.

It is produced by deranged air, bile, and phleg by their combinations, and by external injuries: thus five varieties of this disease are produced.

The symptoms of this disease are ushered in by pain in the loins, of an itching nature, and by a swelling near the anus.

1. *Satapanaka*. This variety is produced by deranged air, from living on bad food, when accompanied by a bad temper. The swelling usually takes place a finger breadth from the

---

शोषाभिवृद्धिस्तम्मूला रुजाश्च वलक्षयः सर्व्वत एव शोथः। क्षतेषु सन्धिष्वचलाचलेषु स्यात् सर्व्वकर्म्मोपरमश्च लिङ्गम्॥ घोरा रुजो यस्य निशादिनेषु सर्व्वास्ववस्थासु च नैति शान्तिम्। भिषग्विपश्चिद्विदितार्थसूत्र स्तन्तस्थिविद्धं पुरुसं व्यवस्येत्॥ यथास्वमेतानि विभावयेच्च लिङ्गानि मर्म्मस्वभिताड़ितेषु। पाण्डुविवर्णः स्पर्शनं न वेत्ति यो मांसमर्म्मण्यभिपीड़ितः स्यात्॥ विसर्पः पक्षघातश्च शिरास्तम्भोऽपतानकः। मोहोन्मादव्रणरुजो ज्वर-स्तृष्णाऽनुग्रहः॥ कासश्छर्द्दिरतीसारो हिक्का श्वासः सवेपथः। षोड़शोपद्रवाः प्रोक्ता व्रनानां व्रणचिन्तकैः॥

anus, by the air deranging the flesh, and producing swelling and pain of different kinds. When not properly treated the swelling suppurates, and is perforated by many holes, through which a copious discharge of matter with air takes place. Sometimes the pain is as if the part was torn, or needles were thrust into it. Towards the termination air, urine, fæces, and semen is discharged from the opening.

2. *Utragraba* is produced by deranged *bile*, which affects the part, and produces a large red swelling resembling the shape of the neck of a camel. It produces a burning and painful sensation, like those produced by deranged bile. When neglected it suppurates, and terminates in ulcers. The parts feel burning, as if it was burnt with fire or caustics, and it discharges a fœtid and hot fluid. If neglected in this state the air, urine, fæces, and semen are discharged.

3. *Parisrábí* is produced by diseased *phlegm*. It is characterized by a white, hard, and itchy swelling near the anus, with the peculiar pain characteristic of diseased phlegm. If not properly treated it suppurates, and passes to ulceration.

अथ भग्ननिदानम्।

भग्नं समासाद्द्विविधं हुताश काण्डे च सन्धौ च हि तत्र सन्धौ। उत्पिष्ट विश्लिष्ट विवर्त्तितञ्च तिर्य्यग्गतं क्षिप्त मधश्च षट् च॥ प्रसारणाकुञ्चनवर्त्तनोग्रा रुक्स्पर्शविद्वेषण मेतदुक्तम्। सामान्यतः सन्धिगतस्य लिङ्गमुत्पिष्टसन्धे श्वयथुः समन्तात्॥ विशेषतो रात्रिभवा रुजा च विश्लिष्टजे तौ च रुजा च नित्यम्। विवर्त्तिते पार्श्वरुजश्च तीव्राः तिर्य्यग्गते तीव्ररुजो भवन्ति॥ क्षिप्तेऽतिशूलं विषमत्वमस्थ्नोः क्षिप्ते त्वधोरुग्विघटश्च सन्धेः।

काण्डे ततः कर्कटकाश्वकर्ण-विचूर्णितं पिच्चितमस्थिच्छल्लिका। काण्डे च भग्नं ह्यतिपातितञ्च मज्जागतञ्च स्फुटितञ्च

This is hard, itchy, and discharges freely a mucilaginous matter, followed by a discharge of air, urine, fæces, and semen.

4. *Sambúkábarta* is produced by the combination of these three humours. It appears first in the form of a swelling, like the great toe, and is accompanied with different kinds of pains. It ulcerates, as in the other kinds, and discharges different coloured fluids.

5. *Unmárga* or the accidental form of fistula-in ano. When an ignorant person eats the bones with fish, or anima-flesh, they are carried to the rectum with the hard fæces, and should they be in a transverse direction in the gut, the bones injure the parts, and produce inflammation, and ulceration Matter is then discharged mixed with blood. When this variety is not properly cleaned, worms form in it, and various openings are formed, and the air, fæces, urine, and semen are discharged from these openings. Sometimes an eruption forms round the anus which is not fistulous. The pain is slight in this disease, and is spontaneously cured. In fistula-in-ano there is much pain accompanied with fever, and the patient feels much inconvenience in walking, or riding, and at the time of the evacuations. He complains likewise of pains in the loins.

वक्रम् ॥ छिन्नं द्विधा द्वादशधापि काण्डे स्रस्ताङ्गता शोथ रुजाति-वृद्धिः। संपीड्यमाने भवतीह शब्दः स्पर्शासह स्पन्दन तोद शूलाः॥ सर्व्वास्ववस्थासु न शर्म्मलाभो भग्नस्य काण्डे खलु चिह्नमेतत्। भग्नन्तु काण्डे बहुधा प्रयाति समासतो नामभिरेव तुल्यम्॥ अल्पाशिनो नात्मवतो जन्तोर्वातात्मकस्य च। उपद्रवैर्वा जुष्टस्य भग्नं कृच्छ्रेण सिध्यति। भिन्नं कपालं कट्यान्तु सन्धियुक्तं तथा च्युतम्॥ जयनं प्रतिपिष्टञ्च वर्ज्जयेद्धि विचक्षणः। असंश्लिष्ट कपालञ्च ललाटे चूर्णितञ्च यत्। भग्नं स्तनान्तरे पृष्ठे शङ्खे मूर्द्ध्नि च वर्ज्जयेत्॥ सम्यक् सन्धितमप्यस्थि दुर्न्निक्षेपनिब-

All the forms of fistula-in-ano are cured with difficulty, more particularly when produced by a derangement of the three humours, and by accidents, as by the gut being transfixed by bones, or the like.

Sores on the genital Organs, (*Upadangsha.*)*

These diseases are supposed to be produced by mechanical injuries of the part, want of cleanliness, and washing with impure water, after sexual intercourse. It is also produced by impure connexion, excessive venery, and the stimulants sometimes employed to enlarge the penis. There are five different forms of these sores, which are distinguished from each other by their colour, and the nature of the discharge. These are :

1. *Bátika*, characterised by the black colour of the pustules (primary), by the lancinating pain, and white discharge.

2. *Paittika* is distinguished by the redness of the pustules, by the burning pain, and bloody discharge from the part.

3. *Shleshmika*. In this form the pustules is larger, and are attended with an itching sensation. The discharge is white, and thick.

न्धनात्। संक्षोभाद्वापि यद्गच्छेद्विक्रियां तच्च वर्ज्जयेत्॥ तरुनास्थीनि नामयन्ते भिद्यन्ते तलकानि च। कपालानि विभजयन्ते स्फुटन्ति रुचकानि च॥

अथ नाड़ीव्रणनिदानम्।

यः शोथमाममिति पक्वमुपेक्षतेऽज्ञो यो वा व्रणं प्रचुर पूयमसाधुवृत्तय। अभ्यन्तरं प्रविशति प्रतिदार्य्यय तस्य स्थानानि पूर्व्वविहितानि ततः सपूयः॥ तस्यातिमात्रगमनाद्गतिरिष्यते तु नाड़ीव यद्वहति तेन मता तु नाड़ी। दोषैस्त्रिभिर्भवति सा पृथगेकशस्च संमूर्च्छितैरपि च सल्यनिमित्ततोऽनया॥

---

* From *upa*, near ; and *dangsha*, biting.

4. *Sannipátika.* This is a complicated form of the disease, in which the above symptoms appear. It is considered incurable.

5. *Agantuka, or accidental injuries* of the organs of generation. In this description no secondary symptoms of syphilis are mentioned. The description is confined entirely to the primary sores. The unfavourable symptoms of this oca disease is confined to the suppuration, sloughing, and destruction of the penis, and to the generation of worms in the sores. In such cases the disease was supposed to be incurable.

It is stated that these sores should be treated by an ignorant person, or should the person continue to have intercourse with women, he will die; from the ...ing of the parts, and the irritative fever which ac...mpanies it.

Another local disease of the genitals is named *Mingubarti* (warts) and consists in excrescences near the vagina, between the scrotum and penis, or corona glandis. They appear crop after crop, and resemble a cock's comb; they are without pain, and are cured with difficulty.

तत्रानिलात् परुषसूक्ष्ममुखी सशूला फेनानुविद्धमधिकं स्रवति क्षपासु। पित्तात्तृषाज्वरकरी परिदाहयुक्ता पीतं स्रवत्यधिकमुष्णमहःसु चापि॥ ज्ञेयो कफाद्बहुघनार्ज्जुनपिच्छिलास्रा स्तब्धा सकण्डुररुजा रजनीप्रवृद्धा॥

दाहज्वरश्वसनमूर्च्छनवक्त्रशोषा यस्यां भवन्त्यभिहितानि च लक्षणानि। तामादिशेत् पवनपित्तकफोप्रकोपाद् घोरामसुंक्षय-करीमिव कालरात्रिम्॥

नष्टं कथञ्चिदनुमार्गमुदीरितेषु स्थानेषु शल्यमचिरेण गतिं करोति। सा फेनिलं मथित मूष्णमसृग्विमिश्रं स्रावं करोति सहसा सरुजा च नितरम्॥ नाड़ी त्रिदोषप्रभवा न सिद्ध्येच्छेषास्च तिस्रः खलु यत्नसाध्याः॥

History of Syphilis.

The history of Syphilis is so peculiar, and various opinions as to its origin has produced so much discussion that I shall here add a few remarks on the subject.

From the above account of these diseases of the genital organs, as given in the ancient Sanskrit writings, it appears that there were only five, or rather six, varieties of local sores to which they were liable. These are stated to have been produced by injuries, or other causes of irritation, such as want of cleanliness, &c.; which are quite sufficient to account for the varieties of these sores, and resemble those recorded by the Jews. They are quite different from the peculiar disease known by the name of syphilis, or the venereal disease. The history of this disease in Europe affords the explanation of these peculiarities.

The venereal disease, as it now appears in its characte istic local and general features, seems to have been unknown befo the return of Columbus to Spain, after the discovery of America (1494), when the sailors introduced the disease into Spain. Astruc asserts, on the authority of Oviedo, the historian, and of

---

अथ भगन्दरनिदानम्।

गुदस्य द्व्यङ्गुले क्षेत्रे पार्श्वतः पिड़कार्त्तिकृत्। [भिन्नो भगन्दरो ज्ञेयः स च पञ्चविधो मतः॥ कषाय रूक्षैरतिकोपिते-ऽनिल स्त्वपानदेशे पिड़कं करोति याम्। उपेक्षणात् पाकमुपैति दारुणं रुजा च भिन्नारुण-फेनवाहिनी॥ तत्रागमो मूत्र-पुरिष-रेतसां व्रणैरनेकैः शतपोनकं वदेत्॥

प्रकोपनैः पित्तमति प्रकोपितं करोति रक्तां पिड़कां गुदा-श्रिताम्। तदाशुपाका हिमपूतिवाहिनीं भगन्दरन्तूष्ट्रशिरोधरं वदेत्॥ कण्डुयनो घनस्रावी कठीनो मन्दवेदनः। श्वेतावभासः कफजः परिस्रावी भगन्दरः॥ बहुवर्णरुजास्रावा पीड़का गोस्त-नोपमा। शम्बुकावर्त्तवन्नाड़ी शम्बुकावर्त्तको मतः॥ क्षताद्गतिः

many contemporary physicians, who flourished a short time after that period, that the disease was communicated to the Spaniards by the Indian women of Hispaniola, when Columbus first arrived in that country ; and they, in their turn, communicated it to their country-women.

In the course of a year or two afterwards (1495) Ferdinand, king of Spain, sent an army under the command of the great Gonsalva de Cordova to the assistance of the Neapolitans, at that time engaged in a war with the French. The Spaniards infected the Neapolitans, who communicated the disease to the French. As they had not had the disease before they attributed it to the climate, and called it the "Mal de Naples." The Neapolitans, as much astonished as the French, and treating them as the hostile power, imagined that they had brought it to the country, and called it the French disease.

During such an age we can easily understand how the disease should be rapidly propagated over Europe when introduced into an army of mercinary soldiers, composed of nearly every nation of Europe, who thus conveyed

---

पायुगता विवर्द्धते ह्युपेक्षणात् सुग्रः क्रिमयो विदार्यते । प्रकुर्व्वते मार्गमनेकधा मुखै र्व्रणैस्तदुन्मार्गि भगन्दरं वदेत् ॥ घोराः साधयितुं दुःखाः सर्व्व एव भगन्दराः । तेष्वसाध्यः त्रिदोषोत्थः क्षतजश्च विशेषतः ॥ वातमूत्रपुरीषाणि क्रिमयः शुक्रमेव च । भगन्दरात् स्रवन्तस्तु नाशयन्तु तमातुरम् ॥

अथोपदंशनिदानम् ।

हस्ताभिघातान्नखदन्तपाता द्धावनादत्युपसेवनाद्वा । योनि-प्रदोषाच्च भवन्ति शिश्ने पञ्चोपदंशा विविधापचारैः ॥ सतोदभेद-स्फुरणैः सकृष्णैः स्फोटैर्व्यवस्येत् पवनोपदंशम् । पीतैर्बहुक्लेदयुतैः सदाहैः पित्तेन रक्तात् पिशितावभासैः ॥ स्फोटैः सकृष्णैः रुधिर-स्रवन्तं रक्तात्मकं पित्तसमानलिङ्गम् । सकण्डुरैः शोथयुतैर्महद्भिः

the infection with them on their return to their respective homes; and explains many circumstances related of its progress in different countries. It was from the great intercourse at that time subsisting between the French and Scots that the disease first appeared in Scotland, and it was not until a year afterwards that it appeared in England. Astruc assigns another cause in the licentious manners of the age, for the rapid spreading of the venereal disease, on its first appearance in Europe.

Soon after the appearance of the disease in Europe its ravages extended over a considerable part of Asia and Africa, as well as Europe. This is stated by Fracastorio, who flourished at the close of the fifteenth century, was an eye witness of the entensive progress of the disease; and from his high medical reputation, and residence almost on the spot of its first appearance, and more largely engaged in the cure of it than . ny physician in his day, had the best opportunities of judging of the nature af the disease. He says, that the disease fi .t appeared in central Europe and extended its ravages from France to Great Britain, where it got the name of the French disease; and still approaching towards the East, at was called "Armani danah;" from which country it extended to Persia,

---

शुक्रे घनस्रावयुतैः कफेन ॥ नानाविधस्रावरुजोपपन्न मसाध्यमाहुस्त्रिमलोपदंशम् ।

विशीर्णमांसं क्रिमिभिः प्रजग्धं मुष्कावशेषां परिवर्ज्जयेच्च ।

संजातमात्रेन करोति मुढ़ः क्रियां नरो यो विषये प्रसक्तः ॥ कालेन शोथक्रिमिदाहपाकै र्विशीर्णशिश्नो म्रियते स तेन ।

अङ्कुरैरिव संघातैरुपर्युपरि संस्थितैः । क्रमेण जायते वर्त्ति स्ताम्रचूड़शिखोपमा ॥ कोषस्याभ्यन्तरे सन्धौ पर्व्वसन्धिगतापि वा । अवेदना पिच्छिला च दुश्चिकित्सा त्रिदोषजा ॥ लिङ्गवर्त्तिरभिख्याता लिङ्गार्श इति चापरे ।

where Mir Bahaú Daula Nur Baxsh was said to have been the first who described and treated the disease. From Persia it advanced into Hindustan, where it is still known by its Persian name; Nár Fársi, Persian pox; or Jumra, blotches; or from its peculiar symptoms A, tshak, nocturnal fire; disease of foreigners, strangers, more especially of Europeans. Soon after (A. H. 950) in the time of Timur Lang, emperor of Persia, Amír Imámdin Muhammad Shirází wrote a short treatise on the venereal disease; in which he declares it to have been of recent origin, and, with the exception of Nur Baxsh is stated to have been the first who wrote correctly on the subject.

The same evidence is afforded by the Hindu writers. We have seen that the early writers gave minute and characteristic descriptions of the usual local diseases of these organs; and what is remarkable, syphilis has not got a Sanskrit name, but is named from the Europeans, who first visited these shores. This was more readily adopted, as the presence of the disease conveyed a feeling of disgust and reproach. It is in the modern Sanskrit compilations, such as *Bhábaprakása*, where the disease is named the "*Faringí Roga*," or Portuguese disease.

अथ शूकदोषनिदानम् ।

अक्रमाच्छेफसो वृद्धिं योभिवाञ्छति मूढ़धीः । व्याधय स्तस्य जायन्ते दश चाष्टौ च शूकजाः ॥ गौरसर्षपसंस्थाना शूकदुर्भुक्त-हेतुका । पिड़का श्लेष्मवाताभ्यां ज्ञेया सर्षपिका तु सा, कठिनै र्विषमैर्भुग्नै र्वायुना ष्ठीलिका भवेत् ॥ शूकै र्यत् पूरितं शश्वद्ग्रथितं नाम तत् कफात् । कुम्भिका रक्तपित्तोत्था जाम्ववास्थिनिभा शुभा तुलग्रजास्तु लजीं विद्याद् यथाप्रोक्तां विचक्षणः ॥ मृदितं पीड़ितं यच्च संरब्धं वातकोपतः । पाणिभ्यां भृशसंमूढ़े संमूढ़पिड़का भवेत् ॥ दीर्घा वह्वश्च पिड़का दीर्यन्ते मध्यतस्तु याः ॥ सोऽधि-

In this work the disease is characterized by all the symptoms of secondary syphilis, as detailed by European authors; such as cutaneous eruptions, and affections of the bones, particularly those of the nose and palate. In these modern works syphilis is divided into three varieties; one of which is characterized by the appearance of cutaneous eruptions, the second by diseases of the bones; and in the third variety both the skin and bones are affected. The disease is attributed to connection with the Portuguese, whether male or female, and it was supposed that it could only be cured by the use of mercury. The same author likewise states that after the mercurial treatment has been completed, *Topchiní*, or China-root, must be administered to complete the cure.

We have thus a disease presenting characteristic appearances, and of peculiar virulence, without a Sanskrit name—not even mentioned by the ancient Hindu medical writers; and still called by the name of the people who first visite these shores from Europe. But as the disease was also introduced into Hindustan from the south-east by the Portuguese,

---

मन्थः कफासृग्भवां वेदना रोमहर्षकृत्। पिड़काचिता या पिड़का पित्तशोणितसम्भवा॥ पद्मकर्णिकसंस्थाना ज्ञेया पुष्करिका तु सा।

स्पर्शहानिस्तु जनयेच्छोनितं शूकदूषितम्। मुद्गमाषोपमा रक्ता रक्तपित्तोद्भवा तु या॥ व्याधिरेषोत्तमा नाम शूकाजीर्णनिमित्ततः। छिद्रैरनुमुखै लिङ्गं चितं यस्य समन्ततः॥ वातशोणितजो व्याधिः स ज्ञेयः शतपोणकः। वातपित्तकृतो ज्ञेय स्त्वक्पाको ज्वरदाहकृत्॥ कृष्णैः स्फोटैः सरक्ताभिः पिड़काभिर्निपीड़ितम्। यस्य वास्तु रुजश्चोग्रा ज्ञेयं तच्छोणितार्बुदम्॥ मांसदोषेण जानीयादर्बुदं मांससम्भवम्। शीर्यन्ते यस्य मांसानि यस्य सर्वाश्च वेदनाः॥ विद्यात्तं मांसपाकन्तु सर्वदोषाकृतिं भिषक्॥

is was called the Portuguese or European (*faringhí*) disease; and likewise from Persia in the north-west, when the disease was named the "Persian pox." It was only after the disease was introduced from the north and south of Hindustan, that an account is recorded of the characteristic disease, by modern compilers, including both the local and constitutional symptoms. Hence it would appear that this disease was introduced from America to Europe and Asia, as the small-pox and measles seem to have first appeared in Asia, from whence they spread, and committed such ravages in Africa, Europe, and America.

The following proofs may be thus adduced of the venereal disease having been brought from America :—

1st. The opinion of ancient authors who have left us minute descriptions of disease, such as *Moses*, *Charaka*, *Sushruta*, *Hippocrates*, *Celsus*, &c., not having mentioned the venereal disease. Local sores on the genitals, and even the occurrence of buboes, &c. being no proof of the presence of this disease, without its specific secondary symptoms. Any irritating cause applied to the genitals would produce local

---

विद्रधिं सन्निपातेन यथोक्तमपि निर्द्दिशेत्। कृष्णानि चित्रा-ण्यथवा सूकानि सविषाणि वा॥ पाचितानि पचन्त्याशु मेढ्रं निरवशेषतः। कालानि भूत्वा मांसानि शीर्य्यन्ते यस्य देहिनः॥ सन्निपातसमुत्थांस्तु तान् विद्यात्तिलकालकान्। तत्र मांसार्ब्बुदं यच्च मांसपाकश्च यः स्मृतः॥ विद्रधिश्च न सिद्ध्यन्ति ये च स्यु स्तिलकालकाः।

अथ कुष्ठनिदानम्।

विरोधीन्यन्नपानानि द्रवस्निग्धगुरूणि च। भजता मागतां छर्द्दिं वेगां श्चान्यान् प्रतिघ्नताम्॥ व्यायाममतिसन्ताप मतिभुक्त्वा निषेविणाम्। घर्म्मश्रमभयार्त्तानां द्रुतं शीताम्बुसेविणाम्॥ अजीर्णाध्यशिनाञ्चैव पञ्चकर्म्मापचारिणाम्। नवान्नदधि

sores, and if not properly attended to would inflame the inguinal glands; as sores on the feet are often found to produce the same swellings.

2nd. The consternation into which all Europe was thrown by the rapid progress of this fearful disease. Like all new diseases, soon after its introduction into Europe, by the followers of Columbus, it spread in the most alarming manner; or like that leprosy from the east, which at one time filled the Lazar-houses of Europe with its victims. Masses, prayers, and alms, were offered up to avert the anger of offended heaven; as the superstitious notions of the age made people believe that it was a dispensation from God, to correct the licentious, and wicked manners of the times. The severity of a new disease when it occurs in a country is seen in the visits of the small-pox, to islands, and distant countries; as occurred in the Mauritius, and committed such dreadful ravages at first, and slowly appeared to wear itself out. Such was the case with Syphilis when it first appeared in Europe, compared with the mittigated symptoms of the present times. This is certainly in part

---

मत्स्याति-लवणाश्च निषेविनाम् ॥ माषमूलकपिष्टान्नतिल-क्षीर-गुड़ाशिनाम् । व्यवायञ्चाप्यजीर्णेऽन्ने निद्राञ्च भजतां दिवा ॥ विप्रान् गुरुन् धर्षयतां पापं कर्म्म च कुर्व्वताम् ।

वातादयस्त्रयो दुष्टा स्त्वग्रक्तं मांसमम्बु च । दूषयन्ति स कुष्ठानां सप्तको द्रव्यसंग्रहः अतः कुष्ठानि जायन्ते सप्त चैकादशैव च । कुष्ठानि सप्तधा दोषैः पृथग् द्वन्द्वैः समागतैः ॥ सर्व्वेष्वपि त्रिदोषेषु व्यपदेशोऽधिकस्ततः । अतिश्लक्ष्णखरस्पर्शस्वेदास्वेद विवर्णताः ॥ दाहः कण्डु स्त्वचिस्वापस्तोदः कोठोऽरतिर्भ्रमः । व्रणानामधिकं शूलं शीघ्रोत्पत्तिश्चिरस्थितिः ॥ रूढ़ानामपि रूक्षत्वं निमित्तेऽल्पेऽपि कोपनम् । रोमहर्षोऽसृजः कार्ष्ण्यं कुष्ठ-लक्षणमग्रजम् ॥

owing to our following a better plan of treatment, but still more to this disease being of a less virulent nature than before.

3rd. The progress of the syphilitic disease indicates that it was first brought to Spain, from whence it spread over Europe, Africa, and Asia.

4th. The analogy of other diseases prove that new diseases may so appear, and spread as the small-pox, measles, &c. from Asia; and perhaps the croup and sweating sickness of Britain, &c.

Paribarttiká—Phymosis. This disease is produced by pressure, or external injuries, by which the prepuce is swollen by the diseased air, and covers the glans. When it remains swollen, hard, and very painful, the inflammation sometimes passes to suppuration.

Abapátiká—Pariphymosis. When much force is used during connection with a young girl, or when the prepuce is forced back with force, it remains there, and is followed with much swelling and pain.

Another variety of the above disease is called *Niruddaprakasha*, or stricture, or diminution of the urethra. In some

---

कृष्णारुणकपालाभं यद्रूक्षं परुषं तनु। कापालं तोदबहुलं तत् कुष्ठं विषमं स्मृतम्॥ रुग्दाहरागकण्डूभिः परीतं रोमपिञ्जरम्। उडुम्बरफलाभासं कुष्ठमौडुम्बरं वदेत्॥ श्वेतं रक्तं स्थिरं स्त्यानं स्निग्धमुत्सन्नमण्डलम्। कृच्छ्रमन्योन्यसंयुक्तं कुष्ठं मण्डलमुच्यते॥ कर्कशं रक्तपर्यन्तमन्तःश्यावं सवेदनम्। यदृष्यजिह्वसंस्थानमृष्यजिह्वं तदुच्यते॥ सश्वेतं रक्तपर्यन्तं पुण्डरीकदलोपमम्। सोत्सेधञ्च सरागञ्च पुण्डरीकं तदुच्यते॥ श्वेतं ताम्रं तनु च यद्रजो घृष्टं विमुञ्चति। प्रायश्चोरसि तत् सिध्ममलाबुकुसुमोपमम्॥

cases this is produced by an adhesion of the prepuce to the glans, impeding the passage of the urine, which in some cases only passes in drops.

Shúkadosha, inflammation of the penis, is produced by the pernicious habit of applying stimulants to enlarge the organ. There are eighteen forms of this disease, *Sarshápiká*, *Ashthíliká*, *Grathita*, *Kumbhíká*, *Aladí*, *Mridita*, *Sammúrhapiraka*, *Abamantha*, *Pushkariká* *Sparshaháni*, *Uttamá*, *Shatápínaka*, *Twakapáka*, *Sanitárbudá*, *Mángsapáka*, *Bidradhi*, *Tilakálaka*, *Mángsárbuda*, &c.

Sarshápiká are small pimples, like mustard seed round the penis, which are produced by the presence of a kind of insect, which is sometimes applied to the part with the intention of increasing the size of the organ.

The other forms of inflammation are produced by the application of other stimulants which cause inflammation of a chronic or acute form. Sometimes abscess and mortification of the part occur so as sometimes to destroy the penis. The other varieties are merely modifications of these inflammations, and their terminations.

यत् काकणन्तिकावर्णं सपाकं तीव्रवेदनम्। त्रिदोषलिङ्गं तत् कुष्ठं काकणं नैव सिध्यति। अस्वेदनं महावास्तु यन्मत्स्यशकलोपमम्। तदेककुष्ठं चर्म्माख्यं बहलं हस्तिचर्म्मवत्। श्यावं किण-खरस्पर्शं परुषं किटिमं स्मृतम्। वैपादिकं पाणिपादस्फुटनं तीव्रवेदनम् कण्डुमद्भिः सरागैश्च गण्डैरलसकं चितम्। सकण्डुरागपिड़कं दद्रुमण्डलमुद्गतम्। रक्तं सशूलं कण्डुमत् सस्फोटं यद् गलत्यपि। तच्चर्म्मदलमाख्यातं संस्पर्शासह मुच्यते। सूक्ष्मावह्वः पिड़काः स्राववत्यः पामेत्युक्ताः कण्डुमत्यः सदाहाः। सैव स्फोटैस्तीव्रदाहैरुपेता ज्ञेया पाण्योः कच्छुरुग्रा स्फिचोश्च॥ स्फोटाः श्यावारुणाभासा विस्फोटाः स्युस्तनुत्वचः। रक्तं श्यावं

Leprosy, *(Kushtha or Kuth.)*

This disease is the most aggravated af all that afflict the body, and when a person dies with it the Hindus believe that the person will be afflicted with it in the next life, unless he performs the *práschitta*, penance. This penance consists of abstinence for a day, shaving the whole hair off the head, presents of a certain number of cowries and other articles to the bráhmans, who perform certain prayers, and to whom the person confesses his sins. This ceremony is now generally performed before entering upon the treatment of any supposed dangerous disease.

The Hindus distinguish three kinds of Leprosy, the black, white, and red varieties, which are produced by various causes. Sometimes the disease is caused by bad air, and drink ; eating substances which do not assimilate, as milk and fish, food of a rancid, salt, and indigestable nature ; or thin oleaginous food : when the person eats immoderately of such food, for some time, it will produce this disease. In other cases irregularity in eating and fasting, mental agitation, violent exercise, exposure

---

सदाहार्त्तिः शतारुः स्याद्बहुव्रनम्। सकण्डुपिड़काः श्यावा बहु-स्रावा विचर्च्चिकाः॥

खरं श्यावारुणं रूक्षं वातकुष्ठं सवेदनम्। पित्तात् प्रकुपितं दाहरागस्रावान्वितं मतम्॥ कफात् क्लेदिघनं स्निग्धं सकण्डु शैत्यगौरवम्। द्विलिङ्गं द्वन्द्वजं कुष्ठं त्रिलिङ्गं सान्निपातिकम्। त्वकस्थे वैवर्ण्यमङ्गेषु कुष्ठे रौक्ष्यञ्च जायते। त्वक्स्वापो रोमहर्षश्च स्वेदस्यातिप्रवर्त्तनम्। कण्डु विपुयकश्चैव कुष्ठे शोणितसंश्रिते। बाहल्यं वक्त्रशोषश्च कार्कश्यं पिड़कोद्गमः। तोदः स्फोटः स्थिरत्वञ्च कुष्ठे मांससमाश्रिते। कौण्यं गतिक्षयोऽङ्गानां संभेदः क्षतसर्पणम्। मेदःस्थानगते लिङ्गं प्रागुक्तानि तथैव च। नासाभङ्गोऽक्षिरागश्च

to fatigue, or too great heat, especially after a full meal; night watching with exposure to the night air, using new rice, milk, curds, fish, and the too frequent use of pulse, radishes, sesaman and treacle, produce leprosy. In others it is produced by checking natural evacuations, or suppressing them when artificially excited; such as vomiting or the expulsion of air, urine or dejections, or the irregularity and alternate use of hot and cold applications. Sometimes it is produced from eating hot or cold articles of food, first at dinner, or after fasting, when the usual food is not eaten, after much perspiration, fatigue, or fear, or when the person bathes or drinks cold water at improper times. In other cases the disease is produced when the food is not digested, or when time has not been given for this purpose, before more is taken into the stomach; when after the use of emetics and purgatives, the usual simple food, &c. is not employed; when the person sleeps during the day with a loaded stomach; or when he visits his wife before the food is digested. The blood and seminal secretions of parents when tainted by leprosy, affects their offspring. Lepers in one life, are born again with the complaint; and the disease is

---

क्षतेषु क्रिमिसम्भवः। स्वरोपघातश्च भवेदस्थिमज्जसमाश्रिते। दम्पतोः कुष्ठवाहुल्याद् दुष्टशोणितशुक्रयोः। यदपत्यं तयोर्जातं ज्ञेयं तदपि कुष्ठितम्॥

साध्यं त्वग्रक्तमांसस्थं वातश्लेष्माधिकञ्च यत्। मेदसि द्वन्द्वजं याप्यं वर्ज्ज्यं मज्जास्थिसंश्रितम्। क्रिमितृड्दाहमन्दाग्निसंयुक्तं यत् त्रिदोषजम्। प्रभिन्नं प्रस्रुताङ्गञ्च रक्तनेत्रं हतस्वरम्। पञ्चकर्म्मगुणातीतं कुष्ठं हन्तीह मानवम्।

वातेन कुष्ठं कापालं पित्तेनौड़ुम्बरं कफात्। मण्डलाख्यं विचर्च्चीं च ऋष्याख्यं वातपित्तजं। चर्म्मैककुष्ठं किठिमं सिध्मालसविपादिकाः। वातश्लेष्मोद्भवाः श्लेष्मपित्ताद्दद्रुशतारुषी। पुण्ड-

supposed to be communicable by contact, by breathing the same air, by eating together, by wearing the clothes, or ornaments, of a person labouring under the disease. Whoever speaks disrespectfully or does any other improper action, or commits sins against his *guru* or *bipra* (pandit bráhman); such as, committing adultery with a bráhman's wife, killing a good man, and robbing a person of his estate, will be liable to be afflicted with this disease. Such causes derange air, bile, and phlegm, by which the skin, blood, flesh, and watery parts of the blood (*ambu*) are deranged, and produce the eighteen forms of leprosy: of these seven are severe, and eleven are mild.

Before leprosy appears the skin becomes glossy, thin, and rough, and of an unnatural colour; there is much perspiration, or a suppression of it, itchiness and occasional horripilation; the body feels hot, parts of the surface become insensible, and the blood in the veins becomes blacker than usual, while other parts of the surface become discoloured, painful, swell quickly, remain so for a long time, and slowly heal. In such a person any injury turns to a sore, is very painful, heals with great difficulty, and a rough cicatrix is left. The person has fits of

---

रीकं सविस्फोटं पामाचर्म्मदलं तथा। सर्व्वैः स्यात् काकणं पूर्व्वत्रिकं दद्रुसकाकणम्। पुण्डरीकर्षजिह्वा च महाकुष्ठानि सप्त तु।

कुष्ठैकसम्भवं श्वित्रं किलासं वारुणं भवेत्। निर्द्दिष्टम परिस्रावि त्रिधातुद्भवसंश्रयम्। वाताद्रुक्षारुणं पित्तात्ताम्रं कमलपत्रवत्। सदाहं रोमविध्वंसि कफाच्छ्वेतं घनं गुरु। सकण्डुरं क्रमाद्रक्तमांसमेदःसु चादिशेत्। वर्णनैवेदृगुभयं कृच्छ्रं तच्चोत्तरोत्तरम्। अशुक्लरोमबहुल मसंश्लिष्टं मिथो नवम्। अनग्नि दग्धजं साध्यं श्वित्रं वर्ज्जमतोऽन्यथा। गुह्यपाणितलौष्ठेषु जातमप्यचिरन्तनम्। वर्ज्जनीयं विशेषेण क्रिलासं सिद्धिमिच्छता।

giddiness, with impaired, or an irregular state of the appetite. The seven severe forms of leprosy are produced by deranged air, bile, or phlegm: they are thus described.

1. *Sidhma,* is produced by deranged phlegm and air, and is characterized by small, white, coppery, or red spots, which spread over large surfaces accompanied with a thin mealy dust. This is the Lepra Vulgaris, or L. Alphos.

2. *Audumbará.* In this form the blotches are livid, and resemble the ripe fig, or Ficus glomerata. This form is accompanied with much pain, and a burning on the surface. The hair becomes tawny; and the morbid humour is bile.

3. *Rishwajihwa*; the patches of tubercles, are shaped like the tongue of a bear; hard and red round their edges, dark in the centre and are accompanied with severe pain. This form is produced by a derangement of the air, and bile.

4. *Kapala*; is covered with black and purplish patches resembling the broken pieces of a black earthen vessel. These blotches are irregular, hard, and dry, and are accompanied with pricking and pain. The *air* is the humour principally affected.

5. *Kákanaka,* resembles the seed of *kunch* (Abrus precatorius), with red and black spots in the centre. The blotches

---

प्रसङ्गाद्गात्रसंस्पर्शान्निःश्वासात् सह भोजनात्। एकशय्यासनाच्चैव वस्त्रमाल्यानुलेपनात्। कुष्ठं ज्वरश्च शोषश्च नेत्राभिष्यन्द एव च। औपसर्गिकरोगाश्च संक्रामन्ति नरान्नरम्।

अथ शीतपित्तोदर्द्दकोठनिदानम्।

शीतमारुतसंस्पर्शात् प्रदुष्टौ कफमारुतौ। पित्तेन सह सम्भुय वहिरन्तर्विसर्पतः। पिपासारुचिहृल्लासदेहसादाङ्गगौरवं। रक्तलोचनता तेषां पूर्व्वरूपस्य लक्षणम्। वरटीदंष्ट्रसंस्थानः शोथः संजायते वहिः। सकण्डुतोदवहुलश्छर्द्दिज्वर-

are extremely painful, and often terminate in suppuration. The three humours are deranged in this variety; which is incurable.

6. *Pundarika.* The patches in this variety are pale red in the centre, with dark dull red edges, and resemble the petals of the lotus, when exposed to the sun. This variety is produced by derangements of the phlegm and bile.

7. *Dadrukushtha.* The patches in this variety are elevated, black, round, and spreading; there are many sorts, which are accompanied with much itching, burning, and pain; and are produced by derangements of the phlegm, and bile. These are the general symptoms of the severe forms of leprosy.

The slighter varieties of leprosy, *Kshudra,* are according to *Sushruta* as follows:

1. *Sthalâruska.*	2. *Mahâkushtha.*	3. *Ekshyukushtha.*
4. *Charmadala.*	5. *Bisarpa.*	6. *Parisarpa.*
7. *Sidhma.*	8. *Bicharchikâ.*	9. *Kitima.*
10. *Pâmâ.*	11. *Rakashâ.*	

Charaka has the following arrangement.

विदाहवान्। उदर्द्दमिति तं विद्याच्छीतपित्त मथापरे। वाताधिकं शीतपित्तमुदर्द्दश्च कफाधिकः। सोतसङ्गैश्च सरागैश्च कण्डुमद्भिश्च मण्डलैः। शैशिरः कफजो व्याधि रुदर्द्द इति कीर्त्तितः।

असम्यग्वमनोदीर्णपित्तश्लेष्मान्ननिग्रहैः। मण्डलानि सकण्डुनि रागवन्ति वहूनि च। उतकोठः सानुवन्धश्च कोठ इत्यभिधीयते।

अथ अम्लपित्तनिदानम्।

विरुद्धदुष्टाम्लविदाहि पित्तप्रकोपि पानान्नभुजो विदग्धम्। पित्तं स्वहेतुपचितं पुरा मत्तदम्लपित्तं प्रवदन्ति सन्तः। अविपाकक्लमोत्क्लेशतिक्ताम्लोद्गारगौरवैः। हृत्कण्ठदाहारुचिभिश्चाम्लपित्तं वदेद्भिषक्।

1. When there is no perspiration, and the patches are very large, and of a dark brown colour, and oblong, like the scales of fish, and rough like an elephant's skin, it is called *ekakushtha*, (Ichthyasis).

2. When it has patches of a dark yellow colour, like the cicatrices of healed ulcers, with a hardness and roughness of the part, it is called *kitima*.

3. When sores and chaps form in the hands and feet, about the nails, accompanied with small tubercles of a red colour, much pain, and itching, it is called *vaipádiká*.

4. When the tubercles are large, of a red colour, and very itchy, they are called *álásaka*.

5. Should the patches be of a slightly dark redish colour, itchy, spreading, and elevated into tubercles, it is called *dadrumanala*.

6. When the spots are of a red colour, with severe pain, and itchiness, the blotches are very sensible, ripen soon, and much matter is discharged, it is called *charmadala*.

तृड्दाहमूर्च्छाभ्रममोहकारि प्रयात्यधो वा विविधप्रकारम्। हृल्लासकोठानलसादहर्ष-स्वेदाङ्गपीतत्वकरं कदाचित्। वान्तं हरितं पीतकनीलकृष्णमारक्तरक्ताभमतीव चाम्लं मांसोदकाभं त्वतिपिच्छिलाच्छं श्लेष्मानुजातं विविधं रसेन। भुक्ते विदग्धे त्वथवाप्यभुक्ते करोति तिक्ताम्लवमिं कदाचित्। उद्गारमेवं विधमेव कण्ठहृत्कुक्षिदाहं शिरसो रुजं वा। करचरणदाहमौष्ण्यं महतीमरुचिं ज्वरञ्च। कफपित्तं जनयति कण्डुमण्डलपिड़काशतनिचितगात्ररोगनिचयम्।

रोगोऽयमम्लपित्ताख्यो यत्नात् संसाध्यते नवः। चिरोत्थितो भवेत्द्याप्यः कृच्छ्रसाध्यः स कस्यचित्॥ सानिलं सानिलकफं सकफं तच्च लक्षयेत्। दोषलिङ्गेन मतिमान् भिषङ्मोहकरं हि

7. Small tubercles in great numbers, of a black or purplish hue, with a copious bloody discharge, accompanied with burning, and itching, it is called *pámá.*

8. When the eruptions are merely larger than the last, and are accompanied with much pain in the palms of the hands, or buttocks, it is called *kachchhú.*

9. When the eruptions are of a dark yellow or red colour, and the skin is dry and thin, the variety is called *bishphotha.*

10. Another form has yellow, or dark redish coloured blotches, accompanied with much heat and pain, and numerous itchy tubercles: it is called *sotárush.*

11. When the tubercles are small numerous and itchy, of a dark yellow colour, and discharge much ichor, blood, &c., the variety is called *bicharchiká.* The four first varieties are supposed to be produced by derangements of the *air* and *phlegm*; and the seven last by derangements of the *bile* and *phlegm.*

When leprosy is in the *skin,* its colour is unnatural, rough, dry, and insensible; and the hairs on the body are generally

---

तत् ॥ कम्पप्रलापमूर्च्छा चिमिचिमिगात्रावसादशूलानि । तमसो दर्शन विभ्रमो प्रमोह हर्षाणामनिलकोपात् ॥ कफनिष्ठीवन गौरवः जड़तारुचि शीतसाद वमिलेपाः ॥ दहनवलसाद कण्डु निद्राचिह्नं कफानुगते । उभय मिद मेव चिह्नं मारुतकफसम्भवे भवतमले ॥ तिक्ताम्ल कटुकोद्गार हृत् कुचि कण्ठदाहक्तत् । भ्रममूर्च्छारुचि च्छर्द्दि रालस्यञ्च शिरोरुजा । प्रसेको मुखमाधुर्यं श्लेष्मपित्तस्य लक्षणम् ॥

अथ विसर्पनिदानम् ।

लवनाम्लकटुष्णादिसंसेवाद्दोषकोपतः । विसर्पः सप्तधा ज्ञेयः सर्व्वतः परिसर्पनात् । पृथक् त्रयस्त्रिभिश्चैको विसर्पा द्वन्द्वजास्त्रयः ।

erected, and the person perspires freely. When *blood* is deranged the body becomes itchy with fetor, and the skin is hard, and pus is discharged.

When *flesh* is diseased it is called *gajacharma* (Ichthyasis Simplex) ; the mouth is often parched, perspiration is defective, the surface of the body is rough, is like the scales of fish, and eruptions form over the body, with pain. Patches of vesicles sometimes form, and terminate in ulcers, which remain for long periods.

When *fat* is affected the hands and feet become stiff, immoveable, and ulcerated, and drop off, with severe pain ; the sores pass from one part of the body to another, and the symptoms of diseased flesh appear also in this form.

When the *bones* and *marrow* are leprous, the nose falls in, the eyes become red, and worms breed in the sores. The voice becomes unnatural, and hoarse. When the leprosy is in the skin, blood, or flesh, or in the air or phlegm, it may be cured. When in the fat, with two of the humours deranged, as air and phlegm, or air and bile, the person will not be cured,

---

वातिकः पैत्तिकश्चैव कफजः सांन्निपातिकः। चत्वार एते विसर्पा वच्यन्ते द्वन्दजास्त्रयः। आग्नेयो वातपित्ताभ्यां ग्रन्थ्याख्यः कफवातजः। यस्तु कर्द्दमको घोरः स पित्तकफसम्भवः। रक्तं लसीका त्वङ्मांसं दूष्यं दोषास्त्रयो मलाः। विसर्पाणां समुत्पत्तौ विज्ञेयाः सप्त धातवः।

तत्र वातात् स विसर्पो वातज्वरसमव्यथः। शोफस्फुरणनिस्तोद भेदायासार्त्ति हर्षवान्। पित्ताद् द्रुतगतिः पित्तज्वरलिङ्गोऽतिलोहितः। कफात् कण्डुयुतः स्निग्धः कफज्वरसमानरुक्। सन्निपातसमुत्थश्च सर्व्वलिङ्गसमन्वितः।

वातपित्ताज्वरच्छर्द्दिमूर्च्छातीसारतृड्भ्रमैः। ग्रन्थिभेदाग्नि सदनतमकारोचकैर्युतः। करोति सर्व्वमङ्गञ्च दीप्ताङ्गारावकीर्णवत्।

nor will it soon destroy the individual. When the bones and marrow are affected and two or three humours are viciated, one of them being the bile, it is incurable.

Fatal symptoms of leprosy occur with worms in the sores, or with the painful disease of the heart (Angina pectoris); with dyspepsia, or with symptoms of diseased air, bile, and phlegm; with sores which discharge copiously; with inflamed eyes, the voice hoarse, and altered, and with weakness so that the person is not able to bear the employment of the five forms of medicine, as purgatives, emetics, &c.

The white, and the red leprosy (*shitra* and *kilása*), are distinguished from the black leprosy by their not being accompanied with any discharge, and only affecting the skin. *charaka* adds, that they sometimes affect the *skin*, *blood*, *phlegm* and *fat*.

When the white leprosy is not produced by burns, and when the hair is not white but remains of the natural colour over the white patches; when the patches are not large and do not join each other, and when recent, the disease may be cured. When produced by burns, and the above symptoms are absent, these kinds of white leprosy are incurable.

यं यं देशं विसर्पश्च विसर्पति भवेत् स सः। शान्ताङ्गारासितो नीलो रक्तो वाशु च चीयते। अग्निदग्ध इव स्फोटैः शीघ्रगतया द्रुतं स च। मर्म्मानुसारी विसर्पः स्याद्वातोऽतिबलस्ततः। व्यथेताङ्गं हरेत् संज्ञां निद्राञ्च श्वासमीरयेत्। हिक्काञ्च सगतोऽवस्थामीदृशीं लभते न ना। क्वचिच्छर्म्मारतिग्रस्तो भूमिशय्यासनादिषु। चेष्टमान स्ततः क्लिष्टो मनोदेहसमुद्भवान्। दुष्प्रबोधोऽश्नुते निद्रां सोऽग्निवीसर्प उच्यते। कफेन रुद्धः पवनो भिन्नं तं बहुधा कफम्। रक्तं वा वृद्धरक्तस्य त्वक्शिरास्नायुमांसगम्। दूषयित्वा तु दीर्घानुवृत्त स्थूलखरात्मनाम्। ग्रन्थीनां कुरुते मालां सरक्तां

When situated about the external genitals, palms of the hands, or lips, the white leprosy is incurable although recent.

The leprosy, with fever, and the drying up or emaciation of the body, and other symptoms of pulmonary consumption (*shosha*) ; a variety of Ophthalmia (*Netrábhishyanda*), and those diseases produced by the influence of the planets, such as small-pox, &c. are contagious.

Urticaria ? (*Sitapita.*)

This disease is called *Sitapita* or *Udordah*, and another form is named *Khatah.* The disease is produced by cold air applied to the body, which deranges the *phlegm*, *air*, and *bile.* These move about on the surface, and within the body, producing thirst, redness of the eyes, nausea, and cause loss of appetite. The body becomes heavy, and the person incapable of work. The disease appears with slight swellings in different parts of the body ; like the sting of the wasp. The part is at first itchy and then very painful, with vomiting, fever, and heat of the body. When the air is much diseased,

---

तीव्ररुग्ज्वराम्। श्वासकासातीसारास्य शोषहिक्कावमिभ्रमैः।
मोहवैवर्ण्य मूर्च्छाङ्गभङ्गाग्निसदनैर्युताम्। इतरं ग्रन्थिवीसर्पः
कफमारुतकोपजः।

कफपित्ताज्ज्वरस्तम्भो निद्रातन्द्राशिरोरुजा। अङ्गावसादविक्षेपौ प्रलेपारोचक भ्रमाः। मूर्च्छाग्निहानिर्भेदोऽस्थ्नां पिपासेन्द्रिय-गौरवम्। आमोपवेशनं लेपः स्रोतसां स च सर्पति। प्रायेणामाशयं गृह्णन्नेकदेशं न चातिरुक्। पीडकैरवकीर्णोऽतिपीतलोहितपाण्डुरैः। स्निग्धोऽसितो मेचकाभो मलिनः शोथवान् गुरुः। गम्भीरपाकः प्राज्योष्मा स्पृष्टः क्लिन्नोऽवदीर्यते। पङ्कवच्छीर्णमांसश्च स्पष्टस्नायुशिरागणः। शवगन्धी च वीसर्पः कर्दमाख्यमुशन्ति तम्।

beyond the other humours it is called *Sitapita*; and when phlegm is much deranged, producing red circles, accompanied with itching, it is called *Udordah.*

It is called *Khata*, when the stomach is deranged. This is more liable to occur if at the commencement the stomach has not been properly cleared by emetics, and when bile and phlegm are deranged. If in such a case an ignorant person does not promote vomiting, but endeavours to cure the deranged *bile* and *phlegm*, the disease will be aggravated. In such cases the body is covered with large and small circular patches which are itchy, elevated, and have a red colour. They appear and disappear on different parts of the body. This form of the disease will also be produced by repressing vomiting when nature is endeavouring to relieve herself of the contents of the stomach.

Acidity of Stomach, Vomiting of Bile, (*Amlapitta.*)

This disease is produced by improper mixtures of food, by bad water, or articles that derange the bile, which is collected, and is discharged producing this disease. It is characterized

---

बाह्यहेतोः क्षतात् क्रुद्धः सरक्तं पित्तमीरयन्। विसर्पं मारुतः कुर्य्यात् कुलत्थसदृशैश्चितम्। स्फोटैः शोथज्वररुजादाहाढ्यं श्यावशोणितम्। ज्वरातीसारौवमथुस्तृड् मांसदरणं क्लमाः। आरोचका विपाकौ च विसर्पाणा मुपद्रवाः। सिद्ध्यन्ति वातकफपित्तकृता विसर्पाः सर्व्वात्मकः क्षतकृतश्च न सिद्धिमेति। पित्तात्मकोऽञ्जन वपुश्च भवेदसाध्यः कृच्छ्राश्च मर्म्मसु भवन्ति हि सर्व्व एव।

अथ विस्फोटनिदानम्।

कट्वम्लतीक्ष्णोष्ण-विदाहिरूक्ष-क्षारैरजीर्णाध्यशनातपैश्च। तथर्त्तुदोषेण विपर्य्ययेण कुप्यन्ति दोषाः पवनादयस्तु। त्वच,माश्रित्य

by dyspepsia, languor, nausea, sour and bitter eructations, and the body is heavy, with burning of the breast and throat. The person has no appetite, is thirsty, complains of syncopy, and the head turns round. A dulness of the intellect may be observed, and the fæces are various in appearance, and hot. The internal heat and pain of body diminishes, and the person sometimes vomits green, yellow, and blue matter. Sometimes it is like blood, and is very sour ; sometimes it is like phlegm, or the washings of flesh, or has a mucilaginous appearance. In other cases jaundice is produced with free perspiration, and the body is of a yellow colour. When phlegm and bile are diseased, the abdomen is very hot when any thing is eaten, and if nothing is taken, the vomited matter and eructations are bitter and sour. The neck, chest, and sides are hot ; there is head-ache, and the hands and feet are burning. The person has a disgust for food, is feverish, and itchy eruptions, and patches appear over the body.

If this disease be recent it may be cured with difficulty ; and if old, it will often be incurable. There are three forms of the disease : when air or phlem are deranged ; when air and

---

ते रक्तमांसास्थीनि प्रदुष्य च। घोरान् कुर्व्वन्ति विस्फोटान् सर्व्वान् ज्वर पुरःसरान्। अग्निदग्धनिभाः स्फोटाः सज्वरारक्तपिज जाः। क्वचित् सर्व्वत्र वा देहे विष्फोटक इति स्मृतः।

शिरोरुक् शूल भूयिष्ठं ज्वर स्तट् पर्व्वभेदनम्। सकृष्णवर्णता चेति वातविष्फोटलक्षणम्। ज्वरदाहरुजास्रावपाकतृष्णाभिरन्वितम्। पीतलोहितवर्णश्च पित्तविष्फोटलक्षणम्। छर्द्द्यरोचकजाड्यानि कण्डुकाठिन्यपाण्डुताः। आवेदनश्चिरात् पाकी स विष्फोटः कफात्मकः। वातपित्तकृतो यस्तु कुरुते तीव्रवेदनाम्। कण्डुस्तैमित्य गुरुभि र्जानीयात् कफवातिकम्। कण्डुर्दाहोज्वरश्छर्द्दिरेतैस्तु कफपैत्तिकः। मध्ये निम्नोन्नतोऽन्ते च

phlegm; or when phlegm alone is deranged, which will be distinguished by the experienced physician.

When *air* is diseased the person speaks foolishly, is affected with syncopy, and his body is languid, with slight uneasiness and pain. The room he is in appears dark; in other cases he is still, is always forgetting, and complains of severe pain of the body.

Phlegm. In this form phlegm is always discharged from the mouth, the body feels heavy, the person is languid, has no appetite, the body is cold, and the person is lazy and vomits. The surface of the body feels as if it was rubbed with something, it is itchy, the patient looses his appetite, and he takes much sleep.

When air and phlegm are deranged in one place, the symptoms of the two above forms of disease are present.

Erysipelas, Carbuncle? (*Bisharpa*).

When *air, bile* and *phlegm* are all deranged in the skin, flesh, or blood, they produce a slight swelling of the whole body,

---

कठिनोऽल्प प्रपाकवान्। दाहरागतृषामोह च्छर्द्दिमूर्च्छारुजा ज्वरः। प्रलापोवेपथुस्तन्द्रा सोऽसाध्यः स्यात् त्रिदोषजः। रक्ता-रक्तसमुत्थाना गुञ्जाविद्रुमसन्निभाः। वेदितव्यास्तु रक्तेन पैत्तिकेन च हेतुना। नते सिद्धिं समायान्ति सिद्धै र्योगशतैरपि। एकदोषोत्थितःसाध्यः कृच्छ्रसाध्यो द्विदोषजः। सर्व्वदोषोत्थितो घोरस्त्वसाध्यो भूर्युपद्रवः।

अथ मसूरिकानिदानम्।

कट्वम्ललवणक्षार-विरुद्धाध्यशनाशनैः। दुष्टनिष्पावशाकाद्यैः-प्रदुष्टपवनोदकैः। क्रुरग्रहेक्षणाच्चापि देहे दोषाः समुद्धताः।

which passes from one part to another. When produced by air, the part becomes black, soft, and unequal; accompanied with pain, as if needles were thrust into the part, and the fever produced by deranged air. When surrounded with vesications it is incurable.

When the disease is produced by bile it spreads quickly, and is accompanied with inflammatory fever. This form is accompanied with redness, and vesications. When the inflammation is deep, the flesh and vessels are destroyed, and it discharges a matter like a mixture of water and clay. Such cases are incurable.

When produced by *phlegm* it spreads slowly, has an oily appearance, and is white. There is little pain in such cases, with considerable itching. When produced by the derangement of the three hurmours the symptoms are of a mixed nature. When this disease passes to suppuration it is incurable. When produced by sharp instruments, or such like injuries, the bile and blood are deranged and produces a swelling of the part; which becomes black and red, and is

---

जनयन्ति शरीरेऽस्मिन् दुष्टरक्तेन सङ्गताः। मसूराकृतिसंस्थानाः पिड़काः स्युर्मसूरिकाः। तासां पूर्व्वं ज्वरः कण्डुर्गात्रभङ्गोऽरतिर्भ्रमः। त्वचि शोथः सवैवर्ण्यो नेत्ररागश्च जायते।

स्फोटाः श्यावारुणारूक्षास्तीव्रवेदनयान्विताः। कठिनाश्चिरपाकाश्च भवन्त्यनिलसम्भवाः। सन्ध्यस्थिपर्व्वणां भेदः कासः कम्पोऽरतिःक्लमः। शोषस्ताल्वोष्ठजिह्वानां तृष्णा चारुचिसंयुता। रक्ताःपीताः सिताः स्फोटाः सदाहा स्तीव्रवेदनाः। भवन्त्यचिरपाकाश्च पित्तकोपसमुद्भवाः। विड़्भेदश्चाङ्गमर्दश्च दाहतृष्णारुचिस्तथा। मुखपाकोऽक्षिरागश्च ज्वरस्तीव्रः सुदारुणः। रक्तजायां भवन्त्येते विकाराः पित्तलक्षणाः। कफप्रसेकः स्तैमित्यं शिरोरुग्गात्रगौरवं। हृल्लासः सारुचिर्निद्रा तन्द्रालस्य समन्विताः।

accompanied with violent inflammatory fever. The affected part is surrounded by a black edge, and eruptions like peas.

The first three forms of this disease are curable, and the two last are incurable.

Boils, Pustules, Erysipelas? (*Bishphotaka.*)

The causes of this form of disease are using too much heating, sour, or acid substances;—heavy and indigestable or salt food;—eating too freely, and exposure to the sun—or to too sudden alterations of the weather. By such cause, *air*, *bile*, and *phlegm* are deranged, which affect the blood, flesh, bones, and skin; and produce large bullæ, accompanied with fever. This part appears as if burnt. Sometimes these bullæ appear over all the body, and in other cases they are confined to particular parts. When the air is much deranged in this disease it is accompanied with head-ache, fever, thirst, pain in the joints, and the bullæ become black, accompanied with much pain. When produced by deranged bile there is much fever, burning of the body, and a large discharge of fluid from the bullæ. They then become red, or yellow.

श्वेताः स्निग्धाभृशं स्थूला कण्डुरा मन्दवेदनाः। मसूरिकाः कफोत्थाश्च चिरपाकाः प्रकीर्त्तिताः।

नीलाश्चिपिटविस्तीर्णा मध्ये निम्ना महारुजाः। चिरपाकाः पूतिस्रावाः प्रभुताः सर्व्वदोषजाः। कण्ठरोधारुचिस्तम्भ प्रलापारतिसङ्गताः। दुश्चिकित्स्याः समुद्दिष्टाः पीड़काश्चर्म्मसंश्चिताः।

रोमकूपोन्नतिसमारागिस्राः कफपित्तजाः। कासारोचक-संयुक्ता रोमान्तरोज्वरपूर्व्विकाः।

तोयवुद्बुदसङ्काशा त्वग्गतास्तु मसूरिकाः। स्वल्पदोषाः प्रजायन्ते भिन्ना स्तोयं स्रवन्ति च रक्ताख्या लोहिताकाराः शीघ्र-पाका स्तनु त्वचः। साध्यानातर्य्थदुष्टाश्च भिन्ना रक्तं स्रवन्ति च।

When produced by deranged phlegm it is accompanied with vomiting, dyspepsia, languor, and the affected parts become itchy, hard, and white, without pain. Suppuration often takes place, and continues for a long time.

When the three humours are deranged the disease is incurable; and also when the bullæ are depressed in the centre and hard. The patient in such cases complains of a burning sensation, thirst, fainting, vomiting, fever, delirium, rigors, and drowsiness. These are unfavourable symptoms, as also when the bullæ become red.

When the disease is produced by blood, the tubercles are like the seed of the *gunja*; (that is red with a black spot). This form is incurable (*Charaka*).

Small Pox, (*Masuriká.*) *

Stimulating and heating substances produce this disease; as also pungent, acid, or saline substances, and improper mixtures

---

मांसस्थाः काठिनाः स्निग्धा स्थिरपाका घनत्वचः। गात्रशूलतृषाकण्डुज्वरारतिसमन्विताः।

मेदोजा मण्डलाकारा मृदवः किञ्चिदुन्नताः। घोरज्वरपरीताश्च स्थूलाः स्निग्धाः सवेदनाः। सम्मोहारतिसन्तापाः कश्चिदाभ्यो विनिस्तरेत्। क्षुद्रा गात्रसमा रूक्षा स्थिपिटाः किञ्चिदुन्नताः। मज्जोत्था भृशसंमोहवेदनारतिसंयुताः। छिन्दन्ति मर्म्मधामानि प्राणानाशु हरन्तिहि। भ्रमरेणेव विद्धानि कुर्व्वन्त्यस्थीनि सर्व्वतः। पक्काभाः पिड़काः स्निग्धाः सूक्ष्माश्चात्यर्थवेदनाः। स्तैमित्यारतिसंमोहदाहोन्मादसमन्विताः। शुक्रजायां मसूर्य्यान्तु लक्षणानि भवन्ति हि। निर्द्दिष्टं केवलं चिह्नं दृश्यते न तु जीवितम्। दोषमिश्रास्तु सप्तैता द्रष्टव्या दोषलक्षणैः।

---

* In Persian it is styled *Chechak*; in Sanskrit *Guti* and *Masúri* or *Masúriká*, resembling a pill or lentil *masúrá*, (Ervum hirsutum and Cicer lens.)

of food ; eating before the former food has been digested : unwholesome meats, and certain roots or fruits ; bad air or water ; and the influence of a bad planet. These causes derange air, bile, and phlegm, &c., which with the bad blood produces an eruption like the *masúra*.

Before small-pox appears, fever occurs, with pain over the body, but particularly in the back ; and itching, lassitude, stretching, restlessness, redness of the face and eyes, with cough. The skin swells slightly, and is of an unusually red colour.

When air is much deranged in this disease the pustules are of a dark-green, and red colour ; or dull, hard, and rough, and are accompanied with severe pain. This variety ripens slowly.

When bile is deranged, in this disease, severe pain is felt in the large and small joints, with cough, shaking, listlessness and languor ; the palate, lips and tongue are dry with thirst, and no appetite. The pustules are red, yellow, and white, and they are accompanied with burning pain. This form soon ripens.

When produced by diseased *phlegm* the pustules are large, white, and shining, with much itching, and less pain than the

---

त्वग्गता रक्तजाश्चैव पित्तजाः श्लेष्मजा स्तथा। श्लेष्मपित्त-कृताश्चैव सुखसाध्या मसूरिकाः॥ वातजा वातपित्तोत्थाः श्लेष्मवात-कृताश्च याः। कृच्छ्रसाध्या मता स्तस्मात् यत्नादेता उपाचरेत्॥ असाध्याः सन्निपातोत्था स्तासां वक्ष्यामि लक्षणम्। प्रवालसदृशाः काश्चित् काश्चिज्जम्बुफलोपमाः॥ लोहजालसमाः काश्चिदतसीफल-सन्निभाः। आसां बहुविधा वर्णा जायन्ते दोषभेदतः॥ कासो-हिक्का प्रमोहश्च ज्वरस्तीव्रः सुदारुणः। प्रलापश्चारतिर्मूर्च्छातृष्णा दाहोतिघुर्णता॥ मुखेन प्रस्रवेद्रक्तं तथा घ्राणेन चक्षुषा। कण्ठे घुर्घुरकं कृत्वा श्वसित्यत्यर्थवेदनम्॥ मसूरिकाभिभुतस्य यस्यै-तानि भिषग्वरैः॥ लक्षणानि च दृश्यन्ते न दद्यात्तत्र भेषजम्।

former kind. They ripen slowly. In this form, some of the general symptoms of small-pox are aggravated. There is catarrh with chilliness, head-ache, fever, heaviness of the body, nausea, loss of the appetite, languor, drowsiness, and the patient sleeps much.

When blood is deranged diarrhœa, lassitude, and stretching occur; with thirst, laziness, want of appetite, burning over the surface, and the mouth becomes ulcerated. The eyes are red, strong fever is present, with the symptoms already enumerated under deranged bile.

When air, bile and phlegm are deranged in this disease the body has a blue colour, and the skin seems studded with rice. The pustules become black and flat, are depressed in the centre, with much pain. They ripen slowly, and the discharge is copious, and very fœtid.

When air, bile and phlegm are thus deranged the patient is always dozing, he has no appetite, breathes with difficulty, and is drowsy, restless and delirious. This form is cured with much difficulty, and it is called *Charma* or fatal form.

मसूरिकाभिभूतो यो भृशं घ्राणेन निश्वसेत् ॥ सभृशं त्यजति प्राणान् तृष्णार्त्तो वायुदूषितः ॥ मसूरिकान्ते शोथः स्यात् कुर्परे-मणिवन्धके। तथांसफलके चापि दुश्चिकित्स्यः सुदारुणः ॥

अथ क्षुद्ररोगनिदानम्।

१। स्निग्धाः सवर्णा ग्रथिता नीरुजा मुद्गसन्निभाः। कफवातोत्थिता ज्ञेया बालानामजगल्लिकाः ॥

२। यवाकारा सुकठिना ग्रथिता मांससंश्रिता। पीड़का कफवाताभ्यां यवप्रख्येति सोच्यते ॥

३। घनामवक्त्रां पिड़कामुन्नतां परिमण्डलाम्। अन्त्रालजीमल्पपूयां तां विद्यात् कफवातजाम् ॥

The following are other varieties of Small-pox :—

1. *Measles (Romántiká, Hám, B.)* is produced by vitiated phlegm and bile, and the symptoms are fever followed by an eruption of small red papellæ, like the roots of hairs; these appear over the body, accompanied with loss of appetite and cough.

2. *Water-pox (Togotoh, Masúriká, Páni-Basanta, B.)* The pustules are large, and full of water. In this form the skin is alone affected.

When the blood is particularly affected in small-pox, the pustules are of a redder colour, have a thinner cuticle than usual, and quickly ripen. They may generally be cured, but on being opened, should blood be discharged, the disease is incurable.

When the pustules proceed from *flesh* they are hard and shining, they ripen slowly, and the skin covering the part is thick. The pain over the body is severe, with listlessness, itchiness of the skin, thirst, and fever.

When the disease is produced by diseased *fat*, the pustules are large, soft, round, and slightly elevated, with severe fever

---

४। विवृत्तास्यां महादाहां पक्वोडुम्बरसन्निभाम्। परिमण्डलां पित्तकृतां विवृतां नाम तां विदुः॥

५। ग्रथिताः पञ्च वा षड् वा दारुणाः कच्छपोपमाः। कफानिलाभ्यां पिड़का ज्ञेया कच्छपिका बुधैः॥

३। ग्रीवांसकक्षा करपाददेशे सन्धौ गले वा त्रिभिरेव दोषैः। ग्रन्थिः सवल्मीकवदक्रियाणां जातः क्रमेणैव गतः प्रवृद्धिम्॥ मुखैरनेकैः स्रुतितोदवद्भि र्विसर्पवत् सर्पति चोन्नताग्रैः। वल्मीकमाहु र्भिषजो विकारं निष्प्रत्यनीकं चिरजं विशेषात्॥

७। पद्मकर्णिकवन्मध्ये पीड़काभिः समाचिताम्। इन्द्रविद्धां तु तां विद्याद्वातपित्तोत्थितां भिषक्॥

and pain. This form is very dangerous, and is accompanied with loss of sense, laziness and stupor. Some strong persons may be cured of this disease.

When the *marrow* is particularly diseased, the pustules are very small, flat, and slightly elevated and dry. The person is insensible, with severe pain of a gnawing kind in the vital parts. This form quickly destroys the person.

When the *bones* are particularly affected in this disease; they feel pained, as if bored by an insect. The pustules appear as if ripe, small, shining and very tender. The person feels chilly, restless, and delirium occurs, with a burning feeling.

When *semen* is affected in this disease, the symptoms are the same as when the bones are affected; and this form is so fatal that as soon as a person is affected with it he dies, so that there is no time for the pustules appearing.

These different forms will be known by an experienced physician. When small-pox is caused by derangements in the skin, blood, bile, or phlegm; or phlegm and bile, it will be quickly cured. When air or bile; or phlegm and air; and when the air, bile, and phlegm are deranged the disease is in-

---

८। मण्डलं वृत्तमुत्सन्नं सरक्तं पीड़काचितं रुजाकरीं गर्द्द-भिकां तो विद्याद्वातपित्तजाम् ॥

९। वातश्लेष्मसमुद्भुतः श्वयथु र्हनुसन्धिजः। स्थिरो मन्द-रुजः स्निग्धो ज्ञेयः पाषाणगर्द्दभः ॥

१०। कर्णस्याभ्यन्तरे जातां पीड़का मुग्रवेदनाम्। स्थिरां पनसिका तान्तु विद्यादन्तः प्रपाकिनीम् ॥

११। विसर्पवत् सर्पति यः शोथस्तनुरपाकवान्। दाहज्वर-करः पित्तात् स ज्ञेयो जालगर्द्दभः ॥

१२। पीड़का मुत्तमाङ्गस्थां वृत्तामुग्ररुजां जराम्। सर्व्वा-त्मिकां सर्व्वलिङ्गां जानीयादिरिवेल्लिकाम् ॥

curable. Of the latter kind the eruptions are sometimes like coral, or like rose-apple (*Jám*), oval, like the iron weight of a fishing net, or like a grain of linseed. The colour of this dangerous form of small-pox varies according to the strength of the individual. The other bad symptoms are cough, hiccough, coma, fever of a severe kind, delirium, listlessness, and thirst. The body remains very hot, blood flows from the mouth, eyes and nose, and there is a gurgling (*gharghari*) noise in the throat, with difficult and sonorous respiration. Such cases of small-pox are incurable; as also those in which great thirst is accompanied with difficulty in breathing, which is performed through the mouth.

Should the elbow, wrists, or axilla swell after the small-pox, the person will be cured with difficulty.

It appears that the Chinese as well as the Hindus were familiar with small-pox many centuries before the Arabian physicians described it. It was probably conveyed westward by the Persian conquerors of Hindustan; which seems to be a further confirmation of the country from which it originally came, and the manner in which it gradually approached and eventually reached Europe. The distance and the hot deserts

---

१३। बाहुपार्श्वांसकचेषु कृष्णस्फोटां सवेदनाम्। पित्त-प्रकोपसम्भूतां कचामित्यभिनिर्द्दिशेत्॥

१४। एकाभिताद्दशीं दृष्ट्वा पीड़कां स्फोटसन्निभाम्। त्वग्गतां पित्तकोपेन गन्धमालां प्रचच्यते॥

१५। कचभागेषु ये स्फोटा जायन्ते मांसदारुणाः। अन्तर्दाहज्वरकरा दीप्तपावकसन्निभाः॥ सप्ताहाद्वा दशाहाद्वा पचाद्वा घ्नन्ति मानवम्। तामग्निरोहिणीं विद्यादसाध्यां सर्व्वदोषजाम्॥

१६। नखमांसमधिष्ठाय वायुः पित्तञ्च देहिनाम्। कुर्व्वते दाहपाकौ च तं व्याधिं चिप्पमादिशेत्॥

through which the only intercourse for so long a period was held, prevented for a time its progress westward ; but, as navigation extended, ships from India would frequently touch at the Arabian ports of the Persian Gulf, and Red Sea, where it seems first to have appeared, A. D. 900.

The description of the small-pox by Rhazes, * the distinguished Arabian physician, first drew the attention of the European physicians to the disease.

Some say it was introduced into Arabia in 572, the year that gave birth to Mohammad ; other testimonies seem to accord with the statement that it was at the siege of Mecca (A. D. 569), by Abraham that the Arabians were first affected with the disease.

The conquests of the followers of Mohammad conveyed the disease to Persia, Syria, and Egypt ; and the successful stand made by the inhabitants of Constantinople, for some time prevented the spread of the disease beyond the Hellespont. So completely does this appear to have been the case, that Honus, a resident physician in that city in the tenth century, states that neither the small-pox nor measles were known in his time in Constantinople.

१७। तद्देवाल्पतरै र्दोषैः परुषं कुनखं वदेत्।

१८। गम्भीरामल्पसंरम्भां सवर्णा मुपरि स्थिताम्। पादस्यानुशयीं तान्तु विद्यादन्तः प्रपाकिनीम्॥

१९। विदारीकन्दवद्वृत्तां कक्षावङ्क्षणसन्धिषु। विदारिकेति तां विद्यात् सर्व्वजां सर्व्वलक्षणाम्॥

२०। प्राप्य मांससिरास्नायुः श्लेष्मा मेद स्तथानिलः। ग्रन्थिं करोत्यसौ भिन्ने मधुसर्पिर्वसानिभं॥ स्रवत्यास्रावमनिल स्तव वृद्धिं पुनर्गतः॥ मांसं संशोष्य ग्रथितां शर्करां जनयेत्ततः।

---

* The translation was printed in England by Dr. Meade, in 1747 : see his Works, page 297.

The whole of the southern coast of the Mediterranean sea had been subdued by the Arabians; but, it was not till the commencement of the eighth century that the disease was introduced into Spain by the Moors. The Victorious Saracens overran Spain, crossed the Pyrenese mountains, and inundated the southern provinces of France. They were driven back by Charles Martel; but they left the small-pox and measles with the conquerors. From this source the diseases quickly spread over Europe.

The Spaniards in their invasion of Hispaniola and Mexico conveyed the same diseases to these countries, where it committed the most extensive ravages. It would thus appear that the small-pox as well as the measles commenced in Asia, and extended to Africa, Europe, and the new World.

Small diseases are arranged under the following heads—(Locales.)

1. *Ajagalliká.*—Small tuberculous eruptions of the form of peas. It occurs in children.

दुर्गन्धि क्लिन्नमत्यर्थं नानावर्णं ततः शिराः । स्रवन्ति रक्तं सहसा तं विद्याच्छर्कराबुर्दम् ॥

२१। परिक्रमणशीलस्य वायुरत्यर्थरूक्षयोः । पादयोः कुरुते दारीं पाददारीं तमादिशेत् ॥

२२। शर्करोन्मथिते पादे क्षते वा कण्टकादिभिः । ग्रन्थिः कीलवदुत्पन्नो जायते कदरं हि तत् ॥

२४। क्लिन्नाङ्गुल्यन्तरौ पादौ कण्डूदाहरुजान्वितौ । दुष्टकर्द्दमसंस्पर्शादलसं तं विभावयेत् ॥

२५। रोमकूपानुगं पित्तं वातेन सह मूर्च्छितम् । प्रच्यावयति रोमाणि ततः श्लेष्मा सशोणितः ॥ रुणद्धि रोमकूपांस्तु ततोऽन्येषामसम्भवः । तदिन्द्रलुप्तं खालित्यं रुह्येति च विभाव्यते ॥

2. *Jabaprakhia* are hard fleshy eruptions, like the grains of barley. They are produced by diseased phlegm and air.

3. *Andálají.*—Round elevated pimples containing matter, produced by diseased phlegm and air.

4. *Bibritá.*—An eruption like the ripe fig with inflammation.

5. *Kachhapiká.*—Five or six tumors of the shape of turtles; produced by diseased phlegm and air.

6. *Balmikí*, are tumors in the soles of the feet or palms of the hand, or in a joint, or in the neck, axilla, and other parts. They increase by degrees, like the hills of white ants; and are surrounded with painful and itchy ulcers, and accompanied with a discharge.

7. *Indrabriddhá.*—Tumors surrounded by small eruptions, like the inside of a water-lily.

8. *Gardhabiká.*—Elevations surrounded by small eruptions with many openings.

२५। दारुणा कण्डुरा रुक्षा केशभूमिः प्रपाटयते। कफमारुतकोपेन विद्याद्दारुणकन्तु तम्।

२६। अरुंषि बहुवक्त्राणि बहुक्लेदीनि मूर्द्धिं तु। कफासृक् क्रिमिकोपेन नृनां विद्यादरुंषिकाम॥

२७। क्रोधशोकश्रमकृतः शरीरोष्मा शिरोगतः। पित्तञ्च केशान् पचति पलितं तेन जायते॥

२८। शाल्मलीकण्ठकप्रख्याः कफमारुतरक्तजाः। युवानपीड़का यूनां विज्ञेया मुखदूषिकाः॥

२९। कण्टकै राचितं वृत्तं मण्डलं पाण्डु कण्डूरम्। पद्मिनीकण्टकप्रख्यं तदाख्यं कफवातजम्॥

३०। सममुत्सन्नमरुजं मण्डलं कफरक्तजम्। सहजं लक्ष्म चैकेषां लक्ष्यो जतुमणिस्तु सः॥

9. *Pásándgar dabhá*—is a hard swelling below the ear, or in the articulation of the lower jaw. It is produced by diseased phlegm, and is hard, painful, and shining.

10. *Panásiká.*—An eruption in the inside of the ear, which suppurates.

11. *Jalagardaba.*—A slight swelling which spreads rapidly, without passing to suppuration. It is accompanied with a strong inflammatory fever.

12. *Jrebilliká.*—A painful eruption over the head, accompanied with much pain and fever.

13. *Kakhia.*—Swellings of the glands in the axilla.

14. *Gundanamá.*—Pustules over the body, like the last.

15. *Agnihini.*—A hard inflammatory swelling in the axilla, with strong fever, and other severe symptoms. It is a dangerous disease when not treated in the first stage.

16. *Chippa.*—Ulceration destroying the nails, (see before.)

17. *Kunakha.*—Discolouration of the nails, which drop off.

३१। अवेदनं स्थिरञ्चैव यस्मिन् गात्रे प्रदृश्यते। माषवत् कृष्णमुत्सन्नमनिलान्माषकन्तु तम् ॥

३२। कृष्णानि तिलमात्राणि नीरुजानि समानि च। वातपित्तकफोद्रेकात् तान् विद्यात्तिलकालकान् ॥

३३। महद्वा यदि वा चाल्पं श्यावं वा यदि वासितम्। नीरुजं मण्डलं गात्रे न्यच्छमित्यभिधीयते ॥

३४। क्रोधायास प्रकुपितो वायुः पित्तेन संयुतः मुखमागत्य सहसा मण्डलं विसृजत्यतः। नीरुजं तनुकं श्यावं मुखव्यङ्गं तमादिशेत् ॥

३५। कृष्णमेवं गुणं गात्रे मुखे वा नीलिकां विदुः ॥

३६। मर्द्दनात् पीड़नाद्वापि तथैवाप्यभिघाततः। मेढ्रचर्म्म यदा वायुर्भजते सर्व्वतश्चरन् ॥ तदा वातोपसृष्टत्वात् तच्चर्म्म परि-

18. *Pádánusoie.*—Small scrofulous tumors in the feet.

19. *Bidariká.*—Large swellings in the axilla and groin.

20. *Shekárárbuda.*—Are bleeding tumors, (see before.)

21. *Cadara.*—Hard swellings like the seeds of the plum in the soles of the feet, produced by external injuries.

22. *Alasa.*—Sores between the toes.

23. *Indralupta.*—Baldness.

24. *Darunaka.*—Scaley eruptions in the roots of the hairs of the head.

25. *Arunsíká.*—Small pustules in the head, which discharge.

26. *Palíta.*—Gray hair.

27. *Mukhadusíká.*—Small eruptions appearing in the face, at the time of puberty.

28. *Pudíníkantaka.*—Rough circular spots on the surface of the body.

29. *Jatumani.*—Black and sometimes red or white spots, in any part of the body.

वर्त्तते। मणेरधस्तात् कोषश्च ग्रन्थिरूपेण लम्वते॥ परिवर्त्तिकेति तां विद्यात् सरुजां वातसम्भवाम्। सकण्डुकठिना वापि सैव श्लेष्मसमुत्थिता॥

२७। अल्पीयः खां यदा हर्षाद्दलाद्गच्छेत् स्त्रियं नरः। हस्ताभिघातादथवा चर्म्मण्युद्वर्त्तिते बलात्। यस्यावपाट्यते चर्म्म तां विद्यादवपाटिकाम्॥

२८। वातोपसृष्टे मेढ्रे वै चर्म्म संश्रयते मणिम्। मणिश्चर्म्मोपनद्धस्तु मूत्रस्रोतोरुणद्धि च॥ निरुद्धप्रकशे तस्मिन् मन्दधारं सवेदनम्॥ मूत्रं प्रवर्त्तते जन्तो र्मणि र्विव्रियते न च। निरुद्धप्रकशं विद्यात् सरुजं वातसम्भवम्॥

30. *Masaka.*—Blackish spots like the figure of *máskalái*, (a kind of pea).

31. *Tílakálaka.*—Very black spots over the body. These are not accompanied with pain, and are like *til* seed.

32. *Nyachchha.*—Spots of grey or dark colour, sometimes covering most parts of the body. These are indolent, and without pain.

33. *Byanga.*—Small circular spots in the face.

34. *Nilika.*—Bluish coloured spots in the face.

35. *Pariburtika.*—Swelling of the prepuce, (Phymosis, see before.)

36. *Abapátika.*—When the prepuce turns backwards, and swells (Paraphymosis, see before.)

37. *Nirudhoprokasa.*—Stricture of the urethra, (see before.)

38. *Sanniradaguda.*—Stricture of the anus, (see before.)

39. *Ahiputana.*—Small eruptions round the anus, particularly in children.

३९। वेगसन्धारणाद्वायु विंहितो गुदसंश्रितः। निरुणद्धि महास्रोतः सूक्ष्मद्वारं करोति च॥ मार्गस्य सौक्ष्म्यात् कृच्छ्रेण पुरीषं तस्य गच्छति। सन्निरुद्धगुदं व्याधि मेतं विद्यात् सुदारुणम्॥

४०। शकृन्मूत्रसमायुक्ते धौतेऽपाने शिशो र्भवेत्। स्विन्ने वा स्नाप्यमाने वा कण्डुरक्तकफोद्भवा॥ कण्डुयनात्ततः क्षिप्रं स्फोटः स्रावश्च जायते॥ एकीभूतं व्रणं घोरं तं विद्यादहि पूतनं॥

४१। स्नानोत्सादनहीनस्य मलो वृषणसंस्थितः। यदा प्रक्लिद्यते स्वेदात् कण्डुं जनयते तदा। कण्डुयनात्ततः क्षिप्रं स्फोटः स्रावश्च जायते। प्राहुर्वृषणकच्छुं तां श्लेष्मरक्तप्रकोपजाम्।

40. *Brisánákuchu.*—Peculiar itch of the scrotum produced by uncleanness.

41. *Gudabhrunsa.*—Prolapsus ani.

42. *Shukárádunstraká.*—Swellings with inflammation of the skin.

43. *Grunthi.*—Tumors and diseases of glands.

44. *Bisharpa.*—Erysipelatous inflammation, (see before.)

Diseases of the Mouth, (*Mukharoga*).

The diseases of the mouth are sixty-five : viz. eight diseases of the lips ; fifteen of the gums ; eight of the teeth ; four of the tongue ; nine of the palate ; seventeen of the throat ; and three general diseases.

Diseases of the Lips.

By using too much food, such as fish, the flesh, of buffaloes, milk, curdled milk, &c. the three humours

---

४२। प्रवाहनातिसाराभ्यां निर्गच्छति गुदं वहि। रुच-दुर्व्वलदेहस्य गुदभ्रंशं तमादिशेत्॥

४३। सदाहो रक्तपर्य्यन्त स्त्वक्पाकी तीव्रवेदनः। कण्डूमान्-ज्वरकारी च स स्याच्छूकरदंष्ट्रकः॥

अथ मुखरोगनिदानम्।

अथौष्ठगतनिदानम्।

आनुपपिशितक्षीर-दाध-मत्स्यातिसेवनात्। मुखमध्ये गदान् कुर्युः क्रुद्धा दोषा स्त्रय स्तथा॥ कर्कशौ परुषौ स्तब्धौ संप्राप्तानिलवेदनौ। दालेप्रते परिपाटेप्रते ओष्ठौ मारुतकोपतः॥ चीयते पिड़काभिश्च सरुजाभिः समन्ततः। सदाहपाकपिड़कौ पीता-

are deranged producing diseases of the Lips. They become rough, hard, and stiff. When the bile is much deranged they are very painful, and small eruptions appear upon the surface. When bile is deranged, there is much inflammation, the lips become yellow, and the eruptions are painful, and of a yellow colour. When phlegm is deranged the lips are covered with a thin oleaginous looking matter, are cold, stiff, and of a dark yellow, white, or mixed colour. The eruptions are likewise of different colours.

When blood is deranged in the lips they become red, swollen, and very painful. They often bleed. When the flesh is affected they become swollen, heavy, sometimes ulceration takes place, and worms form in it. When fat is affected the lips become glistening, like the surface of ghee. They are also itchy and heavy, and the discharge is like pure water. These ulcers do not heal easily.

भासौ च पित्ततः। सवर्णाभिश्च चीयेते पीड़काभि रवेदनौ॥ भवतस्तु कफादोष्ठौ पिच्छिलौ शीतलौ गुरू। सकृत्कृष्णौ सकृत् पीतौ सकृच्छ्वेतौ तथैव च। सन्निपातेन विज्ञेयावनेकपिड़काचितौ॥ खर्ज्जूरफलवर्णाभिः पिड़काभि र्निपीड़ितौ। रक्तोपसृष्टौ रुधिरं स्रवतः शोणितप्रभौ॥ गुरू स्थूलौ मांसदुष्टौ मांसपिण्डवदुद्गतौ। जन्तवश्चात्र मूर्च्छन्ति नरस्योभयतो मुखात्॥ सर्पिर्मण्डप्रतीकाशौ मेदसा कण्डुरौ गुरू॥ अच्छं स्फटिकसङ्काशमास्रावं स्रवतो भृशम्॥ तयो र्व्रणो न संरोहेन्मृदुत्वञ्च न गच्छति। ओष्ठौ पर्यवदीर्य्येते पाट्येते चाभिघाततः।

अथ दन्तवेष्टगतनिदानम्।

शोणितं दन्तवेष्टेभ्यो यस्याकस्माद् प्रवर्त्तते। दुर्गन्धीनि सकृष्णानि प्रक्लेदीनि मृदुनि च॥ दन्तमांसानि शीर्य्यन्ते पचन्ति च परस्परम्॥ शीतादो नाम स व्याधिः कफशोणितसम्भवः॥ दन्तयो

Diseases of the Gums.

There are fifteen diseases described under this head.

Sitáda is when the gums are black and blood is discharged without any external cause. In such cases the gums are separated from the teeth, soft, and putrid. In other cases they slough. This disease is produced by derangements of phlegm, and blood.

Dantapapataka. This disease is produced by derangements of phlegm and blood; and is characterized by painful swelling of the gums, covering two or three of the alveolar processes.

Dantabeshta is produced by deranged blood, and is characterized by a discharge of pus mixed with blood. In this disease the teeth become loose.

Sawesara is characterized by a painful swelling of the gums, which are itchy, and are accompanied with a copious discharge of saliva. This disease is caused by a derangement of phlegm, and blood.

स्त्रिषु वा यस्य श्वयथु र्जायते महान्। दन्त पुप्पुटको नाम स व्याधिः कफरक्तजः। स्रवन्ति पूयरुधिरं चला दन्ता भवन्ति च। दन्तवेष्टः स विज्ञेयो दुष्टशोणित सम्भवः॥ श्वयथु र्दन्तमूलेषु रुजावान् कफरक्तजः। लालास्रावी स विज्ञेयः शैशिरो नाम नामतः॥ दन्ताश्चलन्ति वोष्ठेभ्यः स्तालुश्चापयवशीर्य्यते। यस्मिन् स सर्व्वजो व्याधिर्म्महाशैशिरसंज्ञितः॥

दन्तमांसानि शीर्य्यन्ते यस्मिन् ष्ठीवति चाप्यसृक्। पित्तासृक कफजो व्याधि र्ज्ञेयः परिदरो हि सः॥ वोष्ठेषु दाहः पाकश्च ताभ्यां दन्ताश्चलन्ति च। यस्मिन् सोपकुशो नाम पित्तरक्तकृतो गदः॥ घृष्टेषु दन्तमांसेषु संरम्भो जायते महान्। भवन्ति दन्ता श्चपलाः स वैदर्भोऽभिघातजः॥ मारुतेनाधिको दन्तो जायते तीव्रवेदनैः॥ खलिवर्द्धनसंज्ञोऽसौ जाते रुक् च प्रशाम्यति॥ शनैः

Mahásansira is produced by the derangement of air, bile, and phlegm. In this variety the teeth become loose, with severe pain about the palate. Matter is formed in the gums, and the inside of the mouth is inflamed.

Parídarah is produced by derangement of bile, blood, and phlegm; and is characterized by blood being discharged from the gums; which are flabby, and separate from the teeth.

Apakusa is produced by derangement of bile and blood. In this disease, abscesses form in the gums with little pain; the teeth become loose, and when the gums are touched, they bleed. There is fætor of the mouth, and after the discharge of blood from the gums, they again swell.

Baidurba. This disease is caused by external injury, as by cleaning the teeth with too hard a tooth-brush. In this disease the teeth become loose.

Adidanta. When the air is deranged it produces irregularity in the growth of the teeth, with much pain; such teeth should be extracted, apply the actual cautery, and then treat it as of a caries of the tooth.

घनैः प्रकुरुते वायुर्दन्तसमाश्रितः । करालान् विकटान् दन्तान् करालो न स सिध्यति ॥ हानवेत्र पश्चिमे दन्ते महान् शोथो महारुजः । लालास्रावी कफकृतो विज्ञेयः सोऽधिमांसकः । दन्तमूलगता नाड्यः पञ्च ज्ञेया यथेरिताः ।

अथ दन्तगतनिदानम् ।

दीर्यमानेष्विव रुजा यस्य दन्तेषु जायते । दालनो नाम स व्याधिः सदागतिनिमित्तजः ॥ कृष्णश्छिद्रश्चलः स्रावी ससंरम्भो महारुजः । अनिमित्तरुजो वाताद्विज्ञेयः क्रिमिदन्तकः ॥ वक्रं वक्त्रं भवेद्यस्य दन्तभङ्गश्च जायते ॥ कफवातकृतो व्याधिः स भञ्जनकसंज्ञितः ॥ शीतरुक्षप्रवाताम्ल स्पर्शानामसहा द्विजाः । पित्तमारुतकोपेन दन्तहर्षः स नामतः । मलो दन्तगतो यस्तु कफ-

Adímánsíka is the swelling round the wisdom-teeth, producing much pain and swelling, with the discharge of saliva. It is produced by diseased phlegm.

Diseases of the Teeth.

Tooth-ache (Dálana), in which the tooth becomes very painful. This is caused by the derangement of air. When there is a small black decayed part of the tooth which is painful, and discharges matter with swelling, and much pain, it is called *Krímídantaka*, or worm-eaten tooth.

When the mouth is turned to a side, and the teeth broken, as in spasms, it is produced by phlegm, and is called *Bangana.*

Sensible Teeth. (*Dantaharsa*).

In this disease the person cannot bear cold, or hot applications; cool air, and sour articles produce much pain. Diseased bile and air produce this form of disease.

When bile and blood are deranged, the teeth become of a dark colour, as if burnt in the fire, and the disease is named *Siábadantaka.*

मारुतशोषितः । शर्करेव खरस्पर्शा सा ज्ञेया दन्तशर्करा ॥ कपाले-
ष्विव जीर्यत्सु दन्तानां सैव शर्करा । कापालिकेति विज्ञेया
सदा दन्तविनाशिनी ॥ असृङ्मिश्रेण पित्तेन दग्धो दन्तस्त्वशेषतः ॥
श्यावतां नीलतां वापि गतः स श्यावदन्तकः ॥

अथ जिह्वागतनिदानम् ।

जिह्वानिलेन स्फुटिता प्रसुप्ता भवेच्च शाकच्छदनप्रकाशा ।
पित्तेन दह्यतुपचीयते च दीर्घैः सरक्तैः रपि कण्टकैश्च ॥
कफेन गुर्वी बहुलाचिता च मांसोच्छ्रयैः शाल्मलिकण्टकाभैः ।
जिह्वातले यः श्वयथुः प्रगाढः सोऽलाससंज्ञः कफरक्तमूर्त्तिः ॥

Air when deranged, may produce dislocation of the lower jaw, which is called *Hanamaka*, and the symptoms are the same as the form of the disease named *Ardíta*.

Diseases of the Tongue.

When *air* is deranged in the tongue the person has no sense of feeling or taste in the organ, which is rough and divided into fissures. *Bile.* In this variety there is great heat, long and red papillæ spread over its surface. When *phlegm* is deranged the tongue becomes heavy, thick, and the papill,æ over the surface of the tongue enlarge.

Aláza. This form of disease is produced by deranged phlegm and blood, and is characterized by swelling on the upper surface of the tongue, particularly near its root. In this disease the tongue cannot be moved, and sometimes abscesses form.

Apasiba is produced by diseased phlegm and blood, under the tongue. It is like a second tongue. In this disease there with is a profuse discharge of saliva, accompanied with itchiness and burning pain.

जिह्वां स तु स्तम्भयति प्रवृद्धो मूले च जिह्वा भृशमेति पाकम्।
जिह्वाग्ररूपः श्वयथुर्हि जिह्वा मुन्नम्य जातः कफरक्तमूलः॥
लालाकरः कण्डुयुतः सचोषः सा तूपजिह्वा पठिता भिषग्भिः॥

अथ तालुगतनिदानम्।

श्लेष्मासृग्भ्यां तालुमूले प्रवृद्धो दीर्घः शोथाध्मात वस्तिप्रकाशः तृष्णा कास श्वासयुक्तं वदन्ति व्याधिं वैद्यो गलशुण्डीति नाम्ना शोथः स्थूल स्तोददाहप्रपाकी प्रागुक्ताभ्यां तुण्डिकेरी मता तु॥ मन्दः शोथो लोहितो शोणितोत्थो ज्ञेयो ध्रुवः सज्वर स्तीव्ररुक् च। कुर्म्मोन्नतोऽवेदनोऽशीघ्रजन्मा रोगो ज्ञेयः कच्छपः श्लेष्मणा तु॥

Diseases of the Palate.

1. When the phlegm and blood are deranged in the soft palate, it becomes large, like a full bladder, and is accompanied thirst, cough and difficulty in breathing. This disease is called *Kantasunda* (enlarged tonsils).

In other cases the swelling is accompanied with much pain and heat; suppuration being produced by phlegm, and blood. It is called *Tundikari*.

2. When the part is much swelled, hard, and of a red colour, and is produced by diseased blood it is called *Adussah*, which is accompanied with fever and severe pain. When the swelling is of the shape of a turtle, is without pain, is produced slowly, being caused by diseased phlegm, it is called *Kachhapa*.

3. Sometimes the swelling is like a water-lily, and in the soft palate is called *Raktabuda*, and is produced by a disease of the blood.

पद्माकारं तालुमध्ये तु शोथं विद्याद्रक्तादर्बुदं प्रोक्तलिङ्गम्। दुष्टं मांसं नीरुजं तालुमध्ये कफात् प्रोक्तो मांससङ्घात एषः। अरुक् स्थायी कोलमात्रः कफात् स्यात् मेदोयुक्तात् पुप्पुटस्तालुदेशे। शोषोऽत्यर्थं दीर्य्यते चापि तालुं श्वासश्चोग्रस्तालुशोषोऽनिलाच्च। पित्तं कुर्य्यात् पाकमत्यर्थघोरं तालुन्येवं तालुपाकं वदन्ति॥

अथ कण्ठगतनिदानम्।

गलेऽनिलः पित्तकफौ च मूर्च्छितौ प्रदूष्य मांसञ्च तथैव शोणितम्। गलोपसंरोधकरै स्तथाङ्कुरै र्निहन्त्यसून् व्याधिरियं हि रोहिणी॥ जिह्वा समन्ताद्भृशवेदनास्तु मांसाङ्कुराः कण्ठ-

4. When flesh is swelled in the palate, there is no pain; when produced by phlegm, it is called *Mánsasangáhta.*

5. When swelled like a plum, without pain, and remains in one spot, being produced by phlegm, and mixed with fat it is called *Puputah.*

6. *Tálupáka* is produced by deranged bile, and is characterized by suppuration in the soft palate.

7. *Talushosh.* In this disease the palate is very dry, and is accompanied with difficulty in breathing, and much pain.

Diseases of the Neck.

These diseases consist of 1. Diseases of the throat; 2. Hoarseness; 3. Goitre; 4. Scrofulous swellings; and 5. Tumors of the neck.

विरोधिनो ये। सा रोहिणी वातकृता प्रदिष्टा वातात्मकोपद्रव गाढ़युक्ता॥ क्षिप्रोद्गमा क्षिप्रविदाहपाका तीव्रज्वरा पित्तनिमित्तजा तु। स्रोतोविरोधिन्यचलोद्गता च स्थिराङ्कुरा या कफसम्भवा सा। गम्भीरपाकिन्यनिवार्य्यवीर्य्या त्रिदोषलिङ्गा त्रितयोत्थिता च। स्फोटैश्चिता पित्तसमानलिङ्गा साध्या प्रदिष्टा रुधिरात्मिका तु॥

कोलास्थिमात्रः कफसम्भवो यो ग्रन्थिर्गले कण्टकशूकभूतः। खरः स्थिरः शस्त्रनिपातसाध्य स्तं कण्ठशालूक मिति ब्रुवन्ति॥ जिह्वाग्ररूपः श्वयथुः कफात्तु जिह्वोपरिष्टादपि रक्तमिश्रात्॥ ज्ञेयोऽधिजिह्वः खलु रोग एष विवर्ज्जयेदागतपाकमेनम्। वलाश एवायतमुन्नतञ्च शोथं करोत्यन्नगतिं निवार्य्य॥ तं सर्व्वथैवाप्रतिवार्य्य वीर्य्यं विवर्ज्जनीयं वलयं वदन्ति॥ गले तु शोथं कुरुतः प्रवृद्धौ श्लेष्मानिलौ श्वासरुजोपपन्नम्॥ मर्म्मच्छिदं

Throat.

There are five forms of diseases of the throat.

When air, bile and phlegm are deranged in the throat separately or combined, or when the blood is diseased they form the five varieties of this disease. These produce a swelling in the throat, which shuts up the wind-pipe, and produces sudden death. It is called *Rahini*.

When the *air* is deranged, in the severe forms all the symptoms of deranged air are produced.

Bile. In this form papillæ of flesh quickly enlarge, become hot, and ripen, with severe fever.

Phlegm. The passage of the throat is closed, and the swelling remains long and at length suppurates. Fleshy elevations are formed.

When air, bile and phlegm are deranged at the same time, the swelling suppurates to a great depth in the tongue. It is incurable, and the three forms of symptoms of diseased air, bile, and phlegm appear. When blood is deranged many small

---

दुस्तरमेनमाशुर्वलाससंज्ञं निपुणा विकारम्। वृत्तोन्नतोऽन्तः श्वयथुः सदाहः सकण्डुरोऽपाक्यमृदुर्गुरुश्च॥ नाम्नैकवृन्दः परिकीर्त्तितोऽसौ व्याधिर्वलासक्षतजप्रसूतः। समुन्नतं वृत्तममन्ददाहं तीव्रज्वरं वृन्दमुदाहरन्ति। तच्चापि पित्तक्षतजः प्रकोपात् ज्ञेयं सतोदं पवनात्मकन्तु॥

वर्त्तिर्घना कण्ठनिरोधिनी या चितातिमात्रं पिशितप्ररोहैः। अनेकरुक् प्राणहरी त्रिदोषात् ज्ञेया शतघ्नी तु शतघ्नीरूपा॥ ग्रन्थि गले त्वामलकास्थिमात्रः स्थिरोऽतिरुग् यः कफरक्तमूर्त्तिः। संलक्ष्यते सक्तमिवाशनञ्च सशस्त्रसाध्यस्तु गिलायुसंज्ञः॥ सर्व्व गलं व्याप्य समुत्थितो यः शोथो रुजाः सन्ति च यत्र सर्व्वाः। स सर्व्व

swellings form upon the tongue, and near its root, accompanied with symptoms of deranged bile. This form may be cured.

When a swelling like a plum is situated in the throat, and produces difficulty in breathing, and a hard and rough swelling, it is caused by phlegm, and is named *Kantasáluka*. *Adíjiba* is a swelling at the root of the tongue like a second tongue, (this is probably a swelling of the epiglottis,) and is produced by the phlegm and blood. When it suppurates it is incurable. Various other swellings of the throat are also mentioned, such as *Balása*, a swelling of the throat which prevents swallowing, and is produced by phlegm. It is incurable. Phlegm and air produce the swelling in the throat, which is accompanied with severe pain, and difficulty in breathing. This is also a very dangerous form of disease.

Diseased phlegm and blood produce a swelling in the throat accompanied with itchiness, and a burning sensation. It is soft, heavy, and does not suppurate. It is called *Ekabrinda*. When it is accompanied with fever, it is called *Brinda*. This is an incurable disease.

दोषो गलविद्रधिस्तु तस्यैव तुल्यः खलु सर्व्वजस्य ॥ शोथो महानन्नजलावरोधी तीव्रज्वरो वायुगते र्निहन्ता ॥ कफेन जातो रुधिरान्वितेन गले गलौः परिकीर्त्तते तु । यस्ताम्यमानः श्वसिति प्रसक्तं भिन्नस्वरः शुष्कविमुक्तकण्ठः ॥ कफोपदिग्धेष्वनिलायनेषु ज्ञेयः स रोगः श्वसनात् स्वरघ्नः । प्रतानवान् यः श्वयथुः सुकष्टो गलोपरोधं कुरुते क्रमेण ॥ स मांसतानः कथितोऽवलम्बी प्राणप्रणुत् सर्व्वकृतो विकारः । सदाहतोदं श्वयथुं सुताम्रमन्तर्गले पूतिविशीर्णमांसम् । पित्तेन विद्याद्वदने विदारीं पार्श्वे विशेषात् स तु येन शेते ॥

A thick swelling of the throat, causing difficulty in breathing, and surrounded by small papulæ like piles with much pain, is produced by air, bile and phlegm ; it is called *Satagní*, (or it is like the instrument of this name which at once kills 100 persons :) it is incurable.

Gílin. The swelling in this disease is like the stone of a plum, not painful, but hard ; and is produced by diseased phlegm, and blood.

Sarungna. (Croup ?) When phlegm stops the passage of air, this produces dryness of the throat, hoarseness, difficulty in breathing and great uneasiness. It is incurable.

Mánsatána, is a swelling in the throat which produces suffocation. It is always dangerous.

Bidárí. The swelling is accompanied with great pain, redness, followed by sloughing. This is an incurable disease.

अथ सर्व्वसरानिदानम् ।

स्फोटैः सतोदै र्वदनं समन्ताद् यस्याचितं सर्व्वसरः स वातात् ।
रक्तैः सदाहै स्तनुभिः सपीतै र्यस्याचितञ्चापि स पित्तकोपात् ॥
अवेदनैः कण्डुयुतैः सवर्णै र्यस्याचितञ्चापि स वै कफेन ।

ओष्ठप्रकोपे वर्ज्याः स्युः मांसरक्तत्रिदोषजाः । दन्तमूलेषु वर्ज्यौ च त्रिलिङ्गगतिशौषिरौ ॥ दन्तेषु च न सिध्यन्ति श्याव-दालनभञ्जनाः ॥ जिह्वागतेष्वलासस्तु तालव्येष्वर्ब्बुद स्तथा ॥ स्वरघ्नो बलयो वृन्दो बलाशः स विदारिका । गलौघो मांस-तानश्च शतघ्नी रोहिणी गले ॥ असाध्याः कीर्त्तिता ह्येते रोगा नव दशैव तु । तेषु चापि क्रियां वैद्यः प्रत्याख्याय समाचरेत् ॥

अथ कर्णस्रोतोगतनिदानम् ।

समीरणः श्रोत्रगतोऽन्यथा चरन् समन्ततः शूलमतीव कर्णयोः । करोति दोषैश्च यथास्वमावृतः स कर्णशूलः कथितो

Gullagha, is a large swelling in the throat extending over the throat with great pain, and high fever. The patient cannot swallow food nor drink water. It is produced by phlegm and blood, and is considered incurable.

Diseases of the Ears, (*Karnaroga.*)

The more copious secretion from the external ears, and the most changes of temperature of the air, render diseases of this organ of frequent occurrence in this country. They produce much suffering, and much attention seems to have been paid by the Hindus to their nature and cure.

There are twenty-eight diseases of the ear. The corporeal *air* is the cause of all these diseases. When it is deranged in the ear, and is confined in its passage by the other humours, it produces severe pain in the organ, which is called *Karnashúla,* and is very difficult to cure. When air is deranged in the passages of the ear, several kinds of sounds are heard, like those of certain instruments called *Karnanáda.* When *air* is deranged with phlegm in the ear passages, and if not treated it will produce deafness called *Bádhirjya.*

दुराचरः ॥ कर्णस्रोतःस्थिते वाते शृणोति विविधान् स्वरान् ॥ भेरीमृदङ्गशङ्खानां कर्णनादः स उच्यते । यदा शब्दवहं वायुः स्रोत आवृत्य तिष्ठति ॥ शुद्धः श्लेष्मान्वितो वापि वाधिर्य्यं तेन जायते ॥ वायुः पित्तादिभिर्युक्तो वेणुघोषोपमं स्वनम् ॥ करोति कर्णयोः क्ष्वेडं कर्णक्ष्वेडः स उच्यते ॥

शिरोऽभिघातादथवा निमज्जतो जले प्रपाकादथवापि विद्रधेः । स्रवेद्धि पूयं श्रवणोऽनिलार्दितः स कर्णसंस्राव इति प्रदिष्टः । मारुतः कफसंयुक्तः कर्णकण्डूं करोति च ॥

पित्तोष्मशोषितः श्लेष्मा जायते कर्णगूथकः । स कर्णगूथो द्रवतां गतो यदा विलायितो घ्राणमुखं प्रपद्यते । तदा स कर्णप्रतिनाह

Fatigue, or eating hot or astringent substances, or the frequent use of errhines produce a derangement of the air in the ear passages called *Karnakshyera,* which consist in a peculiar ringing noise. In others the disease is produced by blows on the ear, by bathing in water during which water enters the ears, or by a boil in the part which suppurates. This disease is called *Karnasangsrába.*

When *air* and *phlegm* are deranged in the ear it produces itchiness; and bile being deranged dries up the phlegm, and wax in the ear. This disease is named *Karnagúthaka.* When the wax melts it passes out of the nose (*Susruta*), or mouth *Nidana,* and the disease is called *Pratináha,* and is accompanied with much pain in the head.

If worms form in the ear by flies depositing their eggs in the ear, the disease is called *Krimikarnaka.*

When the ear is wounded or otherwise injured it is called *Bidradhi.* In other cases there is great pain, burning, and tightness in the part, with a discharge of yellow pus or blood ;

संश्रितो भवेद्विकारः शिरसूर्द्धभेदकृत् ॥ यदा तु मूर्च्छन्त्यथवापि
जन्तवः सृजन्त्यपत्यान्यथवापि मक्षिकाः । तदप्रञ्जनत्वाच्छ्रवणो
निरुच्यते भिषग्भिराद्यैः क्रिमिकर्णको गदः ॥ पतङ्गाः शत-
पद्यश्च कर्णस्रोतः प्रविश्य हि । अरतिं व्याकुलत्वञ्च भृशं कुर्वन्ति
वेदनाम् ॥ कर्णो निस्तुद्यते तस्य तथा फरफरायते ॥ कीटे
चरति रुक् तीव्रा निस्पन्दे मन्दवेदना । क्षताभिघातप्रभवस्तु
विद्रधिर्भवेत्तथा दोषकृतोऽपरः पुनः । सरक्तपीतारुणमस्रमास्रवेत्
प्रतोदधूमायनदाहचोषवान् ॥ कर्णपाकस्तु पित्तेन कोथविक्ले-
दकृद्भवेत् । कर्णविद्रधिपाकाद्वा जायते चाम्बुपूरणात् ॥ पूयं
स्रवति यः पूति स ज्ञेयः पूतिकर्णकः । कर्णशोथार्बुदार्शांसि
जानीयादुक्तलक्षणैः ॥

it is then called *Karnabidradhi.* By the derangements of bile abscesses are formed, which is called *Karnapáka.*

When *phlegm* is deranged and dried up by the heat of the bile, it melts, and then is discharged from the ear, with a disagreeable smell. It is called *Pritikarnaka.* There are also four kinds of bloody tumors, seven varieties of other tumors, and four kinds of swellings to which the ear is liable.

In defects of the external ear, *Susruta* recommends the surgeon to prepare a new ear, by removing skin from the neighbouring part, leaving a connection to keep up its vitality.

Diseases of the Nose.

There are thirty-one diseases of the nose. When the nostrils are closed, when one is dry, very dirty, and hot, when matter has formed, and when the patient can neither smell nor taste, the disease is called *Pinasa,* and is produced by a derangement of air and phlegm. When the *air* is stopped in the palate and nostrils, and there is a bad smell which proceeds from the mouth and nose, the disease is called *Putinaska.*

अथ कर्णरोगनिदानम् ।

नादोतिरुक् कर्णमलस्य शोषः स्रावस्तनुश्चाश्रवणञ्च वातात् । शोथः सरागो दरणं विदाहः सपीत पूतिस्रवणञ्च पित्तात् ॥ वैश्रुत्य कण्डुस्थिरशोथशुक्लस्निग्धस्रुतः श्लेष्मभवेऽल्परुक् च । सर्व्वाणि रूपाणि च सन्निपाते स्रावश्च तत्राधिक दोषवर्णः ॥

सौकुमार्य्याच्चिरोत्सृष्टे सहसातिप्रवर्द्धिते । कर्णशोथो भवेत् पाल्यां सरुजः परिपोटवान् ॥ कृष्णारुणनिभः स्तब्धः स वातात् परिपोटकः । गुर्व्वाभरणसंयोगात् ताड़नाद्घर्षणादपि ॥ शोथः पाल्यां भवेच्छ्यावो दाहपाकरुजान्वितः ॥ रक्तो वा रक्तपित्ता-भ्यामुत्पातः स गदो मतः ॥ कर्णं बलाद्वर्द्धयतः पाल्यां वायुः

Bile when deranged in the nose produces small pimples, which quickly suppurate, and are called *Násikápáka.* In this disease a· disagreeable discharge often proceeds from the nose and umbiliacus, for which blood-letting is to be used. When blood flows from the nose it is called *Násа-raktapitta,* in which case *air, bile,* and *phlegm* are deranged. When the vital part of the nose is wounded, deranged air, &c. passes through the nostrils producing a bad smelling secretion mixed with blood, it is called *Puerakta.* When stimulating substances are applied to the nostrils, or by regarding the fire, the air is mixed with phlegm and passes from the nostrils with a noise, this is called *Kabuti* or sneezing. If phlegm thickens, as if prepared by fire, and has a saltish taste, it is called *Bransuti.* If hot air proceeds from the nostrils, and *air* is discharged like smoke or is very hot, it is called *Dipta.* Phlegm when deranged with air so as to close the nostrils is called *Pratinaha.* When *air, bile,* and *phlegm* are deranged in the nostrils it dries. When the discharge is thin like water, and passes from the nostrils, particularly at night, it is called *Pásáparsisrábah.*

प्रकुप्यति ॥ कफं संगृह्य कुरुते शोथं स्तब्धमवेदनम् । उन्मन्थकः सकण्डुको विकारः कफवातजः ॥ संवर्द्धमाने दुर्विद्धे कण्डुदाह-रुजान्वितः । शोथो भवति पाकश्च त्रिदोषो दुःखवर्द्धनः ॥

कफासृक् क्रिमयः क्रुद्धाः सर्षपाभा विसर्पिणः । कुर्व्वन्ति पाल्यां पिड़काः कण्डुदाहरुजान्विताः ॥ कफासृक्-क्रिमिसम्भूतः स विसर्पान्वित स्ततः । लिह्येत् सशष्कुलीं पालीं परिलेहीति स स्मृतः ॥

अथ नासारोगनिदानम् ।

अवघ्राते यस्य विशुष्यते च प्रक्लिद्यते धूप्यति चापि नासा । न वेत्ति यो गन्धरसांश्च जन्तु र्जुष्टं व्यवस्येत्तमपीनसेन ॥ तच्चानिल श्लेष्मभवं विकारं ब्रूयात् प्रतिश्याय समानलिङ्गम् । दोषै विदग्धै

When the nose is very hot and dry, and the passage of air gives great uneasiness, it is called *Násáparisasah.*

Pínasa has an acute and chronic form. In the first the head is heavy, the patient has no appetite, and the discharge from the nose is thin. The voice becomes altered, with occasional vomiting and weakness of the body. When chronic, the phlegm as it is discharged from the nose, thickens, and the voice becomes natural. The colour of the skin is natural, and the discharged phlegm is thick, and very adhesive.

Pritisyaiah resembles *Apinnasa* and is sometimes produced by the neglect in the calls of nature, by eating indigestable food, and allowing the accumulation of dust in the nostrils; speaking or crying much; frequent fits of anger, unusual and sudden alteration in the seasons, such as want of the accustomed rain, and exposure of the sun, watching or sleeping during the day, being wet with very cold water or dew, and excessive venery produce the diseases of the nose; as also hot tears passing into the nostrils. By these causes the humours are

---

गलतालुमूले संमूर्च्छितो यस्य समीरणस्तु ॥ निरेति पूति मुखनासिकाभ्यां तं पूतिनस्यं प्रवदन्ति रोगम्। घ्राणाश्रितं पित्तमरूंसि कुर्य्यात् यस्मिन् विकारे बलवांश्च पाकः ॥ तं नासिकापाकमिति व्यवस्येद् विक्लेदकोऽथावथवापि यत्र। दोषै र्विदग्धै रथवापि जन्तो र्ललाटदेशेऽभिहतस्य तैस्तैः ॥ नासा स्रवेत् पूय मसृग्विमिश्रं तं पूयरक्तं प्रवदन्ति रोगम् ॥

घ्राणाश्रितो मर्म्मनि संप्रदुष्टो यस्यानिलो नासिकया निरेति कफानुजातो बहुशोऽतिशब्द स्तं रोगमाहुः क्षवथुं विधिज्ञाः। तीक्ष्णोपयोगादभिजिघ्रतो वा भावान् कटूनर्क निरीक्षणाद्वा। सूत्रादिभि र्वा तरुणास्थिमर्म्मण्युद्घाटितेऽन्यः क्षवथु र्निरेति ॥ प्रभ्रश्यते नासिकया तु यस्य सान्द्रो विदग्धो लवणः कफस्तु।

deranged in the head, producing the usual symptoms of catarrh; the general symptoms of which are sneezing, heaviness of the head, languor and pain, and stiffness over the body (*Guseska*).

When produced by *air* the nostrils become filled up, there is a thin discharge with dryness of the throat, palate, and lips, with severe throbbing pain of the temples, and hoarseness.

When *bile* is deranged the symptoms are a hot discharge of a yellow colour, the body is weak, of a gray colour, and hot. There is much thirst, and what is vomited is hot, and like smoke.

When *phlegm* is deranged the discharge is white or grayish and is copious and cold. The body becomes pale, eyelids swollen, head very heavy, and the throat, palate, lips, and head, are itchy.

When *air*, *bile* and *phlegm* are deranged the symptoms occur rapidly, disappear, and recur again, whether they be acute or chronic. At one time the nose is clean but it again becomes dirty, dry, and closes with fœtid breath, and loss of smell. This is the bad form of the disease, and is cured with

---

प्राक्सञ्चितो मूर्द्धनि सूर्य्यतप्त स्तं भ्रंशथुं रोग मुदाहरन्ति ॥ घ्राणे भृशं दाहसमन्विते तु विनिःसरेद्धूम इवेह वायुः । नासा प्रदीप्तेव च यस्य जन्तो र्व्याधिस्तु तं दीप्त मुदाहरन्ति ॥

उच्छ्वासमार्गन्तु कफः सवातो रुन्ध्यात् प्रतीनाह मुदाहरेत् तम् । घ्रानाद्घनः पीत सीत स्तनुर्व्वा दोषः स्रवेत् स्राव मुदाहरेत्तम् ॥ घ्राणाश्रिते स्रोतसि मारुतेन गाढ़ं प्रतप्ते परिशोषिते च ॥ कृच्छ्रोच्छ्वसेदूर्द्धमधश्च जन्तु र्यस्मिन् स नासापरिशोष उक्तः । शिरोगुरुत्वमरुचि र्नासास्राव स्तनुः स्वरः ॥ क्षामः ष्ठीवत्यथाभीक्ष्णमामपीनस लक्षणम् । आमलिङ्गान्वितः श्लेष्मा घनः खेषु निमज्जति ॥ स्वरवर्णविशुद्धिश्च परिपक्वस्य लक्षणम् ॥

difficulty. If neglected this disease passes into *Pínasa*. When it has continued for a long time it produces deafness, blindness, loss of smell, cough, and dyspepsia.

When *blood* is deranged, and is discharged from the nostrils, the eyes are reddish. This form is produced by injuries of the chest, and both the mouth and nostrils have a bad smell. He loses the sense of smell, and worms are produced in the nostrils. These worms are small and of a black and white colour. The different forms of *Prahsiáka*, if not seen by the practitioner early, are not curable.

There are five forms of *Arbuda*, or tumors attacking the nose, and four of *Sota* (swellings), four kinds of *Arsa* (Polypus), and *Raktapitta* (Hemorrhage).

Diseases of the Eyes, (*Akírogha*).

It is related that *Janaka Rájá* of Mithilá or Tirhoot, did not perform the usual coremonies and prayers to the sun, for

---

सन्धारणाजीर्णरजोऽतिभाष्य क्रोधर्त्तु वैषम्यशिरोऽभितापैः। प्रजागरातिस्वपनाम्बुशीतै रवश्यया मैथुनवाष्पधूमैः॥ संस्त्यानदोषे शिरसि प्रवृद्धो वायुः प्रतिश्याय मुदीरयेत्तु। चयं गता मुर्द्धनि मारुतादयः पृथक् समस्ताश्च तथैव शोणितम्। प्रकुप्यमाना विविधैः प्रकोपनै स्ततः प्रतीश्यायकरा भवन्ति हि॥ क्षवप्रवृत्तिः शिरसोऽतिपूर्णता स्तम्भोऽङ्गमर्द्दः परिहृष्टरोमता॥ उपद्रवाश्चापरपरे पृथग्विधा नृणां प्रतिश्याय पुरःसराः स्मृताः। आनद्धा पिहिता नासा तनुस्राव प्रसेकिनी। गलताल्वोष्ठशोषश्च निस्तोदः शङ्खयो स्तथा। क्षवप्रवृत्तिरत्यर्थं वक्त्रवैरस्य मेव च॥ भवेत् स्वरोपघातश्च प्रतिश्यायेऽनिलात्मके। उष्णः सपीतकः स्रावो घ्राणात् स्रवति पैत्तिके कृशोऽतिपाण्डुः सन्तप्तो भवेदुष्टाभिपीड़ितः। सधूममग्निं सहसा वमतीव स मानवः॥* घ्राणात्

which he was afflicted with the diseases of the eye. By abstinence and humiliation before the sun, however he was cured of the disease; and since then, by proper offerings he obtained the favour of, and was instructed by, *Surya* concerning these diseases. He afterwards wrote a *Shástra* on the subject, called *Sátáka Tantra*, which is stated to be "in profundity like the ocean."

There are 76 diseases of the eye, of these 10 are air diseases, 10 bile, 13 phlegm, 25 are produced by the derangement of the three humours, 16 by blood, and 2 external diseases. These diseases are again sub-divided into 9 of the joinings of the eye, 21 of the eyelids, 11 of the white part of the eye, 4 of the black part, 17 of the eye in general, 12 diseases of the true organs of vision (*Dristi*), and two external diseases from injuries.

1. *Description of the eye.* After a description of the size of the eye it is stated that it is formed by a combination of all the elements. The flesh being produced by the earth, blood

---

कफकृते शीतः कफः पाण्डुः सवेदङ्गः ॥ शुक्लावभासः शुक्लाक्षो भवेद्गुरुशिरा नरः । कण्ठताल्वोष्ठशिरसां कण्डूभिरतिपीड़ितः ॥

भूत्वा भूत्वा प्रतिश्यायो यस्याकस्मान्निवर्त्तते । संपक्वो वापक्वो वा स सर्व्व प्रभवः स्मृतः ॥ प्रक्लिद्यते पुनर्नासा पुनश्च परिशुष्यति । पुनरानह्यते वापि पुनर्विव्रियते तथा ॥ निश्वासो वातिदुर्गन्धो नरो गन्धान्न वेत्ति च ॥ एवं दुष्टप्रतिश्यायं जानीयात् कृच्छ्रसाधनम् ॥ रक्तजे तु प्रतिश्याये रक्तस्रावः प्रवर्त्तते । ताम्राक्षश्च भवेज्जन्तुरुरोघात-प्रपीड़ितः । दुर्गन्धोच्छ्वासवदनो गन्धानपि न वेत्ति सः ॥ सर्व्व एव प्रतिश्याया नरस्याप्रतिकारिणः दुष्टतां यान्ति कालेन तदासाध्या भवन्ति हि ॥ मूर्च्छन्ति चात्र क्रिमयः श्वेताः स्निग्धा स्तथाणवः । क्रिमितो यः शिरोरोग स्तुल्यं

from the fire, the black part from the air, the white part from the water, and the different canals for the tears are produced by ether or sky. The black part extends over one-third of the eye, and the pupil about one-seventh part of the black part. The tunics are the two eyelids, and of the globe of the eye. The first surrounds the vitreous humour (*Tezajala*, or glistening water), the second is covered with flesh, the third with fat, and the fourth with bone. They distinguish five circles, the eye-lashes, eyelids, the white sclerotic coat, the iris, and the pupil. There are five joinings, the eyelashes with the eyelids, the eyelids and white of the eye (sclerotic), the white with the transparent cornea, and this with the pupil, and the corunculo lachrymalis. The humours are carried into the eye by the vessels, and produce many diseases.

The causes of these diseases are bathing when the body is very hot, intensely regarding minute objects, or those at a great distance, or sleeping at irregular periods, frequent crying, grief, anger, external injuries, excessive venery, constipated or sour articles of food, or a kind of pea (*máskalái*). Irregularities of seasons produce them, retaining the tears in the eye,

---

तेनास्य लक्षणम् । वाधिर्य्यमन्ध्यमघ्रत्वं घोरांश्च नयनामयान् ॥ शोषाग्निसादकासांश्च वृद्धाः कुर्व्वन्ति पीनसाः ॥ अर्व्वुदं सप्तधा शोषा श्चत्वारोऽर्शश्चतुर्व्विधम् । चतुर्व्विधं रक्तपित्तमुक्तं घ्राणेऽपि तद्विदुः ।

अथ नेत्ररोगनिदानम् ।

अथ सर्व्वगतनिदानम् ।

नव सन्ध्याश्रयास्तेषु वर्त्मजास्त्वेकविंशतिः । शुक्लभागे दशै-काश्च चत्वारः कृष्णभागजाः । सर्व्वाश्रयाः सप्तदश दृष्टिजाः द्वादशैव तु ॥ वाह्यजौ द्वौ समाख्यातौ रोगौ परमदारुणौ । भूय एतान् प्रवक्ष्यामि संख्यारूपचिकित्सितैः ॥

smoke and dust, profuse vomiting, or stopping it suddenly. These causes with derangements of air, bile and phlegm or blood, produce diseases of the eye. The deranged humours are conveyed into the eye by the vessels, and produce the different diseases in the different parts of the eye. The general symptoms of diseases of the eye are its changing its natural colour, pain, redness, a discharge of tears, and there is a burning sensation in the eye as if there was an external body in it. The eyelids feel painful, as if thorns were under the eyelid, and there is intollerance of light.

2. *Inflammation.* There are four varieties of inflammation of the eye, produced by derangement in the air, bile, phlegm, and blood. The ten diseases of the air are characterized by severe pain in the eye, which remains immoveable, a feeling of sand in the eye, which is dry, with an inclination to rub it. The patient complains of head-ache, and the tears are cold.

Bile produces inflammation of the eye, which is characterized by burning, with the discharge of blood and pus, and cold applications are grateful. The eye seems to be cover-

---

उष्णाभितप्तस्य जले प्रवेशा द्दूरेक्षणात् स्वप्नविपर्य्ययाच्च। स्वेदाद्रजो धूमनिषेवनाच्च छर्द्दे र्विघाताद्वमनातियोगात् ॥ द्रवात्तथान्नान्निशि सेविताच्च विण्मूत्रवातक्रमनिग्रहाच्च ॥ प्रसक्तसंरोदनकोपशोकाच्छिरोऽभिघातादतिमद्यपानात् ॥ तथा ऋतुनाञ्च विपर्य्ययेण क्लेशाभिघातादतिमैथुनाच्च। वाष्पग्रहात् सूक्ष्मनिरीक्षणाच्च नेत्रे विकारान् जनयन्ति दोषाः ॥

वातात् पित्तात् कफाद्रक्तादभिष्यन्द श्चतुर्विधः। प्रायेन जायते घोरः सर्व्वनेत्रामयाकरः। निस्तोदन-स्तम्भन-रोमहर्ष-संहर्ष-पारुष्य-शिरोऽभितापाः ॥ विशुष्कभावः शिशिराश्रुता च वाताभिपन्ने नयने भवन्ति। दाहप्रपाकौ शिशिराभिनन्दा धूमायनं वाष्पसमुच्छ्रयश्च। उष्णाश्रुता पीतकनेत्रता च पित्ताभिपन्ने नयते

ed with a haze, feels hot, and has a yellow colour. There is likewise a discharge of warm tears.

Cough, when it produces inflammation it is characterized by hot applications being grateful to the eye, which feels heavy, swelled, itchy, and cold. There is also a copious discharge of tears, which are of an oily nature.

Blood produces inflammation which is characterized by the discharge of a copper colour, the eye is red, and the small vessels of the eye become turgid. Before this appears the peculiar symptoms of bile are present. When this inflammation is neglected, or improperly treated, it produces one of the four varieties of severe ophthalmia (*Adimanta*). This aggravated form has the following symptoms: severe pain, as if the eyes were torn; throbbing, which extends to half of the head, and is characterized by the above symptoms of each variety. When this is produced by phlegm it will destroy the eye in seven days; if blood is diseased it will destroy the organ in five days, if air in six days, and if bile in one day. In the acute stage of this ophthalmia the pain is severe, as if a foreign body was in

---

भवन्ति। उष्णाभिनन्दा गुरुताक्षिशोफः कण्डूपदेहावतिशीतता च॥
स्रावो मुहुः पिच्छिल एव चापि कफाभिपन्ने नयने भवन्ति।
पित्तस्य लिङ्गानि च यानि तानि रक्ताभिपन्ने नयने भवन्ति।
वृद्धैरेतैरभिष्यन्दैर्नराणामक्रियावताम्॥ तावन्तस्त्वधिमन्थाः
स्युर्नयने तीव्रवेदनाः। उत्पाट्यत इवात्यर्थं नेत्रं निर्मथ्यते तथा॥
शिरसोऽर्द्धञ्च तं विद्यादधिमन्थं स्वलक्षणैः। हन्याद्दृष्टिं श्लैष्मिकः
सप्तरात्रादधिमन्थो रक्तजः पञ्चरात्रात्॥ षड्रात्राद्वा वातिको
वै निहन्यान्मिथ्याचारात् पैत्तिकः सद्य एव॥ उदीर्णं वेदनं
नेत्रं रागशोकसमन्वितम्॥ घर्षनिस्तोदशूलाश्रुयुक्तं मामान्वितं
विदुः। मन्दवेदनता कण्डूः संरम्भाश्रुप्रशान्तता। प्रशस्तवर्णता
चाक्ष्णोः संपक्वदोषमादिशेत्।

it, with redness and swelling, and a copious discharge of tears from the eye. When merely chronic the pain is less, with itchiness in the part, the discharge of tears is slight, and the eyelids can be opened, and the globe appears healthy. When the inflammation produced by air is neglected, the accessions recur at intervals, and produce pain of different kinds. The eye swells, suppurates, and is red like a wild fig. It suppurates without swelling, when the other symptoms are the same. The eye in such cases is very painful, and the disease is incurable.

Another form of the disease is named *Bátaparjiya*, in which air is deranged, and the eyebrow and eye are painful, so that the person winks, and brings the eyelids forcibly together.

Suskákipáka. When the eyelids are dry, and suppurate, the eye is very painful, the sight is troubled, and the patient cannot shut the eyelids.

Anutágabáta. When the air of the neck and head, ears, cheeks, or vessels of the back of the neck are deranged, and in other situations, the eyebrow and eye are very painful.

In *Amládhasita,* the eye is of a green colour with a red

कण्डुपदेहाश्रुयुतः पक्वोडुम्बरसन्निभः। संरम्भी पच्यते यस्तु नेत्रपाकः स शोथजः॥ शोथहीनानि लिङ्गानि नेत्रपाके त्वशोथजे। उपेक्षणादक्षि यदाधिमन्थो वातात्मकः सादयति प्रसह्य॥ रुजाभिरुग्राभिरसाध्य एष हताधिमन्थः खलु नाम रोगः॥ वारं वारञ्च पर्येति भ्रुवौ नेत्रे च मारुतः॥ रुजश्च विविधास्तीव्राः स ज्ञेयो वातपर्ययः। यत् कूणितं दारुणरुक्षवर्त्म संदह्यते चाविलदर्शनं यत्। सुदारुणं यत् प्रतिबोधने च शुष्काक्षिपाकोपहतं तदक्षि। यस्यावटुः कर्णशिरोहनुस्थो मन्यागतो वाप्यनिलोऽन्यतो वा। कुर्याद्रुजं वै भ्रुवि लोचने च तमन्यतो वात मुदाहरन्ति॥

circumference, from the colour of the blood in the part. It extends over the eye which is hot, swelled, and tears continually flow. This is produced by sour articles of food.

Sirotpáta. It is accompanied with more or less pain in the eye, which becomes red. When neglected this form is called *Siráharsa,* when the discharge is of a copper colour, and the person cannot see. These are the general diseases of the eye.

2. *The diseases of the black part of the Eye. Ulcers of the Cornea,* (*Bruna-sukra.*) In this disease the black part appears spotted, the discharge is very hot, and if it is not near the pupil and there is only one spot, which is without pain and any discharge, it may sometimes be cured.

When the ulcer is of long standing, extensive, and deep-seated, it is difficult to cure. When depressed in the middle and the margin elevated it will destroy vision. When both coats (cornea and iris) are destroyed by the ulcer, which has a red margin, and has been of long standing, it is incurable.

Abruna-sukra. When the inflammation is in the black part of the eye with a burning sensation, it is very white like

---

श्यावं लोहितपर्य्यन्तं सर्व्वञ्चाक्षि प्रपच्यते ॥ सदाहशोथं सास्राव मस्राश्रुषितमस्रतः । अवेदना वापि सवेदना वा यस्याक्षिराजी हि भवन्ति ताम्राः । मुहुः विरज्यन्ति च या स तादृग्व्याधिः शिरोत्पात इति प्रदिष्टः ॥ मोहात् शिरोत्पात उपेक्षितास्तु जायेत रोगस्तु शिराप्रहर्षः । ताम्राभ मस्रं स्रवति प्रगाढ़ं तथा न शक्नोत्यभिवीक्षितुञ्च ।

अथकृष्णागतनिदानम् ।

निमग्नरूपन्तु भवेद्धि कृष्णे सूचीव विद्धं प्रतिभाति यद्वैः । स्रावं स्रवेदुष्णमतीव यच्च तत् सव्रणं शुक्र मुदाहरन्ति ॥ दृष्टेः समीपेन भवेत्तु यच्च न चावगाढ़ं न च संस्रवेद्धि । अवेदनं वा न च युग्म शुक्रं तत् सिद्धिमायाति कदाचिदेव ॥

the moon, it is curable. If of old standing, is white, large, and deep-seated, it will be cured with difficulty.

Pákátiya, or opacity of the cornea following inflammation.

Ajakáyáta, small tumors like the litter of goats, slightly red, which protrudes through the cornea, from which a bloody discharge proceeds mixed with pus.

The *Dristi* (crystalline lens) is the principal part of the organ of vision. It is like the form of a pea (*masuri*), and is produced by a mixture of the essential parts of the five elements. It resembles the firefly, and it is largely supplied with the eternal fire (*Abaytazi*). It is covered by the external tunic of the eye, and has externally an opening (pupil ?). By cold it is kept in a healthy state. Tho diseases of this part of the eye are very tedious in their cure.

3. *Diseases of the membranes of the Eye.* When the first tunic (*Pratarnapatala*) is deranged, the vision is indistinct. When the second tunic is affected the sight is very imperfect, and the person sees an appearance of motes, musquitoes, hairs, and nets. In other cases it is in the

---

स्यन्दात्मकं कृष्णागतं सचोषं शङ्खेन्दुकुन्द-प्रतिमावभासम्। वैहायसाभ्रप्रतिमाप्रकाशं मथाव्रणं साध्य मुदाहरन्ति। गम्भीर जातं बहलञ्च शुक्रं चिरस्थितञ्चापि वदन्ति कृच्छ्रम्। विच्छिन्न-मध्यं पिशितावृतं वा चलं शिरासूक्ष्ममदृष्टिकृच्च। द्विलग्-गतं लोहितमन्ततश्च चिरोत्थितञ्चापि विवर्ज्जनीयम्॥ उष्णाश्रु-पातः पिड़का च नेत्रे यस्मिन् भवेत् मुद्गनिभञ्च शुक्रम्। तदप्य-साध्यं प्रवदन्ति केचिदन्यच्च यत् तित्तिरिपक्षतुल्यम्॥ श्वेतं समाक्रामति सर्व्वतो हि दोषेण यस्यासितमण्डलञ्च। तमक्षिपाकात्य यमक्षिरोगं सर्व्वात्मकं वर्ज्जयितव्यमाहुः। अजापुरीषप्रतिमो रुजावान् सलोहितो लोहितपिच्छिलास्रः। विगृह्य कृष्णं प्रचयोऽ-भ्युपैति तच्चाजकाजातमिति व्यवस्येत्।

form of a circle like spectres, rays, and as every thing were indistinct and immersed in water, or like rain, clouds, and darkness. The person cannot distinguish distance, so that near objects seem at a distance.

When the third membrane is deranged he can neither see above nor below; large objects appear covered, and he cannot distinguish the features of a person placed before him. Such a person has often double vision.

Linganása. In this form the whole crystalline lens (*Dristi*) is affected, and if not very deep the person can see the moon, star, and lightning. When *air* is much increased the patient sees every object red; and when *bile* is affected, he can see the sun, the rainbow, and lightning. In other cases every thing appears black, variegated, and like the feather of a peacock. When affected by *phlegm* every object appears as if covered with oil and white. When the three humours are deranged, every thing appears spotted as of a mixture of different colours. When *blood* is deranged every object appears red and dark. In *Linganása* the colour is made of six different tints.

When the eye is affected with deranged *bile*, it is called *Pittabidagdha dristi*, which is characterized by the yellowness,

---

अथ दृष्टिजनिदानम् ।

प्रथमे पटले दोषा यस्य दृष्ट्यां व्यवस्थिताः । अव्यक्तानि स रूपाणि कदाचिदथ पश्यति ।

दृष्टिर्भृशं विह्वलति द्वितीयं पटलं गते । मक्षिकामशकांश्चापि जालकानि च पश्यति ॥ मण्डलानि पताकांश्च मरीचिं कुण्डलानि च ॥ परिप्लवांश्च विविधान् वर्षमभ्रं तमांसि च ॥ दूरस्थानि च रूपाणि मन्यते स समीपतः । समीपस्थानि दूरे च दृष्टेर्गोचरविभ्रमात् । यत्नवानपि चात्यर्थं सूचीपाशं न पश्यति ॥

and images appearing yellow. If it affects the third membrane he cannot see during the day, but can see at night.

When *phlegm* is affected it is called *Sleshmabidagdha dristi* which is characterized by the white appearance, and every thing seems white. When deranged in the three membranes of the eye it is called *Nyctalopia,* or nightblindness. He can see during the day. Grief, fever, vexation, severe diseases of the head, cause this disease of the eye, in which every object appears enveloped in smoke; hence it is called *Samadarsher.* In other cases the person cannot see small objects during the day, but sees every thing at night. This is called *Rasajáta.*

When air, bile, and phlegm are deranged, and produce a change in the iris like the mungoose eye (which is very red) every thing appears of a mottled appearance during the day. It is named *Nakulándha.*

Gambiraká. When *air* is deranged it produces the disease in which the pupil of the eye is contracted, and it diminishes the size of the eye; and is accompanied with great pain.

Linganása is of two kinds. The first is called *Sanimita* and the second *Animita*: the first is produced by inflammation of

---

ऊर्द्ध्वं पश्यति नाधस्तात् तृतीयं पटलं गते। महान्त्यपि च रूपाणि छादीतानीव चाम्बरैः॥ कर्णनासाक्षिहीनानि विकृतानीव पश्यति। यथा दोषश्च रजेयत दृष्टिर्दोषे बलीयसी॥ अधःस्थिते समीपस्थं दूरस्थं चोपरिस्थिते॥ पार्श्वस्थिते तथा दोषे पार्श्वस्थं नैव पश्यति॥ समन्ततः स्थिते दोषे सङ्कुलपश्च पश्यति। द्विधा स्थिते द्विधा पश्येद्‌बहुधानवस्थिते॥ दोषे दृष्टाश्रिते तिर्यक् स एकं मन्यते द्विधा॥

तिमिराख्यः स वै दोषश्चतुर्थं पटलं गतः। रुणद्धि सर्व्वतो दृष्टिं लिङ्गनाशमतः परम्॥ अस्मिन्नपि तमो भूते नातिरूढ़े महागदे। चन्द्रादित्यौ सनक्षत्रावन्तरीक्षे च विद्युतम्। निर्म्म-

the eye, and the second by the sight of holy sages, by regarding a kind of large snake (*Maharaza*), or luminous objects by which vision is destroyed. The eye in this disease does not lose its natural appearance.

Abigáta hatadristí is produced by accidents or injuries to the eye, by which the person cannot see ; the organ becomes red like coral, and severe pain is felt as if a person was tearing the eye out.

4. Diseases of the white part of the Eye.

Prastárijarma. In this disease there is a thin red or dark-coloured membrane covering the white part of the eye.

Suklárma. The enlargements in this disease are white and soft, and it advances slowly.

Raktárma is characterized by fleshy growths of a red colour.

Adimánsarma (Ptergium) is a liver-coloured thickening of the white part of the eye. It is stationary. Another form is thick, and fleshy, and of a white colour.

Stárjarma is fleshy swelling of the white of the eye.

लानि च तेजांसि भ्राजिष्णून्यथ पश्यति ॥ स एव लिङ्गनाशस्तु नीलिका काचसंज्ञितः ॥ वातेन चापि रूपाणि भ्रमन्तीव च पश्यति। आविलान्यरुणाभानि व्याविद्धानीव मानवः ॥ पित्तेनादित्यखद्योतशक्रचापतडिद्गुणान् ॥ नृत्यतश्चैव शिखिनः सर्व्वं नीलञ्च पश्यति। कफेण पश्येद्रूपाणि स्निग्धानि च सितानि च ॥ पश्येदसूक्ष्माण्यत्यर्थं वभ्रमेवाभ्रसंप्लवम् ॥ सलिलप्लावितानीव परिजाड्यानि मानवः। पश्येदस्रेण रक्तानि तमांसि विविधानि च ॥ स सितानपि कृष्णानि पीतानपि च मानवः ॥ सन्निपातेन चित्राणि विप्लुतानीव पश्यति ॥ बहुधा च द्विधा चापि सर्व्वाण्येव समन्ततः। हीनाधिकाङ्गान्यथवा ज्योतींष्यपि च भूयसः। पित्तं कुर्य्यात्

Sukti, when there are many small spots of a green flesh colour.

Arjana is when there is a red spot.

Pistaka is a round white elevation of the white of the eye like a drop of water.

Jála. The white part in this case is like a net-work, with hard small vessels of a red colour.

Sirája, in which white pimples appear in the white of the eye, surrounded by enlarged vessels.

Balásaka is a silvery copper-coloured spot surrounded by vessels.

5. *Diseases of the joinings of the eyes:—of the eyeball, cornea and sclerotica, eyelids, eyelashes, &c.*

These diseases are nine in number. The parts sometimes swell, suppurate and are painful; the disease is called *Puyalisa.* Blood and thick pus are discharged in these cases. Anothe form swells much, but does not suppurate; is itchy, but without pain. It is called *Upanáha.*

When air, bile, and phlegm are deranged at the joints, and the passage of the tears are discharged over the eyelids in the

---

परिम्लायि मूर्च्छितं पित्ततेजसा ॥ पीता दिशस्तु खद्योतान् भास्करश्चापि पश्यति ॥ विकीर्यमानान् खद्योतै र्वृक्षां स्तेजोभिरेव वा ॥

वक्ष्यामि षड्विधं रागैर्लिङ्गनाशमतः परं। रागोऽरुणो मारुतजः प्रदिष्टो म्लायी च नीलश्च तथैव पित्तात्। कफात् सितः शोणितजः सरक्तः समस्तदोषप्रभवो विचित्रः। अरुणं मण्डलं दृष्ट्यां स्थूलकाचारुणप्रभम्। परिम्लायिनि रोगे स्यान्म्लायि नीलञ्च मण्डलम्। दोषक्षयात् स्वयन्तत्र कदाचित् स्यात्तु दर्शनम्। अरुणं मण्डलं वातात् चञ्चलं परुषं तथा ॥ पित्तान्मण्डलमानीलं कांस्याभं पीतमेव वा ॥ श्लेष्मणो बहलं पीतं

form of tears, it is called *Netranári* (Fistula Lachrymalis), of which there are four varieties according to the nature of their discharges. When pus alone is discharged it is called *Parsásarba.* When phlegm is alone diseased, and the joint suppurates without pain, the discharge is of a white colour, thick, and shining like oil : it is then called *Sleshmásrába.* Diseased blood sometimes produces this disease, and when there is a hot discharge mixed with much blood it is called *Raktasrába.* When bile is diseased, the discharge has a yellow colour, and it is called *Pittasrába.*

When small pimples appear at the joints of the eye, of a red colour, they burn and are painful. They are called *Parbániká.* Sometimes this occurs at the juncture of the cornea and sclerotica, and are accompanied by the same symptoms as the last. They are of a red colour, and are called *Alaghi.*

Krimágranti. Sometimes worms are produced at the juncture of the eyelids, and eyelashes. They produce much itching ; and sometimes they form between the eyelid and the white part of the eye. They are of different colours and forms, and destroy the eye.

शङ्खकुन्देन्दुपाण्डुरम् ॥ चलत् पद्मपलाशस्थः शुक्लो विन्दु रिवाम्भसः। नृतप्रमाने च नयने मण्डलं तद्विसर्पति ॥ प्रवालपद्मपत्राभं मण्डलं शोणितात्मकम् ॥ दृष्टिरागो भवेच्चित्रो लिङ्गनाशे त्रिदोषजे। यथास्वं दोषलिङ्गानि सर्व्वेष्वेव भवन्ति हि ॥

षड्लिङ्गनाशाः* षड्मि च रोगा दृष्ट्याश्रयाः षट् च षड़ेव वाच्याः। पित्तेन दुष्टेन सदा तु दृष्टिः पीता भवेद् यस्य नरस्य किञ्चित् ॥ पीतानि रूपानि च तेन पश्येत् स वै नरः पित्तविदग्धदृष्टिः ॥ प्राप्ते तृतीयं पटलन्तु दोषे दिवा न पश्येन्निशि चेच्यते सः ॥ रात्रौ च शीतानुगृहीतदृष्टिः पित्तात्पभावादपि तानि पश्येत् ॥ तथा नरः श्लेष्मविदग्धदृष्टिः ज्ञानेव

Diseases of the Eyelids.

There are twenty-one diseases of the eyelids. In this class of diseases, air, bile, and phlegm may be diseased in a combined or separate form. In other cases these derangements affect the vessels of the eye, and the blood and flesh, &c. may separately, or when combined, produce diseases of the eyelids.

Atsangani are small eruptions on the external part of the lower eyelids, they often open internally ; and are produced by diseases of the blood.

Kambiká are swellings at the borders of the upper eyelid. When they break, pus and blood are evacuated ; and they are like small castor-oil seeds.

Another form of swelling is of the colour of blood ; of the size of a mustard seed, hard, and itchy ; and water, pus, and blood are evacuated from them. When painful they are called *Pataki.* When numerous clusters of small eruptions, are rough, elevated, and situated on the inner side of the lid, they are called *Bartasarkará.* Another form are small like melon seeds ; have little pain, are situated in the eyelids, are rough to the feel, and are called *Arsabarta* or *Bartársi.* When like the new

---

शुक्लानि तु मन्यते सः। त्रिषु स्थितोऽल्पः पटलेषु दोषो नक्तान्ध्यमापादयति प्रसह्य। दिवा स सूर्य्यानुगृहीतदृष्टिः पश्येत्तु रूपाणि कफाल्पभावात्॥

शोकज्वरायासशिरोऽभितापै रत्याहता यस्य नरस्य दृष्टिः। धुम्रांस्तथा पश्यति सर्व्वभावान् स धुमदर्शीति नरः प्रदिष्टः। यो ह्रस्वजाड्यो दिवसेषु कृच्छ्रात् ह्रस्वानि रूपाणि च तेन पश्येत्। विद्योतते यस्य नरस्य दृष्टि र्दोषाभिपन्ना नकुलस्य यद्वत्॥ चित्राणि रूपाणि दिवा स पश्येत् स वै विकारो नकुलान्ध्यसंज्ञः॥ दृष्टिर्विरूपा श्वसनोपसृष्टा सङ्कुच्यतेऽभ्यन्तरतस्तु याति॥ रुजावगाढ़ा च तमक्षिरोगं गम्भीरिकेति प्रवदन्ति तज्ज्ञाः॥ बाह्यो

shining germ of a plant, the eyelids are long, hard, rough, indolent and irregular, and the patient cannot open the lid, the disease is called *Saskársa*, or dry hemorrhoidal tumors of the eyelid.

Another form is very hot, painful, and of a copper colour; and is soft, and small, with little pain: it is called *Angannanámika*.

Sometimes the eyelids are covered with small eruptions, and all the small swellings have the same appearance and colour, and are stationary. They are called *Bahalabarta*.

Another form of swelling is when the lids are swollen, itchy, and painful, the lids being tight over the eye, and the eyelids do not completely cover the globe of the eye. This disease is called *Bartabanda*.

When the internal part of the eyelid is spungy, hot, painful, of a copper colour, and changes quickly to a red colour, it is called *Klistahbarta*.

If in this disease bile is deranged and affects the blood, much dirty matter is discharged called *Bartahkardama*.

When the swelling of the lids is both external and internal, with burning and itchy pain of a dark yellow colour with a discharge, it is called *Sábabarta*.

पुनर्द्वाविह संप्रदिष्टौ निमित्ततश्चाप्यनिमित्ततश्च। निमित्तत स्तत्र शिरोभितापात् ज्ञेयस्त्वभिष्यन्दनिदर्शनः सः। सुरर्षिगन्धर्व्वमहोरगाणां सन्दर्शने नापि च भास्करस्य। हन्येत दृष्टिर्मनुजस्य यस्य स लिङ्गनाश स्त्वनिमित्तसंज्ञः। तत्राच्चिविस्पष्ट मिवातिभाति वैदूर्य्यवर्णा विमला च दृष्टिः।

अथ शुक्लजनिदानम्।

प्रस्तार्य्यर्म्मस्तनुस्तीर्णः श्यावं रक्तनिभं सिते। सश्वेतं मृदु शुक्लार्म्म शुक्ले तद्वर्द्धते चिरात्। पद्माभं मृदु रक्तार्म्म यन्मांसं चीयते सिते। पृथुमृद्वधिमांसार्म्म बहुलञ्च यकृन्निभम्॥ स्थिरं

When the upper lid is externally swollen, of a red colour, and much matter is discharged in its inner surface, it is called *Prákninabarta.*

When the eyelids are shut, and they cannot be opened without their being previously soaked in water, on account of the secretion, the disease is called *Akhnabarta.*

When the joints of the eyelids become immoveable, and everted it is called *Bátahattabarta* (Entropium.)

When a pendulous swelling forms in the inside of the eyelid without pain, and is caused by blood, it is named *Arbuda.*

When the vessels which move the eyelids are deranged they produce winking, or a continual movement of the eyes, when it is called *Nimassa.*

When the small fleshy excrescences, situated in the eyelids, are of a red colour, soft, painful, and grow again when removed by the knife, they are produced by diseased blood, and are called *Sunitársa.* Another form of tumor forms on the eyelids like a plum, hard, soft, moist, and does not suppurate, but becomes large and knotted it is called *Lagannah.*

When air, bile, and phlegm are deranged the swelling appears above the eyelid, breaks, and blood, water and pus are discharged through many openings. The pain is so severe as

---

प्रस्तारि मांसाढ्यं शुष्कं स्नायुर्म्मपञ्चमम्। श्यावाः स्युः पिशि-
तनिभाश्च विन्दवो ये शुक्ताभाः सितनियताः सतशुक्तिसंज्ञः॥ एको
यः शशरुधिरोपमश्च विन्दुः शुक्रस्थो भवति तमर्ज्जुनं वदन्ति।
श्लेष्ममारुतकोपेन शुक्ले पिष्टं समुन्नतम्॥ पिष्टवत् पिष्टकं विद्धि
मलाक्तादर्शसन्निभम्॥ जलाभः कठिनशिरो महान् सरक्तः सन्तानः
स्मृत इह जालसंज्ञितः। शुक्रस्थाः सितपिड़काः शिरावृतताया
स्त्वाभ्र्यादसित समीपजाः शिराजाः॥ कांस्याभो मृदुरथ वारिविन्दु-
कल्पो विज्ञेयो नयनसिते वलाससंज्ञः॥

to resemble poison, and is called *Bishabarta.* In other cases these derangements contract the eyelids so that the person can not see distinctly. This disease is called *Kuncharna.*

When air is deranged the eyelashes are turned inwards, and inflame the eye, and the person is always rubbing them. It is called *Pakakapat,* (Entropeon,) and is a difficult disease to cure.

Bile when deranged in the eye produces the falling off of the eyelashes; when the eyelids are itchy and hot, the disease is called *Pakakṣáta*

Besides the seventy-six diseases, which are common both to children and to the adult, there is another which is peculiar to the former. This is called *Kukunáka* or purulent ophthalmia. It is caused by the bad milk of the mother, and also by the derangement of phlegm, air, bile, or blood, singly, or collectively. It affects the eyelids. The symptoms are the continual rubbing the eye, as well as the nose and forehead; great intollerance of light, and a copious discharge.

अथ सन्धिजनिदानम् ।

पक्वः शोथः सन्धिजो यः सतोदः स्रवेत् पूयं पूति पूयालसाख्यः ग्रन्थिर्नाल्पो दृष्टिसन्धावपाकी कण्डुप्रायो नीरुज स्तूपनाहः ॥ गत्वा सन्धीनश्रुमार्गेण दोषाः कुर्य्युः स्रावान् लक्षणैः स्वैरुपेतान् । तं हि स्रावं नेत्रनाड़ीति केचित्तस्या लिङ्गं कीर्त्तयिष्ये चतुर्द्धा ॥ पाकात् सन्धौ संस्रवेद् यस्तु पूयं पूयास्रावोऽसौ गदः सर्व्वजस्तु । श्वेतं सान्द्रं पिच्छिलं यः स्रवेत्तु श्लेष्मास्रावोऽसौ विकारो मतस्तु ॥ रक्तास्रावः शोणितोत्थो विकारः स्रवेत् दुष्टं तत्र रक्तं प्रभूतम् । हरिद्राभं पीतमुष्णं जलं वा पित्तास्रावः संस्रवेत् सन्धिमध्यात् ॥

ताम्रा तन्वी दाहशूलोपपन्ना ज्ञेया वैद्यैः पीड़का पर्व्वणीका । जाता सन्धौ कृष्णशुक्लेऽलजी स्यात्तस्मिन्नेव ख्यापिता पूर्व्वलिङ्गैः ॥

Diseases of the Head (*Síraroga.*)

Under this order will be arranged the varieties of Head-ache, and the diseases of the organs of sense.

Head-ache.—There are eleven varieties of head-ache; which are produced by derangements of the air, bile, and phlegm; by the mixture of the three; by diseased blood; by a deranged or diminished state of the humours, by worms, the eighth is named *Súrjyábartta*, the ninth, *Anantabáta*, tenth, *Ardháyabhedaka*, and the eleventh *Sankhaka*.

1. When *air* is diseased in the head, it is suddenly affected with pain, which is severe at night.

2. *Bile.* In this variety, the head is hot, as if burning charcoal was placed over it, and there is an appearance of smoke proceeding from the mouth.

3. *Phlegm.* In this variety the head is heavy and dull, and it cannot be turned about. The head feels cool, and the eyelids and mouth are swollen.

4. When the above three *dhátu* are diseased, the different symptoms are combined.

क्रिमिग्रन्थिर्वर्त्म तः पक्ष्मतश्च कण्डुं कुर्युः क्रिमयः सन्धिजाताः।
नानारूपा कर्त्म शुक्लान्तसन्धौ चरन्तग्रन्तर्लोचनं दूषयन्तः॥

अथ वर्त्मजनिदानम्।

अभ्यन्तरमुखी ताम्रावाह्यतोवर्त्मनश्च या। स्योत्सङ्गोत्सङ्ग पीड़का सर्व्वजा स्थूलकण्डुरा॥ वर्त्मान्ते पीड़काध्माता भिद्यन्ते च स्रवन्ति च। कुम्भीकवीजसदृशाः कुम्भीकाः सन्निपातजाः॥ स्राविण्यः कुण्डरा गुर्व्वो रक्तासर्षपसन्निभाः। रुजावत्यश्च पीड़काः पोथक्य इति कीर्त्तिताः॥ पीड़का या खरास्थुला सूक्ष्माभिरभि संवृताः। वर्त्मस्था शर्करा नाम स रोगो वर्त्मदूषकः॥ एर्व्वारु वीजप्रतीमाः पीड़का मन्दवेदनाः। श्लक्ष्णाः खराश्च वर्त्मस्था

5. When the blood is deranged, producing this disease, the symptoms are the same as when bile is deranged. The pain in this variety is so severe, that the head cannot be touched, or bent forward.

6. When the disease is produced by a diminution of brain, or fat, phlegm, or blood, in the head, it produces great uneasiness and pain.

7. Worms sometimes produce severe pain in the head, of a kind as if an animal was eating, or tearing the head. A watery red or bloody discharge flows from the nose, and the patient's life is to be considered as in danger.

8. *Súrjyábartta.* In this variety, when the sun rises the eyes and brow fe el painful; and it continues, and increases, while the sun is above the horizon. It diminishes in the evening, and towards night. It is produced by derangement in the air, phlegm, and bile.

9. *Anantabáta.* When air, bile, and phlegm are deranged in the vessels of the neck, they produce great pain, particularly in the eyebrows, temples, and cheeks. It also produces shaking of the head, pain in the lower jaw, and diseases of the eyes (*neuralgia*).

स्तदर्शोवर्त्म कीर्त्तितं ॥ दीर्घाङ्कुरः खरस्तब्धो दारुणोऽभ्यन्तरोद्भवः व्याधिरेषोऽभिविख्यातः शुष्कार्शो नाम नामतः। दाहतोदवती ताम्रा पीड़का वर्त्मसम्भवा ॥ मृद्वी मन्दरुजा सूक्ष्मा ज्ञेया साञ्जन नामिका। वर्त्मोपचीयते यस्य पीड़काभि समन्ततः ॥ सवर्णाभिः स्थिराभिश्च विद्याद्बहलवर्त्म तत्। कण्डूमताल्पतोदेन वर्त्मशोथेन यो नरः ॥ नं स संछादयेदक्षि यात्रासौ वर्त्मबन्धकः।

मृद्वल्पवेदनं ताम्रं यद्वर्त्म सममेव च। अकस्माच्च भवेद्रक्तं क्लिष्टवर्त्मेति तद्विदुः ॥ क्लिष्टं पुनः पित्तयुतं शोणितं विदहेद् यदा ॥ ततः क्लिन्नत्वमापन्न मुच्यते वर्त्मकर्द्दमः। यद्वर्त्म बाह्यतोऽन्तश्च

10. *Ardháyabhedaka, (hemiplegia.)* When much dry food is taken it produces this disease ; or eating without an appetite, or too frequent ; exposure to the easterly wind, or to dew, and the abuse of venery. When the urine and bowels are constipated, and the person has been subjected to much grief, or severe exertion, he is liable to the attacks of this disease ; as also by derangements of air, bile, and phlegm. The attack occurs sometimes every fortnight, in other cases every tenth day, or in other cases every day. The half of the neck, brow, temples, ears, eyes, are very painful. When severe, as it often is, like that of poison, or as if burnt, and the sight and hearing become imperfect. This disease is very obstinate, and most distressing ; so that a thousand physicians cannot sometimes cure it.

11. *Sank-haka.* When air, bile, and phlegm, with blood are deranged, it produces severe pain in the temples and head, which becomes hot. This form is dangerous, like poison. When the person cannot swallow, he will die in three days.

श्यावं शूनं सवेदनम्॥ तदाहुः श्याववर्त्मेति वर्त्मरोगविशारदाः। अरुजं वाह्यतः शूनं वर्त्म यस्य नरस्य हि॥ प्रक्लिन्नवर्त्म तद्विद्यात् क्लिन्नमत्यर्थमन्ततः॥ यस्य धौतान्यधौतानि सम्बध्यन्ते पुनः पुनः। वर्त्मान्यपरिपक्वानि विद्यादक्लिन्नवर्त्म तत्। विमुक्तः सन्धिनिश्लेष्टं वर्त्म यस्य न मील्यते॥ एतद्वातहतं वर्त्म जानीयादक्षिचिन्तकः॥ वर्त्मान्तरस्थं विषमं ग्रन्थिभूतमवेदनम्॥ आचक्षितार्व्वुदमिति। सरक्त मविलम्बितम्॥ निमेषिणीः शिरा वायु प्रविष्टवर्त्मसंश्रयाः। चालयत्यक्षिवर्त्मानि निमेष इति तद्विदुः॥

यः स्थितो वर्त्ममध्ये तु लोहितो मृदुरङ्कुरः। तद्रक्ताजं शोणितार्शं च्छिन्नं भिन्नं प्रवर्त्तते॥ अपाको कठिनो स्थूलो

But if he lives beyond this time, medicines may then be given for the cure.

Diseases of the Female organs of Generation.

There are twenty forms of these diseases, which are produced by using bad food, or taking improper exercise. They are also caused by diseased menses, or semen. In other cases they are produced without any apparent causes.

1. *Udábertá.* When the menses are discharged with great pain, and are frothy.

2. *Bandhyá.* Difficult menstruation, Dismenorrhagæa (*nostartoboh*) where the menses are stopped, by the accumulation of unhealthy humours in the part. When the woman is barren, the disease is called *Bandhyá.*

3. *Biplutá.* Continued pain in the genital organs.

4. *Pariplutá.* Severe pain during connection.

5. *Bátalá.* In this disease the vagina is contracted and rough, accompanied with pain. In these five diseases *air* is

---

-ग्रन्थिर्वर्त्मनि भवेदरुजः ॥ नगणो नाम स व्याधिर्लिङ्गतः परिकीर्त्तितः । त्रयो दोषा बहिः शोथं कुर्युश्छिद्राणि वर्त्मनोः ॥ प्रस्रवन्त्यन्तरुदकं विषवद्विषवर्त्म तत् । वाताद्या वर्त्मसंकोचकं जनयन्ति मला यदा ॥ तदा द्रष्टुं न शक्नोति कुञ्चनं नाम तद्विदुः । पक्ष्माशितानि वातेन पक्ष्माण्यक्षि विशन्ति हि । घृष्यन्त्यक्षि मुहुस्तानि संरम्भं जनयन्ति च । असिते सितभागे च मूलकोषात् पतन्त्यपि । पक्ष्मकोपः स विज्ञेयो व्याधिः परमदारुणः । वर्त्मपक्ष्माशयगतं पित्तं रोमाणि शातयेत् । कण्डुं दाहञ्च कुरुते पक्ष्मशातं तमादिशेत् ।

locally deranged, the parts are hard and swollen, with the various seven varieties of pain produced by diseased air.

6. When the menses are discharged very hot, the disease is named *Sanítakara.* When there is an unusual discharge of a red colour from the vagina, accompanied with pain, and followed by lassitude, &c., the disease is named *Prodorah* or *Menorrhagia.* This disease is produced by bad food, diet, or milk, or any improper mixture of food, sleeping during the day, by the use of ardent spirits, or hot food, or eating frequently without being hungry; by abortion, or frequent venery, by severe exercise particularly riding and walking, by grief, by carrying heavy weights, and by external injuries. These causes produce the disease which is accompanied with fever, and pain over the body; and after a time the patient becomes weak, is affected with giddiness, fainting, thirst, great heat, delirium, jaundice, and drowsiness. It is also accompanied with the general symptoms of diseased phlegm, air, and bile separately, or combined.

When *phlegm* is particularly deranged in this disease; the discharge is whitish, mucilaginous, and has the smell of the water in which flesh had been steeped, or of the colour of water in which straw has been immersed.

अथ शिरोरोगनिदानम् ।

शिरोरोगान्तु जायन्ते वातपित्तकफै स्त्रिभिः। सन्निपातेन रक्तेन चयेण क्रिमिभि स्तथा ॥ सूर्य्यावर्त्तानन्तवातार्द्धावभेदक-शङ्खकैः ॥ यस्या निमित्तं शिरसो रुजश्च भवन्ती तीव्रा निशि चातिमात्रम। बन्धोपतापैश्च भवेद्विशेषः शिरोऽभितापः स समीरणेन ॥ यस्योष्णमङ्गारचितं यथैवः भवेच्छिरोधुमवतीव नासा ॥ शीतेन रात्रौ च भवेद्विशेषः शिरोऽभितापः सतु पित्तकोपात् ॥ शिरो भवेद यस्य कफोपदिग्धं गुरुप्रतिष्ठव्ध मतो हिमञ्च ।

When *bile* is particularly deranged, the discharge is sudden, and is of a yellow or reddish, blue or black colour. It is hot, and the other symptoms of diseases of bile appear.

When *air* is particularly affected the discharge is of a red colour, like the washings of flesh, is frothy, is in smaller quantities than the last variety, and is accompanied with more pain.

When the three humours are deranged producing this disease, the discharge is of the colour of honey mixed with ghee, or of a yellow colour like marrow, and has a fœtid smell. In this form a cure is not to be expected, and the practitioner should refuse to attend such a patient.

The unfavourable symptoms of this disease are when it has continued long, is accompanied with a copious discharge, with fever, great thirst, and heat followed by great debility. When the menses occur every month, without pain or burning, are of the natural colour, and neither too copious, nor too scanty, it is advantageous to health. When the discharge is red, like the colour of the blood of a hare, or like a decoction of lac, and does not permanently discolour cloth when it falls upon it, it is healthy.

भ्रूनाक्षि कूटं वदनञ्च यस्य शिरोभितापः स कफप्रकोपात्। शिरोऽभितापे त्रितयप्रवृत्ते सर्व्वाणि लिङ्गानि समुद्भवन्ति। रक्तात्मकः पित्तसमानलिङ्गः स्पर्शासहत्वं शिरसो भवेच्च॥

असृग्वसाश्लेष्मसमीरणानानां शिरोगतानामिह संचयेण। क्षयप्रवृत्तः शिरसोऽभिघातापः कष्टो भवेदुग्ररुजातिमात्रम्॥ संस्वेदन च्छर्द्दनधूमनस्यै रसृग्विमोक्षैश्च विवृद्धि मेति॥ निस्तुद्यते यस्य शिरोऽतिमात्रं संभक्ष्यमाणं स्फुरतीव चान्तः। घ्राणाच्च गच्छेद्रुधिरं सपूयं शिरोभितापः क्रिमिभिः सघोरः॥ सूर्य्योदयं वा प्रतिमन्दमन्द मक्षिभ्रुवं रुक्समुपैति गाढम्। विवर्द्धते चांशुमता

7. *Bámini.* When semen is discharged with the menses.

8. *Srangsini.* When the blood is discharged, and the parts are diseased, so that it prevents easy delivery.

9. *Patragani.* When the infant has died, or abortion has taken place with a great discharge of blood. In all these cases bile is much diseased, and is accompanied with fever.

10. *Pittalá.* When bile is deranged, there is much heat of the part, which suppurates and is accompanied with fever. These five last diseases are the symptoms of bile.

The following are the diseases produced by deranged phlegm.

11. *Atyánandá.* When the woman has no pleasure in the embraces of her husband.

12. *Karníní.* When phlegm and blood are deranged in the vagina, small granulations form, like the grains of rice from deranged phlegm and blood.

13. *Charuná.* When the semen of the male is more copious than that of the female.

14. *Charaná.* When the male semen does not enter the uterus.

15. *Shleshmalá.* It is produced by diseased phlegm with itchiness and coldness, and the part appears as if covered with oil.

सहैव सूर्य्यापवृत्तौ विनिवर्त्तते च। सर्व्वात्यकं कष्टतमं विकारं सूर्य्यापवर्त्तं तमुदाहरन्ति॥

दोषास्तु दुष्टास्त्रय एव मन्यां संपीड्य घाटासु रुजां सुतीव्राम् कुर्व्वन्ति योऽक्षि भ्रुविशङ्खदेशे स्थितिं करोत्याशु विशेषतस्तु॥ गण्डस्य पार्श्वे तु करोति कम्पं हनुग्रहं लोचनजांश्च रोगान्॥ अनन्तवातं तमुदाहरन्ति दोषत्रयोत्थं शिरसो विकारम्। रुक्षाशनाध्यशन-प्राग्वातावश्यायमैथुनैः॥ वेगसन्धारणायास व्यायामैः कुपितोऽनिलः। केवलः सकफोवार्द्धं गृहीत्वा शिरसो बली।

16. *Sandi.* In this variety the menses are not discharged, the breasts do not swell, and the parts are hard, and rough like a file.

17. *Palani.* When a large man has connection with a small, and young female he injures the parts, and produces this disease.

18. *Mahatí.* When the vagina is very large.

19. *Suchibuktra.* When the entrance is very small.

20. *Sarbalingasamutpanná.* Different varieties of pain, &c. produced by the derangement of the three humours in the part.

The five last forms of these diseases are cured with difficulty.

Kanda, (*Utero Vaginal Tumors.*)

These diseases are produced by the person sleeping during the day, by an angry disposition, by great fatigue, and by too much venery. They may also arise from mechanical injuries of the part. These tumors are like the fruit of the *Lakucha* tree, (a kind of Bread fruit tree, *Artocarpus lacucha*, or *Madar.*)

मन्याभ्रूशङ्खकर्णाक्षिललाटार्द्धेऽतिवेदनाम् । शस्त्रारणिनिभां कुर्यात् तीव्रां सोऽर्द्धावभेदकः ॥ नयनं वाथवा श्रोत्रमतिवृद्धो विनाशयेत् । रक्तपित्तानिला दुष्टाः शङ्खदेशे विमुर्च्छिताः । तीव्ररुग्दाहरागं हि शोथं कुर्व्वन्ति दारुणम् ॥ स शिरो विषवद्वेगी निरुध्याशु गलस्तता । त्रिरात्राज्जीवितं हन्ति शङ्खकोनामतः परम् । त्र्यहा-ज्जीवति भेषज प्रत्याख्याय समाचरेत् ॥

अथ स्त्रीरोगनिदानम् ।

अथ प्रदरनिदानम् ।

विरुद्धमद्याध्यशनादजीर्णाद्गर्भप्रपातादतिमैथुनाच्च । यानाध्व-शोकादतिकर्षणाच्च भाराभिघाताच्छयनाद्दिवा च ॥ असृग्दरं भवेत्

When *air* produces the disease the tumor is dry, and is of a dirty or yellowish colour, and has furrows on its surface.

When diseased *bile* produces the tumor it is very hot and red, and is accompanied with fever.

When *phlegm* produces the tumor it is like the colour of the Indigo flower and is very itchy.

When air, bile, and phlegm are diseased, all the separate symptoms are present. When three are so diseased in one part, it is incurable, and when produced by spirit or by phlegm, &c. it is cured with difficulty.

Diseases of Infants, (*Bálaroga.*)

The diseases of infants are supposed to be produced—

1st. By derangement in the air, bile, and phlegm. If the child sucks the mother's milk, affected by deranged air, he becomes affected with the diseases of air. His voice is changed, his body emaciated, bowels costive, and the secretion of urine is diminished.

The diseased bile affecting the milk produces a shining appearances of the body of the infant, as if it was smeared with

---

सर्व्वं साङ्गमर्द्दं सवेदनम्। तस्यातिवृद्धौ दौर्ब्बल्यं भ्रमोमूर्च्छामदस्तृषा। दाहः प्रलापः पाण्डुत्वं तन्द्रारोगाश्च वातजाः॥ तं श्लेष्मपित्तानिलसन्निपातैश्चतुः प्रकारं प्रदरं वदन्ति॥

आमं सपिच्छाप्रतिमं सपाण्डु पुलाकतोयप्रतिमं कफात्तु। सपीतनीलासितरक्तमुष्णं पित्तार्त्तियुक्तं भृशवेगि पित्तात्॥ रूक्षारुणं फेनिलमल्पमल्पं वातार्त्ति वातात् पिशितोदकाभम्॥ सक्षौद्रसर्पिर्हरितालवर्णं मज्जप्रकाशं कुणपं त्रिदोषात्। तच्चाप्यसाध्यं प्रवदन्ति तज्ज्ञा न तत्र कुर्व्वीत भिषक् चिकित्साम्॥

oil. The body is covered with perspiration, it feels hot, the child has great thirst, with looseness, and the body becomes of a yellow colour.

When the diseased phlegm affects the milk it increases the saliva of the infant, with the symptoms produced by diseased phlegm. He is drowsy, the mouth and eyes swell, with sickness and vomiting.

When two of these diseased states act on the milk, they produce the symptoms of the combination. When three are so diseased the three classes of symptoms are present at the same time. It is only by the degree of crying of the infant, that the kind and severity of pain is known.

Purulent Ophthalmia of Infants, (*Kukunaka.*)

Bad milk produces disease of the eyelids, which, with the neighbouring parts, are very itchy; tears flow copiously, the eyes are very sensible to light, and they cannot open their eyelids.

Marasmus, (*Párigarbhika.*)

When a pregnant woman continues to give suck to a child, it produces cough, bad appetite, vomiting, drowsiness, and emaciation. The child loses its vivacity, and the abdomen swells. When phlegm is diseased in the soft palate small pointed elevations form there, by which the fontanell becomes depressed, the soft palate is destroyed, the child cannot suck, and there is a difficulty in swallowing, great thirst, and pain in the

---

सम्वत् स्रवन्ती मास्रावं तृष्णादाहज्वरान्विताम्। क्षीणरक्तां दुर्व्बलाञ्च तामसाध्यां विनिर्द्दिशेत्। मासान्निष्पिच्छदाहार्त्ति पञ्चरात्रानुवन्धि च। नैवातिबहुलात्यल्प मार्त्तवं शुद्धमादिशेत्॥ शशासृक् प्रतिमं यच्च यद्वालाक्षा रसोपमम्। तदार्त्तवं प्रशंसन्ति यच्चापसु च विरज्यते॥

throat and mouth. He cannot sit up, and he vomits. This disease is called *Tálukantaka.* Children are subject to erysipelas, which is always a most dangerous disease, and requires much attention and care.

In other cases the temples swell, like the leaf of a water-lily, and descends to the breast. It is produced by a disease of the air, bile, and phlegm. In other cases it commences in the thorax or abdomen, and descends to the anus. Other diseases, of the class of small diseases, are produced. Fever, and other diseases of adults may occur in infants.

Diseases poduced by Devils.

Infants are supposed to be liable to be affected by nine kinds of spirits or devils, which may assume various forms at will. They are produced from the mother, or the nurse having committed certain improprieties, by which the devil enters their bodies, in order to amuse himself. When a devil distresses an infant, it becomes depressed in spirits, and starts from fear. The eyes of the child swell, he cries, his fingers are contracted, and at other times he tears his body and clothes with his nails, and bites with his teeth, both himself and nurse. The child turns his face to one side, and moves about his eyes; grinds his teeth together, makes a noise like a person who cannot speak from the severity of the disease, and he frequently yawns. His eyelids and eyebrows are in continual movement, and the two foreteeth and lips remain shut, and foam proceeds from the mouth. The child becomes thinner, cannot sleep, his eyes swell,

---

अथ योनिव्यापन्निदानम्।

विंशति र्व्यापदो योनौ निर्द्दिष्टा रोगसंग्रहे। मिथ्याचारेण ताः स्त्रीणां प्रदुष्टेनार्त्तवेन च। जायन्ते वीजदोषाच्च दैवाच्च शृणु ताः पृथक्। सा फेनिलमुदावर्त्ता रजः कृच्छ्रेण मुञ्चति। वन्ध्या नष्टार्त्तवां विद्याद्विप्लुतां नित्यवेदनाम्॥ परिप्लुतायां भवति

has frequent motions, and an unnatural noise proceeds from the throat. The smell of the body resembles that of blood, or flesh; and the child will not take his usual food. These are the usual symptoms indicating the presence of a devil.

Poisons and their antidotes, (Panata.)

The origin of poisons is explained in the following manner. Soon after the creation of the world, *Bramha* was displeased at the violence of *Kaitaba* one of the demons (*Asura*), and in his anger poison was generated and destroyed *Kaitaba*. The poison increased so much that the *debtás* were afraid that it would destroy the whole animated creation. They prayed to *Bramha* to relieve them, and petitioned that he would distribute the poison over the animal, vegetable, and mineral kingdoms. This was done; and when the poison is introduced into the living body it is not digested, and produces languor,* and deranges all the humours of the body.

It is necessary for the practitioner to have a knowledge of the symptoms of the different poisons, and their antidotes. As the enemies of the Rajá, bad women, and ungrateful servants sometimes mix poison with food. On this account the cook should be of a good family, virtuous, faithful, and not covetous, not subject to anger, pride, or laziness. He should also be cleanly, and skilful in his business. The practitioner should have like qualities with an intimate knowledge of poisons; and

---

ग्राम्यधर्म्मेण रुग्भ्रमम्। वातला कर्कशा स्तब्धा शूलनिस्तोदपीड़िता। चतसृष्वपि चाद्यासु भवन्त्य निलवेदनाः॥

सदाहं क्षीयते रक्तं यस्यां सा लोहितक्षया। सवातमुद्गिरेद्बीजं वामिनी रजसा युतम्॥ प्रस्रंसिनी स्रंसते च क्षोभिता दुष्प्रजायिनी॥ स्थितं स्थितं हन्ति गर्भं पुत्रघ्नी रक्तसंक्षयात्।

* Hence the name *Bisak*.

should examine the food to be eaten by a Rajá in the cooking room. This should be large, airy, light, and surrounded with faithful servants, and no one should be allowed to enter unless he is first examined. In the *Mitákshara* shástra there are copious directions regarding the manner of detecting a person who gives poison. He does not answer questions, or they are evasive answers; he speaks nonsense, rubs the great toe along the ground, and shivers; his face is discoloured; he rubs the roots of the hair with his fingers; and he tries by every means to leave the house. The food which is suspected should be first given to certain animals, and if they die, it is to be avoided. The authority the bráhmans assumed, and the confidence they inspired, has no doubt often had the best effect, in making the wicked shrink from perpetrating deeds, which would be detected and exposed by them.

The long account which is given of these poisons, and the means of preventing their bad effects seems to prove the frequency with which they were employed with bad intentions, at a very early period.

All poisons have the following qualities: they are drying, heating, and stimulating; their effects quickly extend over all the body; they destroy very quickly, are not digested, and from the rapidity with which they produce bad symptoms it is difficult to use remedies with sufficient quickness. The following stages of the effects of poisons are observed.

अत्यर्थं पित्तला योनिर्दाहपाकज्वरान्विता। चतसृष्वपि चाद्यासु पित्तलिङ्गोच्छ्रयो भवेत्॥ अत्यानन्दा न सन्तोषं ग्राम्यधर्म्मेण गच्छति। कर्णिनयां कर्णिका योनौ श्लेष्मासृग्भ्याञ्च जायते॥ मैथुनेऽचरणापूर्व्वं पुरुषादतिरिच्यते। बहुशश्चातिचरणा तयोर्वीजं न विन्दति॥ श्लेष्मला पिच्छिला योनिं कण्डूग्रस्तातिशीतला॥ चतसृष्वपि चाद्यासु श्लेष्मलिङ्गोच्छ्रयो भवेत्। अनार्त्त-

1st. The tongue becomes black and rigid, the person faints, and breathes with difficulty.

2nd. Shivering, perspiration, heat, and pain in the stomach, and chest.

3rd. Severe pain in the stomach, the eye changes its colour, becomes yellow and swells, and when the poison has extended to the intestines pain of the part, hiccough, coughing, and a peculiar noise is heard in the intestines.

4th. Heaviness of the head.

5th. Discharge of saliva from the mouth, change of colour of the skin, and pain in the joints and belly.

6th. Insensibility and purging.

7th. Rigidity and death.

Vegetable poisons (*Dushibisha*) when dried by the fire, by the air, or by the sun, may be given in solution, or in any other way in which their effects are less powerful. In this case the poison does not produce immediate death, but remains in the system for a long time; and the first effect is looseness, fœtid smell of the mouth, great thirst, fainting, vomiting, and paralysis of the tongue. These are followed when taken into the stomach by diseases of phlegm and air, and in the intestines, by diseases of the bile and air. The person's hair falls off, and he becomes like a bird without feathers. When mixed

---

वास्तनी षण्डी खरस्पर्शा च मैथुने ॥ अतिकायगृहीताया स्तरु- णायास्त्वण्डुली भवेत्। विवृता च महायोनिः सूचीवक्त्रातिसं- वृता। सर्व्वलिङ्गसमुत्थाना सर्व्वदोषप्रकोपजा। चतसृष्वपि चाद्यासु सर्व्वलिङ्गोच्छ्रयो भवेत्। पञ्चासाध्या भवन्तीह योनयः सर्व्वदोषजाः।

अथ कन्दनिदानम्।

दिवास्वप्नादतिक्रोधाद्व्यायामादतिमैथुनात्। क्षताच्च नखद- न्तादैर्वातायाः कुपिता यदा ॥ पूयशोणितसङ्काशं लिकुचा-

with the humours of the body as chyle, blood, &c., the poison produces diseases of the humours, as leprosy, and various other kinds of symptoms, as languor, weakness of the joints, and pain over the body ; swelling of the legs and face, dropsy, and in other cases vomiting and diarrhœa, intermittent fever, discolouration of the body, madness, impotency, and other like diseases. All these symptoms are aggravated in cloudy and damp weather.

Such effects may be removed by proper treatment, and a year after the person has taken the poison he will either be cured, or get worse. When weak, and the patient does not observe his diet, the poison will destroy him.

Poisons are usually arranged into two classes, the first consisting of vegetable and mineral poisons, are named *Stábarah* ; and the second animal poisons, *Jangamah*. They are not used internally, as medicines.

1. *Vegetable, and Mineral Poisons.*

The general symptoms produced by vegetable poisons are fever, hiccough, grinding of the teeth, suffocation, foaming at the mouth, vomiting, want of appetite, difficulty of breathing and fainting.

कृतिसन्निभम्। उत्पद्यते यदा दोनौ नाम्ना कन्दस्तु योनिजः। सचं विवर्णं स्फुटितं वातिकं तत् विनिर्द्दिशेत्॥ दाहराग-ज्वरयुतं विद्यात् पित्तात्मकन्तु तम्। नीलपुष्पप्रतीकाशं कण्डू-मन्तं कफात्मकम्॥

अथ मूढ़गर्भनिदानम्॥

भयाभिघातात्तीक्ष्णोष्णपानाशन-निषेवणात्। गर्भे पतति रक्तस्य सशूलं दर्शनं भवेत्॥ आचतुर्थात्ततो मासात् प्रस्रवे-द्गर्भविद्रवः। ततः स्थिरशरीरस्य पातः पञ्चमषष्ठयोः॥

The *Mineral poisons* produce drowsiness, languor, burning of the body, indigestion, horripilation, swelling, and dysentery. The dejections of a person who has taken poison are of a black colour, large, and are discharged with wind.

Vegetable poisons are divided into nine varieties, which are derived from the roots, leaves, fruits, flowers, bark, milky juice, gum, and pith of plants.

1. The *Roots* of the following plants are poisonous:—and when eaten they produce pain over the body, delirium, and stupidity.

Klitaka,.(Olibanum,)
Asamása, (Andropogon muricatum,)
Gunja, (Abrus precatorius,)
Sugandá, (Alpinia galanga,)
Gargaraká, (Cissus glauca,)
Karagáta,
Bidyuchchikhá,
Bijayá, (Cyperus difformis.)

2. The *Leaves* of the following vegetables produce gaping, shivering, and difficulty in breathing.

Bisaputriká, (Vangueria,)
Alumbá, (Arum campanulatum,)
Abadáruka, (Sideroxylon spinosum,)
Karamba, (Dalbergia arborea,)
Mahá karamba, (Antirrhinum cymbalaria,)

गर्भोऽभिघात-विषमाशन-पीड़िताद्यैः पक्वं द्रुमादिव फलं पतति क्षणेन। मूढ़ः करोति पवनः खलु मूढ़गर्भं शूलञ्च योनि-जठरादिषु मूत्रसङ्गम्॥ भुग्नोऽनिलेन विगुणेन ततः स गर्भः संख्यामतीत्य बहुधा समुपैति योनिम्। द्वारं निरुद्ध शिरसा जठरेण कश्चित् कश्चिच्छरीर-परिवर्त्तित-कुब्जदेहः॥ एकेन कश्चिदपरस्तु भुजद्वयेन तिर्य्यग्गतो भवति कश्चिदवाङ्मुखोऽन्यः।

3.—The following poisonous *Fruits* cause a loss of appetite, heat of the body, and a swelling of the testicles.

Kamudatí, (Nelumbium speciosum,)
Bínáká,
Karamba, (Dalbergia arborea,)
Mahá karamba, (Antirrhinum cymbalaria,)
Karakataka, (Cleome viscosa,)
Ranaka,
Kudataka,
Charmara, (Viola suffruticosa,)
Ebajandá,
Sarpagata, (Hibiscus populneus,)
Nandana, (Cedrela Tuna,)
Sarapáka, (Nelumbium speciosum.)

4.—The followi[illegible] poisonous *Flowers* when eaten produce vomiting, swelli[illegible] the abdomen, and difficulty in breathing.

Betra, [illegible]henopodium album,)
Kadamba, (Sinapis dichotoma,)
Ballija, (Ocymum,)
Karamba, (Dalbergia arborea,)
Mahá karamba, (Antirrhinum cymbalaria.)

पार्श्वापवृत्तगतिरेति तथैव कश्चिदित्यष्टधा गतिरियं ह्यपरा चतुर्धा ॥ सङ्कीलकः प्रतिखुरः परिघोऽथ वीज स्तेषूर्द्ध्ववाहु चरणैःशिरसा च योनिम् ॥ सङ्गी च यो भवति कीलकवत् स कीलो दृश्यैः खुरैः प्रतिखुरः स हि कायसङ्गी ॥ गच्छेद्भुजद्वयशिराः स च वीजकाख्यो योनौ स्थितः स परिघः परिघेन तुल्यः ॥

अपविद्धशिरा या तु शीताङ्गी निरपत्रपा । नीलोद्गतशिरा हन्ति सा गर्भं स च तां तथा ॥ गर्भास्पन्दनमावीनां प्रणाशः श्यावपाण्डुता । भवेदुच्छ्वासपूतित्वं शूनतान्तर्मृते शिशौ ॥ मानसागन्तुभिर्मातु रुपतापैः प्रपीड़ितः ॥ गर्भो व्यापद्यते कुक्षौ

5, 6, 7.—The following poisonous *Bark*, *Pith*, and *Gums*, produce a bad smell in the mouth, a roughness of the body, head-ache, and a discharge of saliva from the mouth.

Antra Pásaka, (Æschynomene grandiflora,)
Kutanía, (Solanum Jacquini,)
Sauríaka, (Tetranthera quadrifolia,)
Karagáta,
Karamba, (Dalbergia arborea,)
Nandana, (Cedrela Tuna,)
Baerátaka, (Solanum melongena.)

8 —The following poisonous *Milky Juices* produce foaming from the mouth, looseness, and a swelling, and heaviness of the tongue.

Kamadugna, (Carpopogon neveum,)
Stnahu, (Euphorbia antiquorum,)
Jálakirjah,

9.—The poisonous *Bulbous roots* are :

Kálakuta, (Arum colocasia,)
Batsanábha, (Sida cordifolia,)
Sarshapa, (Panicum colonum,)
Kapálaka, (Cucumis utilatissimus,)
Kardamaka,

व्याधिभिश्च निपीड़ितः॥ योनिसंवरणं सङ्गः कुक्षौ मक्कल्ल एव च। हन्युरः स्त्रियं मूढ़गर्भां यथोक्ता सप्तप्युपद्रवाः॥

अथ सूतिकारोगनिदानम्।

वायुः प्रकुपितः कुर्य्यात् संरुद्धरुधिरं स्रुतम्। सूताया हृच्छिरोवस्ति शूलं मक्कल्लसंज्ञकम्॥ अङ्गमर्द्दो ज्वरः कम्पः पिपासा गुरुगात्रता॥ शोथः शूलातिसारौ च सूतिकारोगलक्षणम्॥ मिथ्योपचारात् संक्लेशात् विषमाजीर्णभोजनात्। सूतिकायाश्च ये रोगा जायन्ते दारुणाः स्मृताः। ज्वरातिसारशोथाश्च

Baerátaka, (Solanum melongena,)
Mustaka, (Pistacea lentiscus,)
Sringíbisa, (Betala,)
Prapandurika, (a small herbaceous plant,)
Múlaka. (Tamarind,)
Halahala, (Valisneria octandra,)
Mahábisha, (a species of lily,)
Karkataka, (Cleome viscosa.)

The *Mineral poisons* are :—
Phenáshmabhasma, (white oxide of arsenic,)
Harítála, (yellow sulphurate of arsenic : *Sushruta*.)

Other authors have added the following poisons :—
Tuta, (Sulphurate of copper,)
Tezpatra,
Deámaká, (white oxide of arsenic.)

There are others of the same kind.

These poisons when administered to a person, produce pain in the chest and body, fainting, shivering, followed by a burning and swelling of the body, but particularly of the throat. These symptoms are succeeded by diarrhœa, languor, coma, and

---

सूलानाह बलच्चयम् ॥ तन्द्रारुचि प्रसेकाद्याः कफवातामयोद्भवाः। कृच्छ्रसाध्या ह्वि ते रोगाः चीणमांसबलाश्रिताः। ते सर्व्वे सूतिकानाम्ना रोगास्ते चाप्युपद्रवाः ॥

अथ स्तनरोगनिदानम्।

सचीरो वापयदुग्धौ वा प्राप्य दोषस्तनौ स्त्रियाः। प्रदूष्य मांसरुधिरं स्तनरोगाय कल्पते ॥ पञ्चानामपि तेषां ह्वि रक्तजं विद्रधिं विना ॥ लच्चणानि समानानि वाह्यविद्रधिलच्चणैः।

गुरुभि र्विविधै रन्नै र्दुष्टै र्दोषैः प्रदूषितम्। चीरं धात्र्याः कुमारस्य नानारोगाय कल्पते ॥ कषायं सलिलप्लावि स्तनं

insensibility. When these symptoms are present, the disease will be fatal.

Poisons introduced into a wound, as by a poisoned arrow. The part quickly swells, blood flows, and from time to time pus is evacuated. The wound becomes of a black colour, and dirty round it, with a bad smell and sloughing. The person is very thirsty, faintish, with fever, and the body becomes very hot. The same symptoms will be produced when poison is placed over a sore.

II. Animal Poisons.

Serpents. Poison is found in all parts of the serpent, but when they are irritated the poison collects in the hood like teeth, when they snap with the head erect, they lodge the poison in the wound; but when the head is turned upside down they do not convey the poison into the wound. The poison is very acid and hot.

There are some serpents (*Debya* or heavenly) which poison the air by their breathing, and by their sight. Others are called *Bhauma*, which live in holes in the ground, and the poison is in their teeth.

Sushruta does not mention the symptoms, and cure of the first kind; as they kill by their breathing and sight, and the method

---

मारुतदूषितम्। कट्वम्ल-लवणं पीतराजीमत् पित्तसंयुतम्॥ कफ-दुष्टं घनं तोये निमज्जति स पिच्छिलम्। अदुष्टञ्चाम्बुनिक्षिप्तमेकीभवति पाण्डुरम्॥ मधुरञ्चाविवर्णञ्च प्रसन्नं तत् प्रशस्यते॥

अथ बालरोगनिदानम्।

वातदुष्टं शिशुः स्तन्यं पिबन् वातगदातुरः। क्षामस्वरः कृशाङ्गः स्याद्बद्धविण्मूत्रमारुतः॥ स्विन्नो भिन्नमलो बालः कामला पित्तरोगवान्॥ तृष्णालुरुष्णसर्व्वाङ्गः पित्तदुष्टं पयः पिबन्।

of preventing their effects is not known. The *Básuki, Takhyak,* etc. belong to the first kind of serpents. Of the second class, their names, the symptoms which their bites produce, are as follows :—

There are eighty kinds of *Bhauma,* serpents, which are again divided into five classes.

1. *Dabikara*, or hooded snakes.
2. *Mandalá,* with figures of round arches on their bodies.
3. *Rajalámanta,* with longitudinal lines.
4. *Nirbisa,* without poison.
5. *Quiranja,* or mixed class; which combine the peculiarities of several of the others.

Certain animals have poison in their teeth and nails; such as dogs, monkeys, cats, snub-nosed aligators, frogs, a kind of fish called *páka mucha,* guanas, a shell-fish (*sambuka*), and lizards.

Others have poisonous urine and fæces, as—*Chipita, Phichataka, Kasháyabásika, Sarsapabásika, Totaka,* and *Kaundilyaka.*

Musika or rats have poisonous semen. Spiders (*Luta*) have poisonous saliva, urine, and fæces; and their bites, and scratches are poisonous.

Brischika (centipede), *Bissambara, Rajibámacha* (a fish), *Uchirangá* and *Samudra Brischika* have poisonous stings.

कफदुष्टं पिबन् क्षीरं लालालुः श्लेष्मरोगवान् ॥ निद्रान्वितो जडः शूनो रक्ताक्षश्छर्द्दनः शिशुः । द्वन्द्वजे द्वन्द्वजं रूपं सर्व्वजे सर्व्वलक्षणम् । शिशो स्तीव्रामतीव्रां च रोदनाल्लक्षयेद्रुजम् । कुकूणकः क्षीरदोषाच्छिशूना मक्षिवर्त्मनि ॥ जायते तेन तन्नेत्रं कण्डुरञ्च स्रवेन्मुहुः । शिशुः कुर्य्याल्ललाटाक्षि कुटनासावघर्षनम् । शक्तो नार्कप्रभां द्रष्टुं न वर्त्मोन्मीलनक्षमः ॥

मातुः कुमारो गर्भिण्याः स्तन्यं प्रायः पिबन्नपि । कासाग्निसादवमथु तन्द्राकार्श्यारुचिभ्रमैः ॥ युज्यते कोष्ठवृद्ध्या च तमाहुः

The *Chitrasira*, *Surabakurdi*, *Satadaruka*, *Animadaka*, and *Sarikamukha*, convey poison by breathing, by biting, by urine, and by fæces. The bones of animals killed by poisonous arrows, and the like; the bones of serpents, and of the fish called *Barati*, produce poisonous effects when eaten.

Makkika, a kind of flea, *Kanaba*, and *Juliká* (a kind of leech), are poisonous by biting.

The fishes called *Sákuli*, and *Raktaráji*, have poisonous bile.

General Symptoms.—There are some kinds of serpents that only produce diseases of air, others of bile, and a third kind of phlegm; accordingly diseases of air are produced by serpents of the *Baghis* (*Darbikara*), or hooded kind, the diseases of bile by those of the *Mandalá* kind, and the derangement of phlegm is produced by those of the *Rajalá* kind.

The *Baghi* leaves a black colour in the wound, with the symptoms of various air diseases. They are known by being hooded. The following symptoms are present. The skin, eyes, nails, teeth, urine, and fæces, and the part which is bitten, become black, with roughness of the body and heaviness of the head; pain in the joints, weakness in the loins, back, and neck; gaping, shivering, alteration of voice, languor, hiccough, thirst, foaming and sluggishness of the circulation; and the secretions, and all the external passages are closed.

पारिगर्भिकम्। रोगं परिभवाख्यञ्च युञ्ज्यात्तत्राग्निदीपनम्। तालुमांसे कफः क्रुद्धः कुरुते तालुकण्टकम्॥ तेन तालुप्रदेशस्य निम्नता मूर्ध्नि जायते॥ तालुपातः स्तनद्वेषः कृच्छ्रात् पानं शकृद्द्रवम्॥ तृडक्षिकण्ठास्यरुजा ग्रीवा दुर्व्वलता वमिः॥

विसर्पस्तु शिशोः प्राणनाशनो वस्तिशीर्षजः। पद्मवर्णो महापद्मो वाले दोषत्रयोद्भवः। शङ्खाभ्यां हृदयं याति हृदयाद्वा गुदं व्रजेत्॥

The bites of the *Mandala* serpent produce in the part a yellow colour. It swells, is painful, and soft ; accompanied with the following symptoms : thirst, stupidity, fainting, fever ; blood is discharged from the mouth and anus, and gangrene occurs in the bitten part. These serpents are shining, and are marked with different circles over the body.

The *Rajíla* serpent produces a swelling, a glistering grey-colour of the part, and the blood is thick, accompanied with the various symptoms of diseased phlegm. They are distinguished by the longitudinal lines along their bodies.

There is a fourth kind of serpents called *Nirbísa*, or serpents without poison.

Should a serpent bite a person under the sacred *pipul* tree, near a temple, where bodies are burnt, on a holy hill, on a white-ants nest, during the two hours in the evening and morning when the sun is disappearing, where four roads meet, towards the south of the house, or if the person is bit on his birth-day, in the temples, or in vital parts of the body, he will not recover.

The bites are also dangerous when the food in the stomach is not digested, when the body is labouring under a bilious

---

क्षुद्ररोगे च कथिते त्वजगन्धाऽहिपूतने। ज्वराद्या व्याधयः सर्व्वे महतां ये पुरेरिताः। बालदेहेऽपि ते तद्वद्विज्ञेयाः कुशलैः सदा॥

क्षणादुद्विजते बालः क्षणात्त्रस्यति रोदिति। नखैर्दन्तै र्दारयति धात्री मात्मान मेव वा॥ ऊर्द्ध्वं निरीक्षते दन्तान् खादेत् कूजति जृम्भते। भ्रुवौ क्षिपति दन्तौष्ठ फेनां वमति चासकृत्॥ क्षामोऽति निशि जागर्त्ति शूनाक्षो भिन्नविट् स्वरः॥ मांसशोणितगन्धी च न चाश्नाति यथा पुरा। सामान्यग्रहदुष्टानां लक्षणं सँमुदाहृतम्॥ एकनेत्रस्य गात्रस्य स्रावः स्पन्दनकम्प-

disease, when the person is fatigued and languid from heat, when the person is affected with a discharge from the urethra; in pregnant women, in old, weak, sickly, or hungry persons; and during rainy and cloudy days. In these cases practitioners must be careful in undertaking the treatment of such patients, as they will be rarely cured. This will also be the case when no blood follows cutting the part, and when the person is senseless so that no weals are produced by the strokes of a whip, or horripilation after throwing cold water on the body. The following symptoms are likewise unfavourable: when the tongue is black, the hair falls off, the nose and mouth become changed in their shape, the voice is altered, and the bitten part becomes black and red, or tetanus supervenes; when thick mucus proceeds from the mouth, or when the blood is discharged from the mouth and anus, and there are the wounds of four teeth.

The hooded snakes are quickly fatal in their effects.

When after being bitten the person is insensible with other bad symptoms, as a stoppage of the throat, the body becoming blue, and the feet and hands immoveable, the disease will be fatal.

These poisons first derange the blood, producing a blackness of the part, and a feeling as if ants are moving upon the surface of the body.

नम्। ऊर्द्धदृष्ट्या निरीक्षेत वक्रास्यो रक्तगन्धिकः॥ दन्तान् खादति वित्रस्तः स्तनं नैवाभिनन्दति। स्कन्दग्रहगृहीतानां रोदनञ्चाल्पमेव च॥ नष्टसंज्ञो वमेत् फेनं संज्ञावानतिरोदिति। पूयशोणितगन्धित्वं स्कन्दापस्मारलक्षणम्॥ त्रस्ताङ्गो भयचकितो विहङ्गगन्धिः सास्त्रावव्रण परिपीड़ितः समस्तात्। स्फोटैश्च प्रचिततनुः सदाह पाके विज्ञेयो भवति शिशु क्षतः शकुनग्रा॥

व्रणैः स्फोटैश्चितं गात्रं पङ्कगन्धं स्रवेदसृक्। भिन्नतक्रा ज्वरी दाही रेवतिग्रहलक्षणम्॥ अतीसारो ज्वर स्तृष्णा

2. The poison affects the flesh, and produces a blackness and swelling of different parts of the body.

3. It next affects the fat.

4. It enters the viscera and organs.

5. The bones.

6. The marrow and lastly semen, which is followed by death.

When animals are affected by animal poisons, their bodies become swollen, they are sluggish, and saliva proceeds from their mouths, with pain in the chest. In the third stage there is pain in the head they cannot support; and fourth. The body shivers, they become insensible and die.

Birds when affected with poison first become sluggish, senseless, and die.

Poisons do not affect cats, nor the mongoose.

Poisonous rats. The symptoms of different kinds of these poisons is given in the medical *shástras.* When they discharge their semen upon any part of the body, the blood is affected, and produces different glandular swellings, blutches, and eruptions. In other cases erysipelas accompanied with pain, fever and fainting, followed by debility, loss of appetite, difficult breathing, and vomiting.

तिर्य्यक् प्रेक्षणरोदनम् ॥ नष्टनिद्रस्तथोद्विग्नो ग्रस्तः पूतनया शिशुः । छर्द्दिः कासो ज्वरस्तृष्णा वसागन्धोऽतिरोदनम् ॥ स्तनग्रद्वेषोऽतिसारश्च अन्धपूतनया भवेत् । वेपते कासते क्षीणो नेत्ररोगो विगन्धिता ॥ छर्द्द्यतीसारयुक्तश्च शीतपूतनया शिशुः । प्रसन्नवर्णावदनः शिराभिरभिसंवृतः । मूत्रगन्धी च वह्वाशी मुखमुण्डतिकाग्रही । छर्द्दिस्पन्दनकण्ठास्र शोषो मूर्च्छा विगन्धिता । ऊर्द्ध पश्येद्दशेद्दस्तान् नैगमेयं ग्रहं वदेत् ॥

The Bites of Mad Dogs.

When a dog, a jackal, a fox, a wolf, a bear, or a tiger become mad they foam at the mouth, which remains open, their tails hang down, they do not hear or see well, and saliva flows from their mouths. In such a state they snap and bite each other. The part that is bitten becomes senseless, blood flows from the wound which becomes black, and the other appearances are observed; as when wounded with a poisoned arrow. The person bitten makes the same kind of noise and movements, as that of the animal which has bitten him. When such a person sees the shape of the animal which has bitten him either in water, or in a glass, it is an unfavourable symptom. It is also unfavourable when the person is afraid of water, and dreads either seeing or hearing it. This is called *Jalatrása* or hydrophobia, the fear of water. When the person dreams of the rabid animal, it is unfavourable. Towards the termination of the disease the person is convulsed, becomes insensible, powerless, and dies.

The Poison of Insects.

These poisons are divided into four classes, one of which derange the air, another the bile, a third the phlegm, and a fourth, or a combination of the three former symptoms.

There are 18 insects which derange air ; as a kind of cricket (*Urchingará*,) the centipide (*Satabáhu*), etc

---

अथ विषनिदानम् ।

स्थावरं जङ्गमञ्चैव द्विविधं विषमुच्यते । मूलाद्यात्मकमाद्यं स्यात् परं सर्पादिसम्भवम् ॥

निद्रां तन्द्रां क्लमं दाह मपाकं लोमहर्षणम् । शोथञ्चैवातिसारञ्च जङ्गमं कुरुते विषम् ॥ स्थावरं ज्वरं हिक्कां दन्तहर्षं गलग्रहम् । फेनवम्यरुचि श्वासं मूर्च्छाञ्च कुरुते विषम् ॥

2nd. There are 24 of the second class which derange bile, as the wasp (*Barati*), the bee (*Bhramara*), etc. This class produce great heat and pain in the part wounded.

3rd. There are 13 of this variety, which derange phlegm; such as the bug (*Kutuba*), and other like insects.

4th. There are 12 varieties of this class of insects, the bites of which are very dangerous, as they affect the three humours, such as *Tunginása, Bihilaka,* etc.

The bites of venomous insects thus produce a derangement of the air, bile, and phlegm of the body, and the wounds are inflamed, brown, red, yellow, or black, according to circumstances. They are sometimes followed by fever, diarrhœa, vomiting, thirst, or a burning sensation over the body. Sometimes there is a shivering, the glands proximate swell, and patches of eruptions or erysipelas appear over the body.

Different kinds of flies, gnats, mosquetos, ants, etc, produce a painful itchiness, and swelling of the part bitten.

Scorpions. There are three varieties of these bites, according as they are mild, strong, and very strong. Those which are generated in dunghills are not so poisonous as those generated in bricks, and dry places. Those generated in the putrid carcases of serpents, and other venomous animals, have the most violent poisons. There are twelve kinds of the first class, three of the second, and fifteen of the third, or dangerous kind. The symptoms resemble those produced

---

इङ्गितज्ञो मनुष्याणां वाक्चेष्टामुखवैकृतैः ॥ जानीयाद्विषदातारमेतैर्लिङ्गैः सबुद्धिमान् ॥ न ददात्युत्तरं पृष्टो विवक्षुर्मोहमेति च। अपार्थं बहुसंकीर्णं भाषते चापि मूढवत् ॥ हसत्यकस्मात् स्फोटयेदङ्गुलीर्विलिखेन्महीन्। वेपथुश्चास्य भवति त्रस्तश्चान्योन्यमीक्षते। विवर्णवक्त्रो ध्यामश्च नखैः किञ्चिच्छिनत्त्यपि। वर्त्तते विपरीतञ्च विषदाता विचेतनम् ॥

by the bites of serpents. The weak kinds produce pain, swelling, followed by shivering and fever, with perspiration, and stiffness of the body. The second class produce swelling of the tongue, so as to prevent swallowing, fainting, and much pain.

The third, or most dangerous class, produce delirium, fever, burning of the body, a discharge of black blood from the nose, and other parts of the body. In this case the person soon dies.

Spiders. It is stated that *Bishwámitra* made *Bashistha* angry on some occasion, and the perspiration which fell from his head fell in drops upon the grass, and in it the spiders were generated. These spiders are therefore called *Lutá*, from being generated in grass intended for the cow. There are sixteen varieties, eight are cured with difficulty, and eight are incurable. The names of the first eight are given, and they produce head-ache, itchiness, pain, and swelling of the part, followed by hot fever and diarrhœa, with derangement of phlegm and air. The eight other varieties produce sloughing of the part, discharge of blood, fever, burning, looseness, and diseases of the three humours. The general appearance of these eruptions over the body, are in the form of blotches or swellings. Some of them are large, others are soft or red, and others black. They pass from one part of the body to another. The first day after the bite there is no change of colour in the part, which feels itchy. The second day the part swells, and the third the characteristic symptoms of the poison develope themselves. The constitution is affected on the fourth day, and on the fifth and sixth all the severe symptoms appear. On the seventh day the person dies, when

उद्वेष्टनं मूलविषैः प्रलापो मोह एव च। जृम्भणं वेपनं श्वासो ज्ञेयं पत्रविषेण तु। मुष्कशोथः फलविषे दाहोऽन्नद्वेष एव च॥ भवेत् पुष्पविषैश्छर्दिराध्मानं श्वास एव च॥ त्वक्-सारनिर्यासविषै रुपयुक्तै भवन्ति हि। आस्यदौर्गन्ध्यपारुष्यशिरो-रुक्कफसंस्रवाः॥

the poison is strong. If the poison remains in the upper part of the stomach it produces diseases of phlegm and air; and if in the stomach, the diseases of air and bile, when the hair falls off. Cloudy, windy, and cold weather increase the violence of the poison. The poisons produce drowsiness, languor, and pain in different parts of the body, and indigestion. Blotches appear over the body, the person loses flesh, his hands and feet swell, followed by faintness, vomiting, diarrhœa, sonorous breathing, thirst, fever, spasm, and swelling of the abdomem (*Anáha*) with delirium.

The red lizard produces a black tinge and grey colour, or mottled colour over the body. This is accompanied with delirium and diarrhœa.

Frogs if seized by a serpent and escape, and bite a person, the persons hair stands on end, severe pain is felt over the body, and the part is insensible. The part swells, and small pimples appear on the part, with vomiting and drowsiness.

Fish poison produces great heat, swelling, and severe pain.

Leeches when poisonous produce an itchiness, and swelling of the part, with fever and fainting.

When poisons have been taken and the person gets well, it is known by his feeling well, the different fluids are healthy, his appetite, urine, dejections are of the natural colour, the body has the natural appearance, as also the senses and mind, and they act properly.

फेनागमः क्षीरविषे विड्भेदो गुरुगात्रता। हृत्पीड़नं धातुविषैर्मूर्च्छा दाहश्च तालुनि। प्रायेण कालघातिनी विषाण्येतानि निर्द्दिशेत्।

सद्यः क्षतं पच्यते यस्य जन्तोः स्रवेद्रक्तं पच्यते चाप्यभीक्ष्णम्। कृष्णीभूतं क्लिन्नमत्यर्थपूति क्षतान्मांसं शीर्य्यते चापि यस्य तृष्णा मूर्च्छा ज्वरदाहौ च यस्य दिग्धाहतं तं पुरुषं व्यव-

Weak poisons (*Apabísha.*) There are seven varieties of these poisons.

Vegetable Poisons.

Hemp, (*Gánjá* or *Grinjá.*) A mixture of tobacco and the extract of hemp, (*Gánjá pitu,*) acts as a poison of a very strong kind. The symptoms it produces are fever, insensibility, thirst, swelling of the abdomen, difficulty of breathing, cough, dryness of the mouth, etc.

Spirits are a kind of poison which, when taken in moderate quantities, and with food, produce good effects, being heating, pungent, subtile, light, placid, and drying. They act quickly, and increase semen. When in large quantities these qualities act unfavourably on the humours, and instead of strengthening the body they will destroy it. Spirits, like medicine, when taken in a proper manner, restore appetite and strength to the body. When taken with butter and rice, flesh, or other food, they increase the person's life beyond the period written at the individuals birth by strengthening, and increasing the person's health. When drank in large quantities it increases so much the internal heat, that it deranges the humours, and the person becomes mad. His sense becomes deranged, and whatever he fancies to do he will not desist from; as singing, telling secrets, speaking nonsense, etc. When spirits are not drank according to rule, it produces different effects. There are three stages of

---

स्येत्। लिङ्गान्येतान्येव कुर्य्याद्मित्रै व्रंणे विषं यस्य दत्तं प्रमादात्। सपीतं ग्टह्धुमाभं पुरीषं योऽतिसार्य्यते॥ फेनमुद्वमते चापि विषपीत तमादिषेत्॥

वातपित्तकफात्मानो भोगिमण्डलिराजिलाः। यथाक्रमं समाख्याता द्व्यन्तरा द्वन्द्वरूपिणः। दंष्ट्रो भोगिकृतः कृष्णाः सर्व्ववातविकारकृत्॥ पीतो मण्डलिजः शोथो मृदुः पित्तविकार-

drunkenness. In the first stage the person feels very happy, and strong. The energy of his body is increased, as also the acuteness of the senses, memory, appetite, and sleep. The person can apply to abstruse books, can play on instruments, and sing better than usual.

2nd. After these symptoms, the mind is obscured and memory deficient, the person speaks and works badly, and the person becomes like a fool. At his work his mind is not quiet, he is always lazy, sleepy, and is like a drunkard.

3rd. He goes after woman, or persons that are respected; his father, mother, etc.; unnatural articles are eaten, and the person speaks everything, and takes no care of his body or goods.

4th. He becomes quite foolish, and falls to the earth like a piece of broken wood. He can do nothing, knows nothing, and lives like a dead man. If a good man, he can no longer perform good actions.

When cooling substances are eaten, or such food as does not increase phlegm, as oleaginous substances, the person will not become so easily drunk. Habit diminishes the susceptibility very much, but becomes liable to the attacks of the most fatal diseases, with severe pain. He also becomes passionate, fearful, thirsty, and melancholy. His body becomes covered with sores, etc. is constipated, and he is fond of eating sour things. In weak persons the body becomes hot, and the habit so bad as to produce various diseases.

वान्॥ राजिजोत्थो भवेद्दंशः स्थिरः शोथश्च पिच्छिलः। पाण्डुः स्निग्धोऽतिसान्द्रासृक् सर्व्वश्लेष्मविकारकृत्॥

अश्वत्थदेवायतनश्मशानवल्मीकसन्ध्यासु चतुष्पथेषु। यामेत्र च दष्टाः परिवर्ज्जनीया ऋक्षे च वा मर्म्मसु ये च दष्टाः। दर्व्वीकराणां विषमाशु वाति सर्व्वाणि चोष्णो द्विगुणी भवन्ति।

When nothing is eaten with the spirit, he soon becomes drunk, accompanied with the diseases produced by great grief. When the person is very angry, and drinks spirit; as also when very fearful, severe diseases are produced; when very thirsty, or when there is great grief, or when he is very hungry and spirits alone are taken. When violent exercise, as fencing, etc. is taken, or when fatigued with walking, spirits are very bad; as also when the stomach, urine, etc. are constipated, or when very sour things have been taken, or what has been eaten is not digested, spirits will produce dangerous diseases. When the person is weak, when the body is very hot from the sun, etc. All these produce severe diseases of various kinds. Such as *Pánátya*, *Parammada*, *Pánárjirna* and *Pánárbibhrama*, in which the body is hot and heavy, has no taste, and there is much cough, no appetite, with a constipated state of the dejections and urine. In *Pánárjirna* the body is hot, head-ache, thirst, pain in the joints, swelling of the abdomen, sour belching, etc.

When air is diseased by spirits, there is pain in the limbs, and the mind is deranged, hiccough, noisy breathing, head-ache, and severe pain in the side, such a person has no sleep, becoming delirious. When bile is deranged, thirst, heat of the body, fever, sweating, and *meha* are produced. When urine is deranged, *Atisar* (diarrhœa), *Abaran* (no memory), and the

---

अजीर्णपित्तातपपीड़ितेषु बालेषु वृद्धेषु बुभुक्षितेषु। क्षीण-
क्षते मेहिनि कुष्ठयुक्ते रूक्षेऽबले गर्भवतीषु चापि॥

अस्त्रक्षते यस्य न रक्तमेति राजयो लताभिश्च न संभ-
वन्ति। शीताभिरद्भिश्च न रोमहर्षो विषाभिभूतस्य विवर्ज्जयेत्तु॥
कृष्णाः सरक्ताः श्वयथुश्च दंशे हन्वोः स्थिरत्वञ्च विवर्ज्जनीयः। वर्त्ति-
र्घना यस्य निरेति वक्त्राद्रक्तं स्रवेदूर्द्ध्वमधश्च यस्य॥ दंष्ट्रानि-
पाताः सतुरस्य यस्य तञ्चापि वैद्यः परितर्ज्जयेच्च। उन्मत्तमत्यर्थं

skin becomes of a green colour. In such cases phlegm is vomited, the person has no appetite, with nausea, and dozing. He has cold fits, and the body is heavy.

When the three are deranged, they produce all the symptoms of the separate diseases, with one named *Pánátya.* The secondary effects of ardent spirits are *Parammada* with deranged phlegm, which is discharged from the body, and the mouth. The body feels heavy, and the mouth has a bad taste with constipation, dozing, no appetite, thirst, head-ache, and the joints are pained.

Pánárjirna, or indigestion, it is a consequence of the free use of spirits. The stomach swells, with much vomiting, the body is hot, he complains of head-ache, the spirit is not digested, and *Ajirna,* in all its forms are produced.

Pánárbibhrama. Symptoms of deranged bile ; with pain of the chest and body, vomiting, fever, head-ache, and cough ; mucus is discharged from the mouth and nose ; the trachea feels like smoke to the person, and the body hot. When a person in this disease appears as if drunk he will die of it. When the mouth of such a person is twisted or otherwise unnatural, the body is cold, but is supposed by the person to be hot, the mouth the colour of oil, the tongue, lips, teeth, of a dark colour, or blue, and eyes yellow or red, hiccough, or fever, vomiting,

---

मुपद्रुतं वा हीनस्वरं ब्रापयथवा विवर्णम् । सारिष्ट मत्यर्थ मवेगिनञ्च ज्ञात्वा नरं कर्म्म न तत्र कुर्य्यात् ।

जीर्णं विषघ्नौषधिभि र्हतं वा दावाग्निवातातपशोषितं वा । स्वभावतो वा गुणविप्रहीनं विषं हि दूषीविषतामुपैति । वीर्य्याल्पभावान्न निपातयेत्तु कफान्वितं वर्षगणानुवन्धि ॥

तेनार्द्दितो भिन्नपुरीषवर्णो वैगन्ध्यवैरस्ययुतः पिपासी । मूर्च्छां भ्रमं गद्गदवाक् वमिञ्च विचेष्टमानोऽरतिमाप्नुयाद्वा ॥ आमा-

or shivering, pain in the sides, cough, forgetfulness, he will not recover.

Dáha (Inflammation), spirits producing heat, derange the blood, and bile of the skin and produce this disease. The following varieties are described :

1. The first variety affects the skin.

2. This variety affects the blood ; producing a wrinkled and dry state and copper colour of the skin with thirst. The smell of the body and mouth resembles that of blood, and the body is hot, like that produced by fever.

3. When bile is deranged it is like the fever which this produces when deranged : and the varieties are the same.

4. This resembles the last. The thirst is not gratified from the person's foolishness, the heat of the internal and external surface of the body is increased. The throat, palate and lips are dry, and the tongue is thrust out of the mouth with shivering of the body.

5. When much blood is collected in the abdomen, great heat is produced.

6. When much of the elements are discharged from the body, a form of this disease is produced. When *dáha* occurs

---

शयस्थं कफवातरोगी पक्वाशयस्थोऽनिलपित्तरोगी ॥ भवेत् समु-
द्ध्वस्त-शिरोरुहाङ्गो विलूनपक्षस्तु यथा विहङ्गः। स्थितं रसा-
दिष्वथवा यथोक्तान् करोति धातुप्रभवान् विकारान् ॥ कोपञ्च
शीतानिलदुर्द्दिनेषु यात्याशु पूर्व्वं शृणु तस्य रूपम् ॥ निद्रा-
गुरुत्वञ्च विजृम्भणञ्च विश्लेषहर्षावथवाङ्गमर्द्दः। ततः करोत्यन्न-
मदाविपाकावरोचकं मण्डलकोठजन्म ॥ मांसक्षयं पादकरप्रशोथ
मूर्च्छान्तथा छर्द्दिमथातिसारम्। दूषीविषं श्वासतृषाज्वरांश्च

the person swoons, is thirsty, mucus is discharged from the nose and throat, and he cannot work. In other cases when severe, and a physician does not see the patient, he dies.

7. Sensible parts when wounded or bruised produce a kind of this disease, which is not cured, as blows on the temples. In all the above forms when the interior of the body is hot, and the exterior is cold, the disease is always dangerous.

Dhajabhanga or Claiba, (*Impotence.*)

There are six kinds of Impotency, 1st. It may be produced by dejection of the mind, or connection with distasteful women.

2nd. By eating too dry and pungent food, as black-pepper, capsicum, etc. or too much acid, salt, or stimulating food. By such causes the secretion of semen is diminished.

3rd. Excessive venery, and eating little food.

4th. Old diseases of the organs of generation, or of injuries or diseases of the vital parts.

कुर्य्यात् प्रवृद्धिं जठरस्य चापि। उन्मादमन्यद्ध्वजभङ्गमन्यद्दानाह
मन्यत् क्षपयेच्च शुक्रम्। गाढ़द्द्रुमन्यज्जनयेच्च कुष्ठं तां स्तान्
विकारांश्च बहुप्रकारान्। दूषितं देशकालान्न दिवास्वप्नैरभी-
क्ष्णशः॥ यस्मात् संदूषयेद्धातून् तस्मात् दूषीविषं स्मृतम्। साध्य-
मात्मवतः सद्यो याप्यं संवत्सरोत्थितम्॥ दूषीविषमसाध्यं स्यात्
क्षीणस्याहितसेविनः॥ सौभाग्यार्थं स्त्रियः स्वेदं रजो नानाङ्ग-
जान् मलान्। शत्रुप्रयुक्तांश्च गरान् प्रयच्छन्त्यन्नमिश्रितान्॥
तैः स्यात् पाण्डुः कृशोऽल्पाग्निर्गरश्चास्योपजायते॥ मर्म्म प्रधमना-
ध्मानं हस्तयोः शोथलक्षणम्। जठरं ग्रहणीदोषो यक्ष्मा गुल्मः
क्षयो ज्वरः। एवंविधस्य चान्यस्य व्याधेर्लिङ्गानि दर्शयेत्।

5th. The congenital variety ; and the
6th. Variety is caused by avoiding sexual indulgences.

The fourth and fifth kinds are incurable. The other four kinds may be treated.

Gudabhrangsa, (*Prolapsus Ani.*)

The rectum is prolapsed during the evacuation of the fæces in weak persons ; particularly when affected with long continued diarrhœa, or much straining.

Ahiputana, (*Superficial Ulcer round the Anus.*)

Eruptions sometimes form round the anus, from want of cleanliness. They become itchy, are scratched, and ulcerate, producing this disease. They often occur in children.

Slight diseases of the Extremities.

Painful swellings in the axilla are produced by bile, and phlegm. Deep seated swellings, which produce much heat, inflammation, and fever, like fire, kill after seven or twelve days, or after a fortnight. They are called *Agnirohíní.*

तस्माल्लूनं तृणं प्राप्ता मुनेः प्रस्वेदविन्दवः। तस्माल्लूतान्तु भाष्यन्ते संख्यया ताश्च षोड़श॥ ताभि र्दष्टे दंशकोत्थः प्रवृत्तिः क्षतजस्य च। ज्वरो दाहोतिसारश्च गदाः स्युश्च त्रिदोषजाः॥ पिड़का विविधाकारा मण्डलानि महान्ति च॥ शोथा महान्तो मृदवो रक्ताः श्यावाश्चला स्तथा। सामान्यं सर्व्वलूताना मेतद्दंशस्य लक्षणम्॥ दंशमध्ये तु यत् कृष्णं श्यावं वा जालकाचितम्। अर्द्धाकृति भृशं पाकः क्लेदशोथज्वरान्वितम्॥ दूषीविषाभिर्लताभि स्तं दष्टमिति निर्द्दिशेत्। शोथः श्वेतोसितारक्ता

When the nails are affected with inflammation round the edges it is called *Chipya.* It is produced by derangements of the bile, air, injuries, etc.. The part which is connected to the flesh, especially at its angles swell, become very painful, and then ulcerate, particularly at its angles, when it is called *Upanaka.* When the nails become dry, rough, and discoloured, the disease is called ***Kunakh*** or ***Kulina.***

When the sole of the foot is injured by some external cause, as by thorns, or the like, it produces much pain, and is called *Dari.* When the swelling is hard, indolent, and like the seed of plumbs, accompanied with much pain, and a considerable discharge, it is called *Kadara.* When the space between the toes ulcerate (*Rhagas*) the disease is called *Alasa.* The other diseases of the leg are described under *Bádobadí.*

Sometimes ulcers form near the axilla or groin, which become hard, red, and sinuous; in such cases the deepseated parts are so affected that when opened they discharge frothy matter like a mixture of honey and ghee. The part then becomes dry, irregular, and discharges fœtid matter of different

---

पीता वा पिड़का ज्वरः। प्राणान्तिकाश्च जायन्ते श्वासहिक्काशिरोग्रहाः॥

आदंशाच्छोणितं पाण्डु मण्डलानि ज्वरोऽरतिः। लोमहर्षश्च दाहश्चाप्याखुदुषीविषार्द्दिते। मूर्च्छाङ्गशोथवैवर्ण्यं क्लेदशब्दाश्रुति ज्वराः। शिरोगुरुत्वं लालासृक् छर्द्दिश्चासाध्य मूषिकैः॥

कार्ष्ण्यः श्यावत्वमथवा नानावर्णत्व मेव वा। मोहोऽथवर्च्चसो भेदो दष्टः स्यात् क्रककण्टकैः॥ दहत्यग्निरिवादौ च भिनत्तीवोर्द्ध्वमाशु च। वृश्चिकस्य विषं याति दंशे पश्चात्तु तिष्ठति। दष्टोसाध्यस्त्व हृद्घ्राणरसनोपहतो नरः। मांसैः पतद्भि रत्यर्थं

colours with blood. Sometimes the hemorrhage is sudden and great. This disease is called *Sharkarárbuda*, (*Ṣarkara*, a piece of earthen pot, and *Arbuda*, tumor.) This is probably an aneurismal tumor.

Emaciation, (*Kársa.*)

If a person takes dry food which does not contain much nourishment, as astringent and pungent kinds of food, much exercise, and venery, they produce emaciation; if he indulgeas in too much study, fer, grief, thinking, watching at night, or food in small quantities, the chyle is formed and absorbed in small quantities, does not circulate and nourish all parts of the body, and produces emaciation. In such a state the person becomes weak and cannot bear hunger or thirst,

---

वेदनार्त्तोजहात्यसून् ॥ विसर्पः श्वयथुः शूलं ज्वरश्छर्द्दि रथापि च। लक्षणं कर्णभेदंष्ट्रे दंशश्चैवावसीदति ॥ हृष्टलोमोच्चिटिगेन स्तब्धलिङ्गो भृशार्त्तिमान् ॥ दष्टः शीतोदकेनेव सिक्तान्यङ्गानि मन्यते। एकदंष्ट्रार्द्दितः शूनः सरुजः पीड़कास्तृषा ॥ छर्द्दिर्निद्रा च स विषैर्मण्डूकै र्दष्टलक्षणम्। मत्स्यास्तु स विषाः कुर्युर्दाहं शोथं रुजं तथा। कण्डुं शोथं ज्वरं मूर्च्छां स विषास्तु जलौकसः। विदाहं श्वयथुं तोदं स्वेदञ्च सहगोधिका। दंशे स्वेदं रुजं दाहं कुर्य्याच्छतपदीविषम् ॥

कण्डूमान मशके विषं शोथस्यान्मन्दवेदनः। असाध्यकीटसदृश मसाध्यं मशकक्षतम् ॥ सद्यः प्रस्राविणी श्यावा दाहमूर्च्छा ज्वरान्विताः। पीड़का मक्षिकादंशे तासान्तु स्थगिकाऽसुहृत्।

heat or cold, currents of air, or rain. Such a person is liable to the attacks of nervous diseases, or diseases of air, and will die of asthma, consumption, acitis, dyspepsia, *gúlma* hæmatemesis, or hæmopysis. Such a person has severe attacks of diseases.

Unhealthy (*Costiveness*) *Discharges*, (*Amaha.*)

When the fæces are not properly prepared for expulsion, but are discharged in small quantities, with pain, it forms this disease. It is accompanied with great pain in the epigastric region, thirst, a discharge of mucus from the mouth and nose, accompanied with head-ache and heaviness of the body, particularly in the chest. The person has no eructations, complains of pain in the loins and back ; the urine and fæces are constipated with severe pain, and there is difficulty in breathing, fainting, and stercorous vomiting. These two last symptoms are only present when the *Pákasia* (the large intestines) are affected.

चतुष्पद्भि र्द्विपद्भिश्च नखदन्तविषञ्च यत् ॥ पूयते पच्यते वापि स्रवति ज्वरवत्यपि । प्रशान्तदोषं प्रकृतिस्थं धातुमन्नाभिकामं समसूत्रविट्कम् । प्रसन्नवर्णेन्द्रियचित्तचेष्टं वैद्योऽवगच्छेदविषं मनुष्यम् ।

दर्शन-स्पर्शन-प्रश्नैः परीक्षा त्रिविधा मता । वयोवर्णशरीराणा मिन्द्रियानाञ्च दर्शनात् ॥

इति श्रीमाधवकरप्रणीतं निदानं समाप्तम् ।

FINIS.